Nelson Yuan-sheng Kiang

The Developmental Neuropsychology of Sensory Deprivation

Contributors

Leo Ganz
Albert Globus
R. L. Kelley
Karl Konrad
Ronald Melzack
Austin H. Riesen
Seth K. Sharpless
J. P. Walker
Judith Boas Walker
Dale E. Zilbert

The Developmental Neuropsychology of Sensory Deprivation

Edited by

Austin H. Riesen

Department of Psychology
University of California
Riverside, California

ACADEMIC PRESS

New York San Francisco London 1975

A Subsidiary of Harcourt Brace Jovanovich, Publishers

Figures used in this text that are from other sources are cited in the legend which is keyed to the references.

Figure 2-11 is reproduced with permission from The Dorsey Press.

Figures 6-1 (1971), 6-4 (1967), 6-11 (1967), and 6-12 (1967) is copyrighted by the American Association for the Advancement of Science.

Figures 6-5 and 6-13 (1965), 8-4 (1970), and 9-1 (1972) is copyrighted by the American Psychological Association and reprinted by permission.

Figures 8-5 (1968) and 8-7 (1968) is reprinted by courtesy of Charles C. Thomas, Publisher, Springfield, Illinois.

Figure 8-10 (1965) is reprinted by permission of Grune & Stratton, Inc.

ACADEMIC PRESS, INC.
111 Fifth Avenue, New York, New York 10003

United Kingdom Edition published by
ACADEMIC PRESS, INC. (LONDON) LTD.
24/28 Oval Road, London NW1

Library of Congress Cataloging in Publication Data

Riesen, Austin Herbert.
The developmental neuropsychology of sensory deprivation.

Includes bibliographies.
1. Developmental psychobiology. 2. Sensory deprivation. I. Title.
RJ131.R54 612'.8 73-18989
ISBN 0-12-588550-4

PRINTED IN THE UNITED STATES OF AMERICA

Contents

List of Contributors ix
Preface xi

CHAPTER I

The Sensory Environment in Growth and Development
Austin H. Riesen

I. Stimulation and Adaptive Growth 1
II. What Environments Supply to Growing and Behaving Organisms 3
III. Adaptive Significance of Innate Stimulus Preferences 4
IV. Subnormal and Supernormal Sensory Systems 6
References 6

CHAPTER II

Brain Morphology as a Function of Presynaptic Morphology and Activity
Albert Globus

I. Introduction 9
II. Results 13
III. Discussion 62
IV. Summary 81
References 82

CHAPTER III

Neurochemical Correlates of Sensory Deprivation
J. P. Walker, Judith Boas Walker, R. L. Kelley, and A. H. Riesen

I. Introduction 93
II. Glycolysis and the Phosphogluconate Pathway 95
III. The Tricarboxylic Acid Cycle 97
IV. Pyridine Nucleotide Oxidation-Reduction 98
V. Nucleic Acids: Synthesis and Turnover 99
VI. Protein Synthesis and Turnover 102

VII. Phosphatases 106
VIII. Neurotransmitters and Related Enzymes 107
IX. Histological, Cytological, and Circulatory Changes 112
X. Nonvisual Modalities 116
XI. Discussion of Issues 117
References 119

CHAPTER IV

Disuse Supersensitivity

Seth K. Sharpless

I. Disuse Supersensitivity: The Phenomenon 125
II. Disuse versus Denervation as Causative Factors in the Development of Supersensitivity in Effector Organs 127
III. Disuse Supersensitivity: Mechanisms 132
IV. Effects of Disuse and Denervation on Neurons 136
V. Conclusions 145
References 146

CHAPTER V

Electrophysiological Changes after Sensory Deprivation

Austin H. Riesen

I. Problems of Neural Function after Deprivation 153
II. Effects along the Visual Pathway 154
III. Changes in Cortical Responses 157
IV. Subcortical Effects, Brain Excitability 162
V. Human Findings and Implications 163
VI. Evoked Potentials after Auditory Deprivation 164
References 164

CHAPTER VI

Orientation in Visual Space by Neonates and Its Modification by Visual Deprivation

Leo Ganz

I. Binocular Pattern Deprivation 171
II. Monocular Pattern Deprivation 188
III. Deprivation of Visual–Motor Correlations 194
IV. Conclusions 206
References 206

CHAPTER VII

Behavioral Consequences of Variations in Early Sensory Environments

Austin H. Riesen and Dale E. Zilbert

I.	The Scope of Behavioral Studies	211
II.	Studies of Visual Deprivation	213
III.	Studies of Auditory Deprivation	232
IV.	Studies of Tactual, Motor, and Somatosensory Deprivation	233
V.	Studies of Multisensory Enrichment and Deprivation	235
VI.	Conclusions	244
	References	246

CHAPTER VIII

Novelty-Enhancement Effects Associated with Early Sensory–Social Isolation

Karl Konrad and Ronald Melzack

I.	Introduction	253
II.	Novelty Enhancement: Comparative Data	255
III.	Novelty Enhancement: An Information Processing Approach	264
IV.	Novelty Enhancement: Interaction with Other Effects of Isolation Rearing	268
V.	The Nature of Sensory–Social Isolation	272
	References	274

CHAPTER IX

Interpretations and Implications

Austin H. Riesen

I.	Function and Structural Development of the Nervous System	277
II.	Neural Metabolic Processes in Sensory Deprivation	278
III.	Competition for Synaptic Space	280
IV.	What Structures Interact with Which Functions?	281
V.	Sensory–Motor and Motor–Sensory Integrations	283
VI.	Discriminative Responding to Complex Sensory Patterns	284
	References	285

Author Index 287
Subject Index 298

List of Contributors

Numbers in parentheses indicate the pages on which the authors' contributions begin.

Leo Ganz (169), Department of Psychology, Stanford University, Stanford, California

Albert Globus (9), Department of Psychiatry, University of California, Davis, California

R. L. Kelley (93), Department of Psychology, University of California, Riverside, California

Karl Konrad (253), Department of Psychology, Saint Mary's University, Halifax, Canada

Ronald Melzack (253), Department of Psychology, McGill University, Montreal, Canada

Austin H. Riesen (1, 93, 153, 211, 277), Department of Psychology, University of California, Riverside, California

Seth K. Sharpless (125), Department of Psychology, University of Colorado, Boulder, Colorado

J. P. Walker (93), Andrus Gerontology Center, University of Southern California, Los Angeles, California

Judith Boas Walker (93), Andrus Gerontology Center, University of Southern California, Los Angeles, California

Dale E. Zilbert (211), Division of Adult Services, Clark Institute of Psychiatry, Toronto, Canada

Preface

Psychological development depends initially upon the growth of bodily structures. This dependence shifts quite early to interdependence; behavior begins to influence structure and then the rising spiral of the structure–function relationship becomes the central subject matter of developmental neuropsychology.

How does use affect neural structure? After scattered and faltering beginnings in the last century, with almost no progress in the period from 1900 to 1950, scientific effort has, in two decades, produced more basic information than can be comprehended within the traditional confines of one given discipline or even two or three.

Psychology, physiology, anatomy, and biochemistry are the research compartments from which there has come a sudden rush of new data. Each of these disciplines is using sensory deprivation and controlled stimulation as a common class of experimental variables. The dependent measures vary with the discipline or the interdisciplinary alliances of research teams. By now the scattering of references across many journals and symposium reports has made the problem of cross-disciplinary communication nearly overwhelming. This volume is offered in order to bring the hundreds of articles into view and to focus on key problems and their partial answers.

The experimental studies that have provided the data for this book were selected by the several authors to emphasize early growth and development, to focus on mammalian nervous systems, and to provide a full coverage of animal experimentation that is significant for behavioral development. The wealth of data has significance for clinical departments as well as for those in the basic sciences. Neurology, ophthalmology, otolaryngology, pediatrics, and psychiatry are facing structure–function issues to which the data from sensory deprivation studies are directly relevant.

If use promotes growth and function of the nervous system and disuse retards development or even induces atrophy, when and how are such effects occurring? To what extent are behavioral deficiencies related to early sensory deprivation? Can biochemical and neuroanatomical correlates of the behavioral effects be identified? Quite clear and specific answers to these questions are given in the chapters of this book. Further problems in urgent need of answers are also identified.

Although most of the research has of necessity been done with animals, more human conditions are directly implicated with each new step in the research. When sensory relay nuclei are affected by birth injury or anoxia, the result is sensory deprivation. Monkey studies have identified delayed cortical atrophy of disuse even when behavior, as a whole, has been improving. Amblyopia, cerebral palsy, congenital cataract, and epilepsy have associated conditions in the central nervous system that now have identifiable relations to deprived sensory nuclei. Useful animal models are being experimentally developed and the causes as well as the conditions for remediation of these afflictions of the central nervous system are unraveling before the research onslaught. Although some of the lessons that we have learned are sobering, the possibilities for preventing or causing major improvements in sensory deprivation syndromes can but renew our dedication to search for the facts, and to let those facts lead us on to the next set of experiments.

Hyperactivity as well as perceptual learning deficiencies will need further investigation with a view to relating these to brain changes that may require early remedial programs. Although critical or optimal periods have been approximately demarcated for some visual functions, much more work is needed to bring about an adequate knowledge of the time dimensions in the effects of sensory deprivation.

The authors of the several chapters in this book have worked with patience and dedication in their efforts to present as complete and well organized an account as possible of what we now know. Even as we were writing, new reports challenged us. The work is, as it should be, never ending. We hope that the present effort at taking inventory and appraising progress will assist the forward march of scientific and clinical understanding. The complex interrelations between stage of development, environmental stimulation or lack of it, and the kinds of social and physiological motivations that are influencing the infant or the juvenile, both animal and human being, have proved to be a major, continuing challenge to biobehavioral investigation.

The assistance of students through calling to question, discovery, and daily chores of animal care and observation can be acknowledged only inadequately. Their challenge continues to broaden the scope of the research effort. Their concerns for procedure and for the health of the experimental subjects have contributed much to what can be said now in this book. Specific mention should include the names of Martin Balaban, Kenneth T. Brown, Jerry Hogan, Lisa Kim, Helen Hendy Neely, Carol Riesen Nelson, Hiroshi Odoi, Dale Schissler, and Jacquelyn La Velle Tamplen.

In the design and construction of testing equipment for behavioral and electrophysiological studies Mr. Diofanto Garro, Dr. Glenn Grandfield, and Mr. Robert Ramsey invested much time and ingenuity.

In the preparation of manuscript, I wish to acknowledge the assistance of Elizabeth Hatch, Ruth H. Jewell, and Lucy Johnson. For constant support, patience, advice, and encouragement I thank my wife, Helen Haglin Riesen.

My co-authors and research collaborators have exercised both patience and impatience in needed times and amounts. To all of them I am most grateful and indebted. Without initial interest and support from Professors Herbert G. Birch, Donald O. Hebb, Karl S. Lashley, and Henry W. Nissen the history of research on the neuropsychology of sensory deprivation would lack the studies that launched its forward thrust in mid-twentieth century. Hebb's 1949 book, *Organization of Behavior*, was the documentation of that launching.

The Developmental Neuropsychology of Sensory Deprivation

CHAPTER I

The Sensory Environment in Growth and Development

Austin H. Riesen

Department of Psychology
University of California, Riverside

I. Stimulation and Adaptive Growth

The higher primates and certain of the other vertebrates are born into and develop in complex and highly varied environments. Human beings are supreme in the capacity to live under qualitatively distinct and quantitatively extreme conditions. Whether highly flexible, or less so, in its environmental requirements as a newborn of a given species, the individual begins immediately to adapt to the more circumscribed conditions of a particular environment. As development proceeds the individual begins to lose degrees of freedom for morphological, physiological, and behavioral adaptations while becoming adapted to the limited range of conditions of a given niche.

Growth in all of its manifestations will depend upon the ranges as well as the average values of conditions that prevail and the sequences of these through the various developmental periods. Individuals are products of inheritance and of environments. As often as this general statement is made and accepted, the biological and behavioral sciences are just beginning to discover how much and why environments make differences among organisms of a given species.

Results of experiments on some effects of sensory deprivation (reduced or simplified stimulation) on morphological, physiological, and behavioral development have opened surprising new vistas for the bio–behavioral sciences. The implications of "early experience" experiments tell us that we are only at the beginning of the revelations that studies of growth under unusual environments will yield. Without environmental demands for their "use" some neural organizations are lost, their structural substrates diminished, and the brain chemistry altered. When certain sensory requirements are imposed, exaggerated neural growth patterns and restructuring of function beyond the ordinary occur. Compensations of structure and of functional capacities result from a shift of environmental demands away from one modality and toward others. The age dependence of these modifications are both very strong and quite weak, depending upon the systems in question. Plasticity is sometimes a critical period phenomenon, as in stereoscopic visual processes and in compensation for lesions in a sensory system, but it also may be general through a major portion of the life span, as in sensory–motor coordination or in those brain changes that result from a broad spectrum of environmental enrichment.

Organisms normally seek and select from the environment many essentials under the dictates of inheritance. Nutritional requirements and sensory preferences are revealed in considerable measure by early choice behaviors. Assuming their availability, the appropriate nutriments, physical supporting media, temperature values, sensory energy levels, and even patterns of sensory stimulation are "wisely" selected. A genetic memory functions prior to individual experience to guarantee that some essentials to organismic growth become available components of environments, internal as well as external. Appetite serves to insure that blood and brain will contain arrays of selected constituents. The behavioral responses of infant organisms are instrumental in supplying a few of the required nutrients. Other dietary needs are only selected appropriately after learning (Nachman & Cole, 1971).

Food preferences in "cafeteria" experiments with infant organisms (Davis, 1928; Richter, Holt, & Barelare, 1938) proved that human and animal infants develop specific hungers at an early age. The newborn is neurophysiologically programmed to seek certain dietary essentials. Looking beyond taste preferences, science is discovering other behaviorally supported and preprogrammed stimulus seeking and selecting activities and discriminative abilities. Some of these have been revealed by recent studies in sensory deprivation but we are discovering at the same time that not all needs are behaviorally supported at an early age.

II. What Environments Supply to Growing and Behaving Organisms

Chemical nutrients are the most extensively studied, both in terms of sources and biological processing, of the essentials to growth that must come from the environment. Specific hungers of the newborn provide for selection of needed quantities of sodium and sugars in those mammals that typically seek foods that taste salty or sweet. Most other taste preferences appear to be learned on the basis of physiological consequences of the ingestion of foods that are available to the individual organism (Nachman & Cole, 1971). The requirements for calcium or for vitamins A and D and thiamine are normally met by the eating of a varied diet. No associated innate taste preferences support the selection of these essential dietary components. Only after a deficiency state has developed do some species learn to prefer a taste that has been associated with the presence of the essential nutrient (Rozin, 1969).

The need for bodily support against gravity is in some part behaviorally provided for at birth or hatching. The postural reflexes and the touch receptors, combined in many species with visual depth avoidance responses, all function to support behaviors of clasping, the seeking of contact, and withdrawal from visual "cliff" situations. Strong emotional components energize these responses. All of these are innately organized (see Chapter VI by Ganz). Beyond the early innate organization is a developmental phase during which the environment supports the improvement and elaboration of more specialized postural skills. Cooperation between the environment and the behavioral propensity of the species is necessary for the perceptual—motor learning of advanced patterns of posture and locomotion.

The physical environment must provide an appropriately limited range of temperatures, oxygen at partial pressures that are physiologically supportive, and a total atmospheric pressure having limited range and variability. Toxic gases must be absent or present in only minute quantities. Which of these factors are effective as stimuli, and which, if any, are subject to control by the organism's preferences or aversions, are questions of developmental significance.

Very young birds and mammals show some capacities for selecting appropriate temperatures by seeking warmth or avoiding extremes of heat and cold. Although breathing space may be fought for, this behavior is controlled primarily by the needs to eliminate excessive CO_2, and no behavior or emotional distress makes it clear that sensory information results from dangerous deviations of O_2 partial pressures or of total atmospheric pressures. Carbon monoxide in the atmosphere is a notoriously insidious hazard. Furthermore, the just cited atmospheric dangers provide no associated stimuli or physiological consequences that will support learning. Evolution has not been called upon to select for such mechanisms of adaptation. In this respect, the biological problem is similar to that in which many essential nutrients (amino acids and minerals as well as vitamins) have been so intermingled and pervasive in nature that no mechanisms for highly selective behavioral choices have developed in the genetic heritage.

III. Adaptive Significance of Innate Stimulus Preferences

Innate stimulus preferences and aversions are clearly related to the various categories of physiological needs. The temporary reduction or satiation of stimulus seeking behavior often occurs too quickly to be accounted for by the delayed reduction of a blood, tissue, or organ requirement. The sensory events appear in themselves to result in an immediate partial satiation, and this supports the interpretation that it is a need for stimulation that is satisfied in the immediate poststimulation period. Other need reducing consequences have independent effects on subsequent behavior. Learned aversions and other long-lasting changes in preference behaviors constitute a topic for special study. Questions that concern the astonishing degree of effectiveness of long-delayed reinforcements remain to be answered (Garcia & Ervin, 1968; Hogan, 1973; Nachman, 1963).

Although some animals, the domestic cat among them, do not respond to a sweet taste, any substance that is sweet tasting to man is initially attractive to most primates, other mammals, and birds. The need for water, as expressed by thirst, and the appetite for salt are highly responsive to fluid or sodium deficiency states. Behaviors of drinking or licking occur prior to reinforcing consequences and upon initial occasions following the onset of water or sodium need states (Falk & Herman, 1961; Nachman & Cole, 1971).

Behavioral expressions of preferences for certain food objects depend on visual stimulation as well as on taste, at least in some species. The pecking response of newly hatched chicks is released by targets having certain shapes, sizes, and colors. Fantz (1957) showed that small visual forms brought forth significantly more frequent pecking if they were round or oval shapes than if they were pointed or angular. This preference persisted in the absence of any rewards for pecking and with all differential tactual cues eliminated. Hess and Gogel (1954) used the same technique to demonstrate initial preferences for objects differing only in color. The innate color preference varies with breed or species of bird. Ducklings are found to initiate pecking when the target objects are green (Hess, 1956). Domestic chicks peck very little at green objects and prefer colors that are more typical of ripe seeds. Work remains to be done to clarify the contributions of odor cues to feeding behaviors prior to conditioning although it is common observation that aversive odors discourage eating in human infants and young animals. Tactual–kinesthetic cues are important in the support of pecking or sucking and of swallowing behaviors. A bitter taste induces prompt rejection of grains pecked at or of nipples that are already in position to stimulate the tongue. Sucking and swallowing, "fixed action patterns," require an appropriate combination of stimuli from several modalities.

Functions of the pituitary and adrenal hormone systems are dependent upon both specific effects of light and summative effects of all stimuli that support a diurnal rhythm of sleep and wakefulness. Growth hormone levels are fluctuating in response to and at the same time are chronically dependent upon daily schedules of stimulation. Weight and skeletal growth are partially independent measures of the adequacy of such schedules of stimulation. Rearing litters of rats in total darkness results in slower growth, but Eayrs and Ireland (1950) suggest that this is due to deficiency in the mother's lactation.

The utilization of calcium and the appearance of new ossification centers during skeletal growth has in one mammalian species or another been variously related to length of daylight, total stimulus deprivation, and to deprivation of normal mother–infant interactions. These three categories of environmental events are obviously not mutually exclusive. As a consequence, the evidence is still far from clear regarding the degree to which they may be interchangeable. Human data and experimentation with animals support a concept of "deprivation dwarfism" as a syndrome that combines emotional disturbance, abnormal diurnal sleep patterns, pituitary–adrenal insufficiency, and retarded growth. A disordered family environment is often the underlying cause (Gardner, 1972; Patton & Gardner, 1969). Stimulation directly affects the structures stimulated. An optimum schedule and degree of use results in optimum growth and efficient functioning of organ systems and their cellular units. Much remains to be discovered about the supporting role of stimuli that somewhat indirectly mediate the satisfaction of physiological needs of organs other than the nervous system, that is, muscles, digestive tracts, liver, blood, skeletal system, and others.

A crucial and still controversial area of study is that which deals with the central issue of this book: the problem of how the sensory system and the central nervous system are supported in optimum growth by their use. Recent history of the neurosciences shows that the visual system, while one of the first to yield evidence that disuse leads to developmental failures, is not unique in its susceptibility. Auditory and tactual sensory functions, and presumably also the cortical projections of these systems, are left in underdeveloped condition when these senses are deprived during early growth periods. All indications are that morphology of the central nervous system interacts with the uses to which the components of that system are put. Documentation of such changes in neural microstructures is the subject of Chapter II by Globus.

IV. Subnormal and Supernormal Sensory Systems

The maximum development of a sensory system including its central projections has been regarded as normal by some workers in the neurosciences. The position taken is that enrichment studies are in truth only studies in which deficient environments have been brought up to normal environmental support of demand characteristics. This presupposes a "normal" that has never been adequately identified, whereas a more defensible position would be that we can best study neuropsychological development when we define environments in terms of their qualitative and quantitative characteristics. Some fine work is already described in the scientific literature that states rather clearly that maximum development of one system may only occur at the expense of others. The general view of what is normal may have to be couched in terms of a healthy balance rather than in the maximizing of all modes of sensory processing. Some individual organisms do have many or even all systems working at below average capacity. These may have suffered a broad spectrum of environmental deprivation, assuming that genetic deficiencies are not the primary source of weakness.

Imbalance of environmental impact during a critical stage of early development may subsequently be found to have produced uneven functioning from which recovery is difficult or impossible. In the chapters to follow this principle of competition will be seen to be exemplified in structural as well as functional deviations. Within limits, diversities that are environmentally encouraged or even mandated are clearly advantageous to species that must adapt to wide variations in the environment.

References

Davis, C. M. Self-selection of diet by newly weaned infants. *American Journal of Diseases of Children,* 1928, **36**, 651–679.

Eayrs, J. T., & Ireland, K. F. The effect of total darkness on the growth of the newborn albino rat. *Journal of Endocrinology,* 1950, **6**(4), 386–397.

Falk, J. L., & Herman, T. S. Specific appetite for NaC1 without postingestional repletion. *Journal of Comparative and Physiological Psychology,* 1961, **54**, 405–408.

Fantz, R. L. Form preferences in newly hatched chicks. *Journal of Comparative and Physiological Psychology,* 1957, **50**, 422–430.

Garcia, J., & Ervin, F. R. Gustatory-visceral and telereceptor-cutaneous conditioning-adaptation in internal and external milieus. *Communications in Behavioral Biology, Part A,* 1968, **1**, 389–415.

Gardner, L. I. Deprivation dwarfism. *Scientific American,* 1972, **227,** (1) 76–82.

Hess, E. H. Natural preferences of chicks and ducklings for objects of different colors. *Psychological Reports,* 1956, **2**, 447–483.

Hess, E. H., & Gogel, W. C. Natural preferences of the chick for objects of different colors. *Journal of Psychology,* 1954, **38**, 483–493.

Hogan, J. A. Development of food recognition in young chicks. II. Learned associations over long delays. *Journal of Comparative and Physiological Psychology,* 1973, **83**, 367–373.

Nachman, M. Learned aversion to the taste of lithium chloride and generalization to other salts. *Journal of Comparative Physiological Psychology,* 1963, **56,** 343–349.

Nachman, M., & Cole, L. Role of taste in specific hungers. In L. M. Beidler (Ed.), *Handbook of sensory physiology,* Vol. IV, Part 2, *Taste.* New York: Springer–Verlag, 1971. Pp. 337–362.

Patton, R. G., & Gardner, L. I. Short stature associated with maternal deprivation syndrome: Disordered family environment as cause of so-called idiopathic hypopituitarism. In L. I. Gardner (Ed.), *Endocrine and genetic diseases of childhood.* Philadelphia: Saunders, 1969. Pp. 77–89.

Richter, C. P., Holt, L. E., Jr., & Barelare, B. Changes in fat, carbohydrate appetite in vitamin B deficiency. *American Journal of Physiology,* 1938, **122,** 734–744.

Rozin, P. Adaptive food sampling patterns in vitamin deficient rats. *Journal of Comparative and Physiological Psychology,* 1969, **69,** 126–132.

CHAPTER II

Brain Morphology as a Function of Presynaptic Morphology and Activity

Albert Globus

Department of Psychiatry
University of California, Davis

I. Introduction

> Die Untersuchungen haben ergeben, dass sich eine Hirnrinde mit den materiellen Spuren von Empfindungen ganz wesentlich von einer solchen ohne dieselben unterscheidet und vor Allem messe ich diesen Ergebnissen eine principielle Bedeutung insofern bei, indem sie zeigen, dass die Reize der Aussenwelt in der Hirnrinde, dem Organ der Psyche, dauernde Veränderungen zurücklassen, wie dies die Lehre von dem psycho-physischen Parallelismus von jeher annimmt. [These investigations have demonstrated that the brain which has received stimulation is significantly different in a material way from the brain which has not received any. Also, these findings have their major significance insofar as they reveal that external stimulation leaves lasting changes in the brain—the organ of the psyche (Berger, 1900, p. 567).]

A. Scope

Many brain structures are dependent on presynaptic morphological integrity and function. In this chapter, I hope to elucidate what is known about the nature of this dependence and to specify morphological changes which take place when presynaptic morphological integrity or function are disrupted. Presumably the changes that take place in learning are a special case of this dependence. It is for this reason that the investigative area of deafferentation and sensory deprivation is of great scientific interest. A thorough understanding of the morphological effects of these experimental findings would delineate the morphological features involved in learning. The effects of learning are certainly within physiological limits, but certainly less pronounced than those of sensory deprivation or deafferentation. Even if qualitatively different, they probably involve the same morphological features.

Reported morphological responses to altered presynaptic integrity or function are principally concerned with neurons and glia. Occasionally, data are reported relative to the extracellular space, synaptic cleft, vascular system, choroid plexus, pia, and ependyma. Most neuronal studies have used light microscopy to study brain volume, cellular volume, dendritic branching and length, and dendritic spines. Recently an increasing number of electron microscopic studies have appeared focusing on size and density of synaptic sites.

The scope of this review includes the morphological effects of deafferentation and sensory deprivation on the postsynaptic neurons or the surrounding structures of the brain. It does not include the effects of surgical section on the terminal portion of the axon. It does include the effects on postsynaptic neurons of such surgery. The specializations of the central nervous system coincident with life styles of animals such as moles where incident light is reduced and in animals such as bats with rudimentary visual systems are not within the purview of this chapter. An attempt has been made to make the bibliographic coverage as complete as possible from 1890 onward.

B. Other Review Articles

Various review articles bearing on this subject include Cowan (1970), Globus (1971), Krech, Rosenzweig, and Bennett (1966), Mann (1894–1895), Mendelson and Ervin (1963), Riesen (1961, 1963, 1965a, b, 1966), Rosenzweig (1966), and Scheibel and Scheibel (1968). Cowan (1970) reviewed the effects of anterograde and retrograde transneuronal degeneration in both the central and peripheral nervous system. Riesen's (1966) review article on sensory deprivation included neurochemistry, neurophysiology, and behavior, as well as morphological correlates. Riesen (1961, 1965a, b) also reviewed the morphological effects of sensory deprivation selectively. Articles by Riesen concentrated on the interaction of adequate stimulation on growth of neuronal structures and maturation of function. Mendelson and Ervin (1963), and Globus (1971) focused on the relation of the postsynaptic structures to presynaptic function and integrity. Scheibel and Scheibel (1968) led and summarized a workshop which included the relation of the dendritic spine to presynaptic integrity and function. Krech *et al.* (1966) and Rosenzweig (1966) reviewed the anatomical findings in the cortex as consequence of differential experience. Mann (1894–1895) reviewed neuronal morphology following excessive stimulation, fatigue, and depression due to metabolic and vascular insult in a number of species including invertebrates. This last article has an excellent bibliography.

C. Principal Hypotheses

The principal hypotheses are all related to the nature of the dependence of a given morphological feature (such as a synapse, endoplasmic reticulum, synaptic vesicle, etc.) on presynaptic structure and function. There are three possible dependencies:

1. Structural dependence on the morphological integrity of the presynaptic structures—studied by morphological disruption.
2. Metabolic dependence on the physiological events taking place during information processing—studied by disturbing, that is, increasing, decreasing, or abolishing, the production of presynaptic action potentials and thus changing the frequency of postsynaptic potentials.
3. Informational dependence on the processing of coherent information —studied by disordering the production of presynaptic action potentials or by making incongruent two or more sets of afferent volleys. This does not involve an increase or decrease in total number of action potentials arriving at the synaptic site.

These hypotheses are applicable to any morphological feature. They are hierarchical in the order listed. Experiments involving informational dependence specify a set of morphological features that must include those involved in learning.

The inferences, experimental methods, and types of dependence are given in Scheme I.

D. Definitions

The terminology used will follow Cowan's (1970) definitions in his review. They are:

1. Anterograde transneuronal degeneration means degeneration or atrophy due to deafferentation, i.e., degeneration in mammalian lateral geniculate body following enucleation.
   a. Primary: changes found in the next synaptic level.

SCHEME I. Inferential Tree, Experimental Methods, Type of Dependence

Presynaptic structures, synapses

- **Present**
  - **Synaptic function normal**
  - **Synaptic function altered**
- **Absent**
  - **Deafferentation–loss of presynaptic structures**
    1. Congenital absence
    2. Lesion
    3. Transneuronal morphologic dependence

						Increased:	
1. Presynaptic action potentials	None	Reduced* within informational limits	Increased* within informational limits	Disordered single afferent	Incongruence of two or more afferent systems	Periodically to jamming	Continually to jamming
2. Release of Transmitter	Markedly reduced, possibly absent	Reduced*	Increased*	Same amount	Same amount	Increased amount	Very much increased
3. Postsynaptic potentials	None	Reduced*	Increased*	Same in type and amount, temporally chaotic	Same in amount but incongruent	Increased	Increased
4. Information processing	Little or none	Reduced in amount	Increased	None or purely accidental	Unknown	Slightly reduced	Reduced to almost nothing
5. Example experiments	Novocaine block	Reduced stimulation Impoverished environment Social isolation	Complex environmental Handling	Jamming	Cut extrocular muscles producing strabismus	Different patterns of hyperstimulation	
6. Type of dependence	Metabolic	Metabolic	Metabolic	Informational	Informational	Metabolic and informational	

* The Change effect (1952) might suggest that these parameters would be increased rather than decreased, or vice versa. See Chapter IV on physiological effects of sensory deprivation and discussion of this review, pp. 62 ff.

b. Secondary: changes found two synapses from the lesioned neuron.
c. Tertiary: changes found three or more synapses from the lesioned neuron.

2. Retrograde transneuronal degeneration means degeneration or atrophy following section of the axon, that is, changes in the retinal ganglion cells following lesions in the visual cortex.

Sensory deprivation refers to the reduction of the total number of adequate stimuli delivered to the receptors of a sensory system. Jamming refers to the disruption of the normal or usual statistical properties of action potential trains of an afferent system.

II. Results

A. Experimental Procedures

1. Absence of Presynaptic Structures

The complete absence of presynaptic structures may be effected by surgical procedures, transneuronal degeneration, chemical toxicity, and congenital agenesis. Examples of surgical procedures include cortical slab production (Benhamida, Ruiz de Pereda, & Hirsch, 1970; Burns, 1951, 1958; Colonnier, 1964) suction of cortical areas, and electrolytic lesions (Ghetti & Wisniewski, 1972; Hamlyn, 1954; Levi-Montalcini, 1949; Loewy, 1972; Matthews, 1964; Penman & Smith, 1950; Pinching & Powell, 1971). Transneuronal degeneration (Dzidzishvili, 1963; Globus & Scheibel, 1966; Hess, 1958) is often used to study the cortex following enucleation. An example of chemical toxicity is the production of retinal receptor cell degeneration following the administration of 1,5-di-(p-aminophenoxy) pentane dihydrochloride (Burke & Hayhow, 1968). Examples of congenital agenesis include anophthalmia (Chase, 1945; Gyllensten & Lindberg, 1964; Recordon & Griffitsh, 1938).

2. Absence and/or Partial Absence of Presynaptic Action Potentials

The absence and/or partial absence of presynaptic action potentials might be produced in short-term experiments by novocaine block without producing significant axon degeneration. I know of no studies of the morphological effects of this or of similar procedures.

3. Reduction in the Total Number of Action Potentials

A variety of procedures is used to reduce the total number of action potentials coursing along an afferent system. They often involve the visual system. Examples are pattern deprivation due to translucent occluders (Chow, Riesen, & Newell, 1957; Wiesel & Hubel, 1965a), eyelid suture (Berger, 1900; Dzidzishvili, 1963; Fifková, 1968; Schüpbach, 1905), limiting the amount of incident light totally (Brattgård, 1952; Bloom, 1920; Cragg, 1970; Globus & Scheibel, 1967a; Goodman, 1932; Rasch, Swift, Riesen, & Chow, 1961; Riesen, 1965b; Schimke, 1959; Valverde, 1971), limiting it to a few hour per day (Chow *et al.,* 1957; Cragg, 1967), and limiting it to a particular frequency band (Chow, 1955; Le Gros Clark, 1943). A number of attempts have been made to study recovery in morphological structures following prolonged periods of sensory deprivation in young animals (Chow & Stewart, 1972; Dolley, 1913; Fifková, 1970b; Fifková & Hassler, 1969; Hubel & Wiesel, 1970; Rasch *et al.,* 1961; Wiesel & Hubel, 1965).

Other sensory systems theoretically subject to this approach include the auditory, in which I have found no references, and proprioception, in which casting the leg or tenotomy may be done (Tower, Howe, & Bodian, 1941). The latter is a physiological study.

More generalized and more subtle approaches include impoverished and enriched environments (Altman & Das, 1964; Bennett, Diamond, Krech, & Rosenzweig, 1964; Diamond, Gray, & Yasargil, 1970; Diamond, Cosenza, & Johnson, 1973; Rosenzweig *et al.,* 1969; West & Greenough, 1972), as well as social isolation (Volkmar & Greenough, 1972).

4. *Increase in the Total Number of Action Potentials*

A variety of means are utilized to increase the activity within an afferent system: electrical stimulation of hypoglossal nerve (Barr & Bertram, 1949) and other parts of the nervous system (Liu, Bailey, & Windle, 1950; Mann, 1894–1895; Mikeladze, 1969); increased presence of adequate stimuli in the visual system by intense light (Gomirato & Baggio, 1962); in the vestibular system (Hamberger & Hydén, 1949; Hydén & Pigon, 1960); increased stressful stimulation (Kocher, 1916; Schapiro & Vukovich, 1970); increased handling (Altman & Das, 1964; Altman, Das, & Anderson, 1968); and increased environmental stimulation (Bennett *et al.,* 1964; Diamond, Krech, & Rosenzweig, 1964; Globus, Rosenzweig, Bennet, & Diamond, 1973; Holloway, 1966; Krech, Rosenzweig, & Bennett, 1966; Rosenzweig *et al.,* 1969; West & Greenough, 1972). I know of no reports of morphological changes due to increased stimulation by a particular frequency of light or sound.

5. *Jamming or Disruption of the Train of Afferent Action Potentials*

There are two modes of jamming. The first is to alter the statistical properties of the action potential volleys of a single afferent system without altering the total number of action potentials arriving at the synaptic site. This method has not been attempted. The other method is to produce an incongruence of two or more afferent systems carrying identical information. The first method becomes the second if there is only one fiber disrupted among many afferent fibers within the same system. Examples of the second method are unilateral eyelid suture (Berger, 1900; Chow & Stewart, 1972; Fifková, 1972; Kupfer, 1965; Maraini, Carta, Franquielli, & Santori, 1967; Sherman & Sanderson, 1972; Wiesel & Hubel, 1965a, b) and section of the extraocular muscles (Wiesel & Hubel, 1965a, b).

B. Results of Deafferentation: Surgical

1. Disruption of Cellular Organization

There are a few studies that show little or no effect following deafferentation, but most studies show striking reduction in overall dimensions and in cellular organization.

Terry, Roland, and Race (1962), studying mice enucleated from birth, showed no difference from controls in the lateral geniculate and visual cortex. This study, like Goodman's (1932) study of visual deprivation, was done without quantitative methods and utilized gross comparison of protein stains such as hematoxylin–eosin and Nissl methods. In fetal guinea pigs, enucleation reduced fiber content in the lateral geniculate body, optic nerve, and superior colliculus. Nuclear structures of the superior colliculus were affected, but no significant effect was found in the neurons of the lateral geniculate body or visual cortex. No quantitative data were reported (Hess, 1958).

Destruction of the vibrissae pad in mice produces a striking disorganization of cortical structures. There are highly structured groups of neurons in somatosensory cortex called "barrels." Each barrel corresponds to a larger mystacial hair in the vibrissal pad. Destruction of these hairs at birth results in a loss of whatever stimulus it is that initiates and maintains the neuronal organization of barrels (Van der Loos & Woolsey, 1973). This effect is achieved through at least two synaptic relays: principal nucleus of the trigeminal nerve and arcuate division of the ventrobasal complex.

Umrath (1965), studying rabbits with Nissl stain following enucleation at eight days, showed reduction in cells of Layers 4 and 5 of the visual cortex (Areas I and II), particularly in the more rostral, binocular area. There was also a loss of fibers and cellular processes in the superior colliculus.

Of great interest is the clinical case of Laura Bridgman (Donaldson, 1890; Donaldson, 1891). Laura contracted scarlet fever at 2 years of age. She lost sight in the left eye and retained some sight in the right eye until the sight of the right eye was lost at 8 years of age. Hearing, taste, and smell were severely impaired. Comparing the results of her brain examination performed when she was 60 to the results of Hubel and Wiesel's (1970) experiments in cats is valuable. Apparently, the little vision left in the right eye of Laura Bridgman until 8 years of age preserved at least the gross structures of vision on the contralateral side of the brain. However, complete loss of function in the left eye before 2 years of age resulted in poor development of the right occipital pole and the cuneus. Thus, the "critical age" for sensory input to save a structure from atrophy, as suggested and defined in cats by Hubel and Wiesel (1970), might well be somewhat between 1 and 7 years of age in man.

2. *Cellular Loss*

There are a great number of studies showing a reduction in neuronal density following varying degrees of deafferentation. Usually the effects are more pronounced the earlier the deafferentation is accomplished, the more complete the deafferentation, and the higher the species' position on the phylogenetic scale. Furthermore, growth and development of the postsynaptic neuron is unaffected if the deafferentation occurs before arrival of the developing afferent fibers until the time when they normally achieve synaptic continuity. Thereafter the growth and development of the postsynaptic neuron is markedly reduced. If deafferentation is effected after the period of time when synaptic continuity is achieved, it normally produces a much less pronounced transneuronal effect. Growth and development of the neuron is apparently under local or contiguous control until the period of time when synaptic continuity is achieved. Thereafter, growth and development depends to a great extent on synaptic continuity for a relatively short period of time. After this time, transneuronal degeneration does not proceed to neuronal death and disintegration unless the vast majority of afferent fibers are disrupted (see Fig. 1).

Enucleation in larvae of *Rana catesbiana* is followed by a reduction of cell division in the optic lobes (Terry & Gordon, 1960). Enucleation in frog larvae results in loss of neurons in the optic lobes at the stage of metamorphosis. In the later experiment enucleation was performed after arrival of developing afferents (Larsell, 1929).

Tsang (1937) demonstrated pronounced reduction in nuclear volume in rats enucleated at birth to adulthood. Quantitative effects were more pronounced in the superior colliculus than the lateral geniculate nucleus and only slight thinning occurred in the visual cortex. He suggested this effect is due to the "functional intimacy" of the retinal fibers to the visual centers. This hypothesis is hardly tenable, as the superior colliculus receives col-

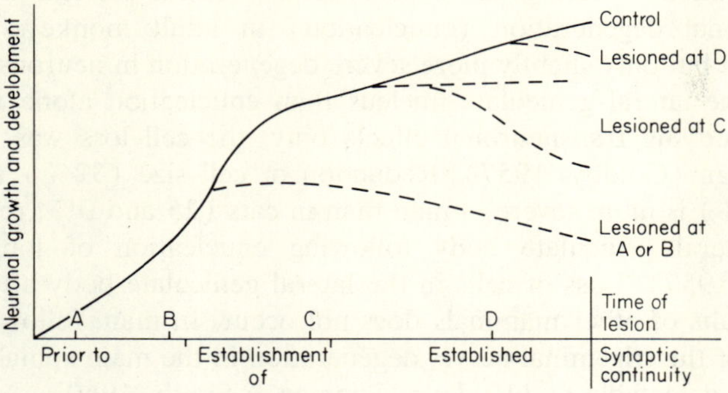

Fig. 1. Graphic summary of the effect of deafferentation. Lesions producing massive deafferentation have the same effect if performed at A or B prior to the establishment of synaptic continuity. Lesions at the end of the period of synaptic continuity (C) produce a variable effect depending on the completeness of deafferentation. Lesions in the mature animals (D) may be described by the same generalization as for C except that, at least for the visual systems, deafferentation produces a greater effect in animals higher on the phylogenetic scale.

laterals from the retinal ganglion axons projecting to the lateral geniculate nucleus. By use of thymidine in enucleated rats it was possible to show that many neurons degenerate and many glial cells fail to form in the superior colliculus (DeLong & Sidman, 1962). In rats with combined dorsal rhizotomy and section of the corticospinal tract, neurons of the ventral horn degenerate (Barron, 1933).

In rabbits following section of the sympathetic trunk, there is a reduction in cell size that is slower and less pronounced than a similar transneuronal degeneration in the lateral geniculate nucleus of the cat (Hamlyn, 1954). Receptors of the olfactory mucosa undergo striking and rapid degeneration following lesions of olfactory bulb. Normally this is thought to be due to retrograde degeneration owing to destruction of axon terminals. Nevertheless, transneuronal degeneration following interruption of axonal endings coming from the region of the olfactory bulb to the olfactory epithelium can not be considered fully excluded (Le Gros Clark, 1957).

In young cats, the enucleation causes no change in the neurons in general but causes some small loss of cells of the visual area in Layer IV. In adult cats there seems to be no change (Umrath, 1965). Transneuronal effects in kittens include cell loss in the inferior olive and pontine nuclei (Torvik, 1956). In dogs, enucleation shows a loss of ganglion cells in Layer IV of the visual area. Umrath (1965) reports an apparent increase in size in the anterior part of the contralateral visual area and a small decrease in the gyrus marginalis.

Combination of retrograde degeneration (ventral cortical lesion) with transneuronal degeneration (enucleation) in adult monkeys effected a more rapid but only slightly more severe degeneration in neurons (14–20% loss) of the lateral geniculate nucleus than enucleation alone (Matthews, 1964). Studying transneuronal effects only, the cell loss was less severe than in man (Goldby, 1957). Reduction of cell size (32%) and loss of cells (50%) is more severe in man than in cats (25 and 0%, respectively) in the lateral geniculate body following enucleation of long duration (Goldby, 1957). Loss of cells in the lateral geniculate body after enucleation in adults of other mammals does not occur. In man, following alcohol injection of the trigeminal nerve, degeneration in the main spinal V nucleus was easily detectable at 110 days (Penman & Smith, 1960).

3. *Changes in the Soma of Neurons*

A variety of changes in the soma are reported, including somal shrinkage in light microscopy, as well as changes in somal organelles in electron microscopy. The generalizations applicable to cell loss are, for the most part, true of the somal shrinkage.

At the 18–26 somite stage, the otocysts of chicks were removed. Development of the cochlear nuclei was unaffected until after 11 days when afferent fibers normally appear. Thereafter, cellular atrophy and loss was prominent (Levi-Montalcini, 1949). This author concludes that not only is the development of neurons dependent on afferent integrity, but that there is a quantitative correlation between the degree of hypoplasia and the number of synaptic connections to be established.

As early as 1894, von Bach reported changes in Nissl substance similar to chromatolysis and disappearance of the nuclei in the lateral geniculate body following the destruction of retinal neuropil in rabbits surviving 3 months before sacrifice. Changes in the Nissl substance of neurons within the dorsal horn following dorsal rhizotomy were reported (Foerster & Gagel, 1934). No measurements were given. In adult cats, following dorsal rhizotomy and/or isolation of the spinal cord, there is severe "chromatolysis." That includes loss of dendritic fields, Nissl body deterioration, and changes in the nucleus. These effects were more rapid and severe when cord isolation was also accomplished (Young & Rowley, 1968). On the other hand, more recent studies call these results into question on technical grounds. In adult cats, dorsal rhizotomy shows degenerative changes in the dorsal horn ipsilateral to the lesion. Changes in the contralateral Clarke's column, which should show transneuronal effects without risk of vascular interference, are not observed (Loewy, 1972). Thus, this author believes that transneuronal degeneration as measured in Nissl preparations does not occur. Similar experiments in kittens (2–6 weeks) do show change in the contralateral Clarke's column. The author concludes that these effects are due to an arrest of maturation and that the effects previously observed in adult animals are secondary to vascular deficit due to the complicated and difficult surgery.

In the lateral geniculate body, folding of the nuclear membrane, as well as cytoplasmic spaces and shrinking, occur in adult monkeys following enucleation (Glees, Hasan, & Tischner, 1967). Cell shrinkage in the lateral geniculate body following enucleation and an increased number of double nucleoli in monkeys have been reported 4 months after enucleation (Matthews, Cowan, & Powell, 1960). In adult man, spinothalamic tractotomy is followed by reduction in cell size, nucleoli blurring, and hypochemia (Bowsher, 1957).

In chromatolysis following axotomy there is a recovery phase. In contrast, transneuronal degeneration leads to a progressive, apparently irreversible loss of cytoplasmic organelles. Another difference is that glial reaction was reported as conspicuously absent.

4. Changes in Dendrites

In most studies, deafferentation is reported to result in some loss of dendritic branching and loss of subsynaptic organelles. These results occur in all species studied and are often effected through several neurons. They depend on transneuronal degeneration.

One of the few negative reports is that of Haddara (1955), who used the Golgi technique to study dendritic branching in the visual cortices of mice following enucleation at birth. Haddara reported no significant change. It is not clear whether short axon or pyramidal cells were studied, nor are there any quantitative data reported.

Studying enucleated mice, Ruiz-Marcos and Valverde (1970), using a computerized analysis of dendritic fields of pyramids called ACRON or "Average Computed Neuron," showed a reduction in basal branches. The branches affected were within 45° of a line descending from the apical dendrite. This effect tended to disappear in older animals. In mice enucleated at birth, and sacrificed at 18 days of age, the dendrites of stellate cells are reported to be oriented away from Layer IV of the area striata (see Fig. 2) (Valverde, 1968, 1971). This finding must be considered tentative as it is the first report of such reorientation, as it is based on relatively few camera lucida drawings, and as it is derived from Golgi material. Nevertheless, the finding is both interesting, plausible, and should be replicated.

Loss of dendritic branching and spines on the remaining dendrites has

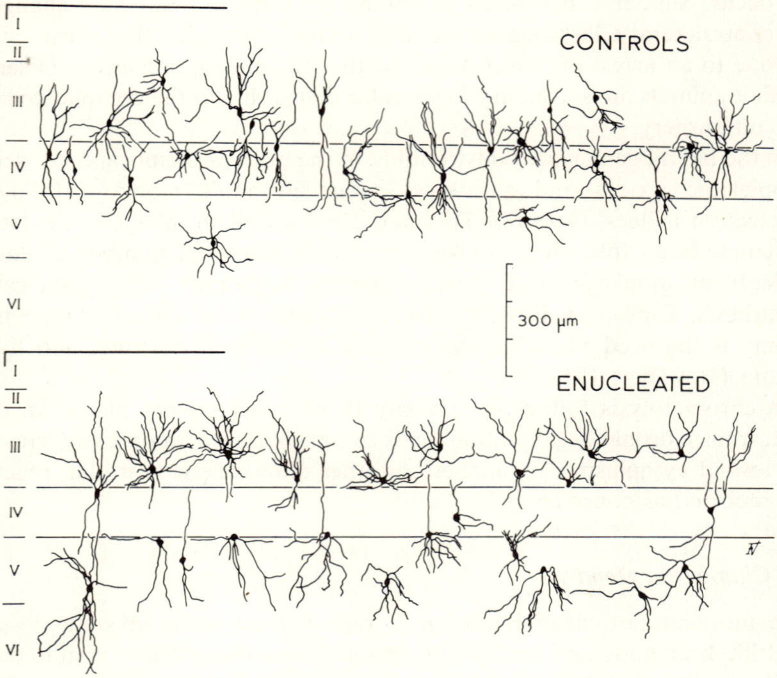

Fig. 2. Composite drawing of stellate cells with ascending axons in the area striata from mice 48 days old. Stellate cells in normal mice appear with bodies and dendrites distributed randomly through Layers V, IV, and III (controls). In mice enucleated at birth the orientation of dendrites outside Layer IV is evident (enucleated). The axons were not traced. The Golgi method, triple impregnation, was used. These are camera lucida drawings. (From Valverde, 1968.)

been shown in Golgi preparations to follow lesions of the olfactory bulb in rats (White & Westrum, 1964). This effect is ascribed to deafferentation. In adult rats with sectioned olfactory bulbs, there was a striking reduction in branching of higher order dendrites. Of course this effects a reduction in total dendritic length (see Fig. 3). In EM studies, persistence of the postsynaptic thickening occurs up to 84 days following resection of the olfactory mucosal membrane in rats. Evidence of change in metabolic activity based on the formation of cisternae was also observed (Pinching, 1969). Nuclear shrinking and detachment of the nuclear membrane, as well as extensive changes in the endoplasmic reticulum and loss of the postsynaptic thickening, were observed in the olfactory bulb and olfactory cortex following resection of the olfactory mucosa (Pinching & Powell, 1971). In study of rats 25–150 days after either optic nerve section or

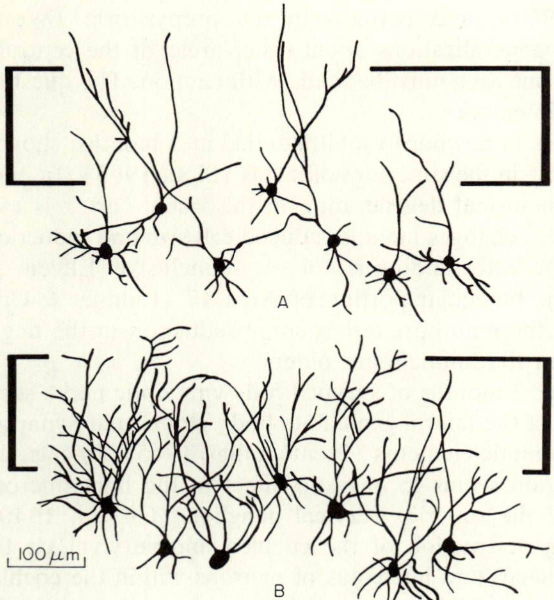

Fig. 3. Reconstruction of the prepiriform cortex of the rat to show the pyramidal cell bodies, synthesized from microprojector tracings: (A) following 91 days deafferentation; (B) normal. The plexiform layer of the prepiriform cortex is indicated by square brackets. (From Jones & Thomas, 1962, p. 378.)

enucleation, electron microscopy of the lateral geniculate body shows striking changes in subsynaptic organelles as well as increased electron density of the synaptic plasma membrane. Dense granules and circular profiles appear within the dendritic cytoplasm (McMahan, 1967).

In studying the rabbit olfactory bulb undergoing transneuronal degeneration following removal of the olfactory mucosa, Powell (1967) reports a reduction in dendrites. He ascribes this to a resistance to Golgi impregnation. He bases this conclusion on the fact that the effect is coincident with the cell body shrinkage (17 days) and that the dendrites are discernible under electron microscopy and Bodian stain. The coincidence with cell body shrinkage, while interesting, is not proof of causation. Bodian stain shows primary and proximal dendrites where the effect reported in Golgi studies is minimal or absent. Furthermore, Bodian stain does not show spines. Presence of dendrites and spines in electronmicrographs does not exclude the possibility that these structures are deafferented. It also ignores EM evidence of spine degeneration following deafferentation in the cortex (Colonnier & Gray, 1962), and in the cerebellum (Mouren-Mathieu &

Colonnier, 1969), and perhaps in the prepyriform (Westrum, 1966). Furthermore, generalizations about other areas of the central nervous system based on one area must be made with caution. The question is open for further experimentation.

Enucleations in newborn rabbit, studied at 2 months, show reduced dendritic branching in the superior colliculus (Siou, 1963). In enucleated adult rabbits, transneuronal degeneration in the visual cortex is evident in only 2–3 days. These changes include reduced cell size and reduction in dendritic branching. The latter finding is not very conclusive. Effects are more pronounced in the binocular portion of Area 17 (Lindner & Umrath, 1955). Furthermore, these authors report some reduction in the degree of change observed when the animals are older.

In cats, after 2 months of survival following optic nerve section, the dendritic portion of the lateral geniculate body glomerular synapse is lost along with the presynaptic elements (Szentágothai, 1965). In cats, deafferentation of short duration seems to have no effect in the light microscopic picture of neurons of the superior cervical ganglion (Gibson, 1940). In mature cats following destruction of the cochlea and survival up to 1 year, the cytoplasm, nucleus and nucleolus of neurons within the cochlear nuclei are all reduced in size. The greatest degree of change is in the cytoplasm. Comparison of time course and severity of degeneration of cells to types of afferents and size of cell body indicates that these two factors do not influence the transneuronal degenerative process (Powell, 1962). They conclude that the shrinkage in transneuronal degeneration of the above mentioned parameters is a function of the number of fibers lost due to deafferentation. This effect is mediated through the hypothesized loss of dendritic volume.

In enucleated monkeys, Le Vay (1971) has shown that the dendrites of the P neurons of the lateral geniculate nucleus (those that project to the visual cortex) withdraw from the neuropil, leaving a few somatodendritic synapses on the I neurons (those that may be inhibitory and that have either no axon or a short axon). The I cell is thought to be the presynaptic element.

In a 56-year-old woman, who underwent enucleation two years previously, the relevant layers of the lateral geniculate body showed shrunken somas and reduced dendritic branching (Le Gros Clark, 1932).

5. *Changes in Dendritic Spines and Synaptic Sites*

Since 1962 there have been varied reports in the literature relative to the atrophy or phagocytosis of the dendritic spines following deafferentation.

The weight of evidence seems to be towards loss of spines both in young and adult animals. There may well be exceptions in certain systems within the central nervous system. Another problem rests on the technique used. Electronmicrography studies show everything within a very small section of tissue, but leave the overall picture in doubt. Golgi studies probably show everything on a particular neuron, but not all neurons in that area. Furthermore there is some question that a Golgi impregnated neuron does show all dendritic specializations. It may be that spines, which are deafferented, fail to impregnate, while the rest of the cell does. The position I have taken for purposes of discussion is that the Golgi picture is complete. That is, if the dendritic spine is not visible in Golgi, it is not there. The reader should keep in mind that this is not yet an area of complete agreement among the investigators in this field.

In adult frogs with preganglionic section, the subsynaptic specializations remain intact to 12 postoperative days. At that time the boutons are replaced by glial processes but the cleft between the glia and postsynaptic membrane is of the same order of magnitude as before (Sotelo, 1968).

Utilizing isolated slabs of rat visual cortex, Colonnier (1964) and Colonnier and Gray (1962) demonstrated that the postsynaptic process and the presynaptic terminal are engulfed by glia as a consequence of deafferentation. This process is the basis of the Golgi technique involving spine counting. It permits the localization of the afferent systems as well as the estimation of the number of synapses on the dentritic processes. It is thus an anatomical index of the afferent system's influence on neurons with spines (Fifková, 1968; Globus & Scheibel, 1966; Globus & Scheibel, 1967a, b, c; Illera, 1968; Mouren-Mathieu & Colonnier, 1969; Valverde, 1967). Although it is possible that this is an effect of retrograde degeneration, it is perhaps more likely a transneuronal effect. The latter proposition is supported by the normal EM appearance of the other postsynaptic structures. Laminar lesions in rat cortex produced by heavy ionizing particle irradiation yield suggestive evidence (Kruger & Hámori, 1970) on an EM level that supports earlier work (Colonnier, 1964) showing that spines degenerate following surgical deafferentation. In adult rats after removal of the olfactory mucosa, spines occasionally undergo phagocytosis by astrocytes (Westrum, 1966).

Most transneuronal changes follow distinct decrease in postsynaptic thickening in both rabbit and rat (Pinching *et al.,* 1971). Under conditions of enucleation or lateral geniculate body lesion at birth, a 30% reduction in spines is observed along the apical dendrite of pyramidal neurons (Globus & Scheibel, 1967).

EM studies of degeneration in the somatosensory cortex show that terminals of the commissural, thalamocortical, and corticocortical fibers synapse mainly on spines (75%). These synapses are of the asymmetrical type (Gray, 1959; Jones & Powell, 1970a, b, c). In the adult cat neocortex, 6 days following lesions of the thalamus or cortex, degenerating axonal terminals were observed. Postsynaptic structures including spines were observed intact. Thus, it appears that deafferentation does not result in deafferentation of the dendritic spines in the somatosensory cortex of mature cats (Jones & Powell, 1970b). Electronmicrograph studies of axodendritic synapses in the cat visual cortex following lateral geniculate body lesions have shown glial engulfment of not only the presynaptic elements but also the synaptic cleft and postsynaptic membrane (Ghetti & Wisniewski, 1972). Reduced numbers of spines (25%) in dendrites of stellate cells of the caudate following cortical lesions or thalamic lesions have been reported (Kemp & Powell, 1971). Distribution was not altered, and was similar in both types of lesions. The effect was additive. The heads of the remaining spines were smaller as well. Whether the lesions were made in a kitten or an adult did not alter the effect. In adult cats, following deafferentation of the lateral cervical nucleus, a loss of dendritic spines was observed. This author does not suggest a specific mechanism for loss, but leans towards microglia as the phagocytizing cell (Westman, 1969). In cat inferior olive, following deafferentation, dendritic multivesicular inclusion bodies were observed adjacent to degenerating boutons. The dendritic surface was marked by pits that were in contact with the degenerating boutons. This is taken as evidence that dendritic pinocytosis of the degenerating terminal occurs (Walberg, 1963). Walberg (1966) studied the effect of lesions of the dorsal columns and of the somatosensory cortex on the cuneate nucleus in adult cats. Although the morphology of the dendrites and soma were described, no mention was made of changes in the postsynaptic surface as the consequence of deafferentation. However, he did mention that as the axodendritic synapse undergoes degeneration, the opposed surfaces remain in contact, and in adult cat cerebellum, following section of parallel fibers, there is a loss of spines due to deafferentation. This result was confirmed both in electron and light microscopy (Illera, 1968). Suggestive evidence is presented that many spines and presynaptic terminals are engulfed by glia although some may simply shrink away (Mouren-Mathieu & Colonnier, 1969). This experiment has the advantage of reducing the possibility of retrograde effects. Cortical slab studies always suffer from problems in distinguishing retrograde from transneuronal degeneration.

Spine or postsynaptic engulfment in adult cat and monkey following deafferentation of the visual cortex by lesions of the lateral geniculate body was not observed by Garey and Powell (1971). The authors believe that specific afferent radiations terminate in stellate neurons with spines in Layer IV of Area 17 as well as in pyramidal neurons.

Axon terminals can be used as a measure of synaptic frequency and, perhaps, size. For instance, Cragg (1968, 1970) sectioned the optic tract in adult monkeys and showed a reduction in frequency and an increase in size of axon terminals in the contralateral visual cortex.

6. *Changes in Axons*

As far as I know there have been no studies of the effect of deafferentation on the axons of the postsynaptic neuron. Mention is made by Pinching and Powell (1971) of axonal shrinkage and increased packing density of neurotubules in rats following surgical resection of the olfactory mucosa. It is not altogether clear whether they are referring to axons of the postsynaptic neurons or axons that have been interrupted by surgical resection of the olfactory mucosa. Surely this is both an important and easy area of investigation.

7. *Changes in Glia*

As far as I know there has been only one study of the glial reaction within the postsynaptic structure following its deafferentation. There are, of course, many studies of glial response to degenerating terminals. Whether there is a long term change in the glia/neuronal ratio following deafferentation is unknown. In my opinion, this is another important area of research awaiting investigators. Attention to long term effects of partial deafferentation would surely shed light on the relation between glia and neurons and would delineate further areas of investigation. Kupfer (1965) reported no increase in glial elements in the lateral geniculate body following enucleation in man. Neuronal loss was observed two years after the enucleation.

Tables I and II are summaries of studies using surgical deafferentation.

C. Results of Deafferentation: Congenital Absence

A critical factor for research design in this area is whether the deafferentation occurs before, during, or after the afferent system effects synaptic continuity. The event of effecting synaptic continuity may be thought of as a period of time in which morphological continuity is first established, ending when the action potentials within the afferent synapse effect mature, and following postsynaptic potentials. There are relatively few studies beginning before synaptic continuity is established. Perhaps studies of congenital absences qualify. This area of investigation has just been broached with a few light microscopy studies. These are summarized in Table III.

TABLE I

Deafferentation in the Visual System: Surgical Interruption[a]

Procedure	Species	Began	Ended	Structure studies and/or interruption	Reference
Enucleation	Frog (*Rana catesbiana*)	40–70 mm larvae	34–52 days	Optic tectum: fewer dividing ependymal cells, reduced cells in extraependymal layers. Optic lobe showed hypoplasia.	Terry and Gordon (1960)
Enucleation	Frog (*Hyla regilla*)	Larvae	Metamorphosis	Optic lobes: reduced in thickness and cells.	Larsell (1929)
Enucleation	Chicken	Hatching	17 days	Arrested development contralateral optic lobe, in weight, protein content, acetylcholinesterase activity. Both light and dark reared similar but smaller effects in cerebral hemisphere if kept in light.	Bondy and Margolis (1971)
Optic nerve section	Chicken	Adult	30 days	Optic tectum: postsynaptic thickening disappeared, occasionally intact with glial process covering synaptic site.	Gray and Hamlyn (1962)
Unilateral enucleation	Mice	Birth	19, 24, 60 days	The younger animal, the more reduced dendritic branching in visual cortex. Basal dendrites enclosed in 45% angle from a line extending from the apical dendrite. Layer IV and V pyramids chosen.	Ruiz-Marcos and Valverde (1970)
Unilateral enucleation	Mice	Birth	24, 48 days	Spines on apical dendrite in Layer: III—8% reduction of area striate IV—25% reduction of area striate—24 days 18% reduction of area striate—48 days V—No change (see Fig. 2).	Valverde (1968)

Unilateral enucleation	Mice	Birth	24, 48 days	Left peristriate cortex: spines on the apical dendrite — no change. Right peristriate cortex: statistically significant reduction of spines in upper Layer III segment of 48 day mice.	Valverde and Estéban (1968)
Enucleation (thymidine-H^3)	Mice	Birth	Adult	Superior colliculus: 40% of neurons disappeared between days 4 and 7. Perikaryon volume of survivors reduced by 5%. 45% of glial cells failed to form, of those that formed 25% were lost later.	DeLong and Sidman (1962)
Unilateral enucleation	Mice	4–6 days	3–11 weeks	Optic nerve, optic tract, chiasma, and stratum griseum of superior colliculus reduced in volume. LGB, striate cortex: no change.	Terry *et al.* (1962)
Enucleation	Mice	Birth	Adult	Golgi Cox method in visual cortex. No effect on dendritic branching.	Haddara (1955)
Enucleation and/or optic nerve section	Rat	25–150 days	1–300 days	LGB subsynaptic organelle extended deeply into dendritic cytoplasm. Increased dense granules.	McMahan (1967)
Slab	Rat	Adult	1, 3, 5, 7, 9, 11, 15 days	Visual cortex: Loss of terminals with postsynaptic processes. Often seen invaginated with large clear processes (dendrites) or glial cell bodies.	Colonnier (1964)
Blinding ECT and IC	Rat	Weaning	3 months	Brain weight 5% greater and cholinesterase activity 3% greater in ECT than in IC.	Krech *et al.* (1963)
Enucleation	Rat	Birth, 13 days, adult	3–7 months	Optic nerve: ⅓–1/5 of normal size (7 month degeneration from birth), ½–⅓ of normal size (3 month degeneration from adult age). LGN: reduction in size 55–65% of normal. Loss of cells. Visual cortex: thinned. Superior colliculus: reduction in size 76% of normal.	Tsang (1937)

TABLE I *(continued)*

Procedure	Species	Began	Ended	Structure studies and/or interruption	Reference
Enucleation	Guinea pig	Gestation 35–55 days	1–9 days removed from uterus	Reduced fibers in LGB, superior colliculus and visual cortex. Reduced stratum opticum in superior colliculus. No change in nuclear content of LGB and visual cortex.	Hess (1958)
Unilateral enucleation	Rabbit	Birth	30 days	Decrease spines on apical dendrite.	Globus and Scheibel (1966)
Enucleation	Rabbit	9 days	5 months	Layer V, Area 17, reduction of cell body size, apical dendrite coiled.	Dzidzishvili (1963)
Enucleation	Rabbit	Birth	87 days	Arrest of development of neuron within the superior colliculus, including a reduction in dendritic branching.	Siou (1963)
Unilateral enucleation	Rabbit	Adult	2 days–several months	Nissl, Visual Areas I, II, 17, 18, and binocular area thoroughly studied Layers II and III rows disturbed. Layer IV cells lost in lower part. Loss of multipolarity. Histological changes same in cell areas. Changes in binocular area most severe. Claimed reduction.	Lindner and Umrath (1955)
Unilateral enucleation	Rabbit	Adult	3–313 days	LGB: decreased nucleus, nucleolus, cytoplasm—2 months. Slow loss of Nissl substance, vaculation—8–10 months. Siow and less pronounced in rabbit.	Cook, Walker, and Barr (1951)
	Cat	Adult	3–313 days		

Unilateral enucleation	Rabbit	8 days	10–26 days	Decreased cell density. Crossed Layer IV and V of Visual Areas I and II. Binocular and monocular loss of fibers in superior colliculus, more pronounced than when enucleated.	Umrath (1965)
		Adult	10–26 days	Same as above.	
	Dog	8 days	10–26 days	Same as above.	
	Cat	8 days	10–26 days	Decreased cell density in anterior part of Layer IV.	
		Adult	10–26 days	Same as above.	
Lesion of LGB	Cat	Adult	4–180 days	Striate cortex: axodendritic synapses studied. Presynaptic membrane still attached to postsynaptic membrane and engulfed by glial cytoplasm.	Ghetti and Wiśniewski (1972)
Slab or deafferentation	Cat	Adult	2 months	LGB: increased axoaxonic contacts. Increase (controls 3–8%, experimental 8–20%) of total synaptic contacts. Cerebellum: loss of spines and dendrites.	Hamori (1968)
Section of optic nerve	Cat	Adult	2 months	LGB: the dendritic protrusions in the complex glomerular synapse are lost.	Szentagothai (1965)
Unilateral enucleation	Cat	5 weeks	2–60 days	LGB: rapid and severe transneuronal atrophy of neurons in appropriate laminae. Decreased activity in TPN-diaphorase, DPN-diaphorase, cholinesterase, and the dehydrogenases of 6-phosphogluconate, succinate, and lactate-DPN.	Kupfer and Palmer (1964)
Lesion of LGB	Cat	Adult	3–5 days	Visual cortex: no post synaptic elements engulfed. Most synapses on spines, 80% on stellate cells, 17% on dendritic surface, 3% on somata.	Garey *et al.* (1971)
	Monkey	Adult	3–5 days		

TABLE I *(continued)*

Procedure	Species	Began	Ended	Structure studies and/or interruption	Reference
Enucleation	Monkey (*Macaca mulatta*)	Adult	11–600 days	LGN: "P" cells, neurons projecting to cortex "withdraw" dendrites. 29 months little or no dendrites left. Some necrosis.	Le Vay (1971)
Section of optic tract	Monkey	Adult	4 months	Striate cortex: axon terminals enlarged (13.5%) but less numerous (23%).	Cragg (1968)
Enucleation	Monkey (*Macaca nemestrina*)	Adult	6–443 days	LGB: cytoplasmic shrinkage and folding of nuclear membranes, later empty spaces with irregular boundaries.	Glees *et al.* (1967)
Unilateral enucleation	Monkey (*Macaca mulatta*)	Mature	1 year	LGN: loss of 14–20% of cells in involved laminae. If combined with retrograde degeneration (visual cortical lesion), early degeneration was more severe.	Matthews (1964)
Enucleation	Monkey (*Macaca mulatta*)	Adult	4 days–4 months	LGN: neurons shrink and staining intensity of Nissl substance decreased. Cytoplasm shrinks more than nucleus. 4 months, increased density of neurons with two nucleoli. Shrinkage reached peak in crossed laminae at 4 days (9–17% control, same animal), and on uncrossed laminae at 8 days (24–30% of control). 4 months mean area of atrophied neuron, 60% of control. Slight loss of neurons in lamina 6.	Matthews *et al.* (1960)

Bilateral enucleation	Rhesus monkey	Adult	4–170 days	LGB: soma, distention of Golgi, dilatation of endoplasmic reticulum, later vacuoles at periphery, proliferation of microtubules. Dendrites, watery dendrites and dendrites with tubulovesicular profiles, reduction in number of dendrites (170 days). Axon terminals phagocytosis accompanied by postsynaptic membrane.	Ghetti, Horoupian, and Wiśniewski (1972)
Unilateral enucleation or macular degeneration	Man	Adult (one subject lost vision at 18 months)	1 month–73 years	LGN: unimodal disturbution in all laminae. No increase in glial elements. After 2 years cell loss occurred in atrophied laminae.	Kupfer (1965)
Unilateral enucleation	Man	18 years	59 years	LGB: ½ cells lost in effected laminae. In Laminae 1 and 2, 32% decrease in area. In Laminae 3–6, 48% decrease in area.	Goldby (1957)
Corneal opacity	Man	Childhood	62, 49, 52 years	Optic nerve reduced by ⅔. Atrophy in LGB. No change in visual cortex.	Hechst (1933)
Enucleation	Man	54 years	56 years	LGB relevant layers: no normal cells. Cells shrunken. Reduction in dendritic branching.	Le Gros Clark (1932)
Scarlet fever Loss of sight (left eye entirely, right eye to 8 years) Loss of hearing, taste, smell	Man (Laura Bridgman)	2 years	Some sight in right eye to 8 years. Died at 60 years.	Brachium of superior and inferior colliculus absent. Pulvinar reduced in size. Flattened occipital pole. Right cuneus poorly developed. Reduced thickness of cerebral cortex. Superior and inferior colliculus reduced in size or absent.	Donaldson (1890–1891)

[a] The abbreviations used in this table are as follows: LGB, lateral geniculate body; ECT, environmental complexity in training; IC, impoverished condition; LGN, lateral geniculate nucleus.

TABLE II

DEAFFERENTATION IN OTHER SYSTEMS: SURGICAL INTERRUPTIONS

Procedure	Species	Began	Ended	Structure studied and/or effected	Reference
Section of abdominal sympathetic chain	Frog	Adult	7–12 days	Axosomatic synapses of sympathetic ganglion: subsynaptic structures (postsynaptic differentiation and subsynaptic formation) remains intact.	Sotelo (1968)
Surgical extirpation of otocyst	Chicken	Stage of 18–26 somites	4–21 days of incubation	Cochlear centers: development not effected until 11 days. After 11 days nucleus angularis severely effected, magnocellularis slightly less, nucleus laminaris uneffected. Vestibular centers: not effected.	Levi-Montalcini (1949)
Removal of mystacial hairs	Mice	Birth	12–43 days	Somatosensory field (S1): disruption of "barrels" of neurons in Layer IV.	Van der Loos and Woolsey (1973)
Removal of olfactory mucous membrane	Rat	Adult	Up to 84 days	Increased density of postsynaptic thickening. Presynaptic membrane parts from postsynaptic membrane. No change in structure. Subsurface cisternae form which are continuous with agranular reticulum.	Pinching (1969)
Removal of olfactory bulb	Rat	Adult (?)	6 hr–3 months	Prepyriform cortex: phagocytosis "apparently by astrocytes" occurs within 48 hr of both spines and synaptic sites.	Westrum (1966)
Resection of olfactory bulb	Rat	Adult (?)	4–8 days	Prepyriform layer: dendrites denuded of spines and shortened.	White and Westrum (1964)
Resection of olfactory bulb	Rat	Adult	91–492 days	Dendritic branches of pyramid cells of prepiriform cortex reduced (see Fig. 3).	Jones and Thomas, (1956, 1962)

Dorsal rhizotomy, section of cortico/spinal tract	Rat	Adult	15–20 days	Motoneurons degenerate "become structurally altered."	Barron (1933)
Destruction of olfactory mucosa	Rat	5–7 weeks	10–250 days	Little change to 150–200 days. Findings similar to rabbit, except no sign of transneuronal change in mitral and tufted cells—possibly due to low sampling.	Pinching and Powell (1971)
	Rabbit	5–7 weeks	10–90 days	Two-thirds of mitral and tufted cells show increased electron density, cellular boundaries are irregular, nucleus shrunken, nuclear membrane detached. Mitochondria, endoplasmic reticulum, Golgi apparatus, and multivesicular bodies swollen and vacuolated. Dendrites shrunken, endoplasmic reticulum swollen. Increased packing of microtubules. Loss of postsynaptic thickening. Spines shrink. Some changes in pyriform cortex. Axon shrinkage, terminals show increased packing, mitochondria and multivesicular bodies. 24 days complete.	
Removal of olfactory mucosa	Rabbit	6 weeks	10–49 days	Few mitral, tufted, and periglomerular cells. Reduced density of dendrites and recurrent collaterals of the external plexiform layer in olfactory bulb.	Powell (1967)
Section of corpus callosum	Rabbit	Birth	30 days	Parietal cortex: reduced number of spines on oblique dendrite.	Globus and Scheibel (1967b)
Removal of olfactory mucosa	Rabbit	Adult	6–200 days	Decreased dendrites of mitral, tufted, periglomerular cells. Decreased areas in mitral and tufted cells. Decreased Nissl in dendrites of tufted cells.	Matthews and Powell (1962)

TABLE II *(continued)*

Procedure	Species	Began	Ended	Structure studied and/or effected	Reference
Preganglionic section of superior cervial ganglion	Rabbit	Adult	40–160 days	Decreased Nissl substance. Decreased cross-sectional area of neurons (40 days, 9%; 100 days, 17%; 160 days, 18%).	Hamlyn (1954)
Dorsal rhizotomy	Cat	2–6 weeks Adult	15 days 15 days	Cellular and nuclear shrinkage. Clarke's column showed no change.	Loewy (1972)
Lesions of cortex, thalamus	Cat	Young, adult	6–52 weeks	Caudate: reduced spine counts over entire dendritic trees (25%). Altered heads—shrunken. No difference in distribution with cortical and thalamic lesion and similar amount of reduction. No difference related to age of animals. Combined lesions roughly doubled effect.	Kemp and Powell (1971)
Lesions of cortex, thalamus	Cat	Adult	2–6 days	Somatic sensory cortex: postsynaptic structures are not detached. Spines are intact but surrounded by glia.	Jones and Powell (1970a)
Cortical slab	Cat	Adult	Adult	Suprasylvian gyrus: decrease of spine density on basilar, oblique, apical dendrites. Dendrites in Layer IV show greater effects.	Benhamida and Ruiz de Pereda (1969)
Cutting of parallel fibers in cerebellum	Cat	Adult	60 days	Loss of spines on Purkinje dendrites. Loss of dendrites later.	Mouren-Mathieu and Colonnier (1969)

Transection of spinal afferents to the lateral cervical nucleus	Cat	Adult	2 days–2 years	Lateral cervical nucleus: decrease in medium size of the neurons. Reduction in the amount of dendritic spines.	Westman (1969)
Total deafferentation of spinal cord and dorsal root section	Cat	Adult	7 days	Perikaryonal hyalinization, eccentric displacement of nucleus, accentuation of satellite cell nucleoli. Increase lysosomal size and activity.	Young and Rowley (1968)
			29 days	Peripheral chromatolysis, uniform Nissl stain, some decrease in cell size.	
			42 days	Increase in DNase activity.	
Section of dorsal rhizotomy, isolated cord segment	Cat	Adult	7 days–several months	Spinal cord population of motoneurons reduced in number and size. Severe chromatolysis, more rapid response in isolated segments. DNase and acid phosphatase activity decreased. Eccentric nuclear displacement, perinuclear caps, nucleolar cysts. Dendritic branching diminishes.	Young and Rowley (1968)
Bilateral section of dorsal root	Cat	Adult	7 days	Chromatolysis. Increase peripheral density, with satellite cells with increased nucleoli.	Young and Rowley (1968)
			28 days	Nuclear cysts, microaggregation of Nissl material, perinuclear Nissl cap formation.	
			30 days	Peripheral chromatolysis.	

TABLE II *(continued)*

Procedure	Species	Began	Ended	Structure studied and/or effected	Reference
Unilateral section of dorsal root	Cat	Adult	7 days	Ventral horn decreased cell size and population, assume spherical shape, decreased dendritic arborization.	Young and Rowley (Continued)
			14 days	No change in satellite cells, increased Golgi and perinuclear aggregate of TPPase. Increased acid phosphotase activity.	
			42 days	Increased DNase activity. Increased TPPase activity. Increased pseudocanalicular pattern.	
Cortical slab[a]	Cat (?)	Adult (?)	60 days	Electron microscope: reduced number of spines on pyramidal cells.	Szentágothai (1965)
Lesions of mesencephalic, periaqueductal gray substance, and adjacent reticular formation	Cat	Adult	7, 14, and 36 days	Inferior olive: multivesicular inclusion bodies in normal dendrites adjacent to degenerating boutons. Pits on the surface of some dendrites.	Walberg (1963)
Destruction of cochlea	Cat	Adult	30–359 days	Ventral cochlear nucleus cell mass reduced 34%. Superior olivary nucleus cell mass reduced 10%. Reduced cell mass in preolivary, medial trapezoid, and lateral lemniscal nuclei. No cell mass loss in auditory relay nuclei and spindle cell layer of dorsal cochlear nucleus.	Powell and Erulkar (1962)

Unilateral cortical lesions	Cat	8–21 days	3–13 days	Pontine nuclei: extensive nerve cell loss, slight loss in reticular tegmental nucleus of Bechterew.	Torvik (1956)
Hemidecerebrations at mesencephalic and thalamic levels				Inferior olive: loss of nerve cells. Intense microglial reaction.	
Unilateral removal of motor cortex and dorsal root segments, L6, L7, S1	Cat	Adult	3, 10, 35, 90, 120, 150, 180 days	No change in spinal cord.	Cook *et al.* (1951)
Preganglionic sympathetic trunk along carotid sheath	Cat	Adult	24 hr	No evidence that the ganglion cells suffered.	Gibson (1940)
Tractotomy (for relief of pain)	Man	Adult	17–50 days	Nucleus ventralis posterolateralis of thalamus: reduction of cell size, hypochromia, blurring of the outline of the neucleolus.	Bowsher (1957)
Transection of olfactory tracts	Man	Adult	2 years	Prepyriform cortex: shrinkage and pyknosis of pyramidal cells.	Allison (1954)
90% alcohol injection into right trigeminal	Man	73 years	110 days	Degeneration of neurons within the main sensory and spinal V nuclei.	Penman and Smith (1950)

[a] Method developed by Burns (1951, 1958).

TABLE III

DEAFFERENTATION IN THE VISUAL SYSTEM: CONGENITAL ABSENCE

Procedure	Species	Began	Ended	Structure studied and/or effected	Reference
Inherited retinal dystrophy	Mice	Birth–10 days	20, 30, 60 days	Striate cortex: retarded growth of cell nuclei in internal granular and supragranular layers.	Gyllensten and Lindberg (1964)
Congenital absence of eye and optic nerve	Mice	Before birth (?)	Birth, 10 days, 5–6 months	Reduction in the volume of the lateral geniculate body, the stratum griseum of the superior colliculus, and of Layer II and III of the striate cortex.	Chase (1945)
Congenital absence of both eyes	Man	Birth	55 days	No optic nerve, lateral geniculate body absent; superior colliculus was normal; cortex seemed normal.	Recordon and Griffitsh (1938)

In mice with inherited retinal dystrophy, where the photoreceptors degenerate between the tenth and twentieth day of life, there is retardation of the growth of cell nuclei in the visual cortex (Gyllensten & Lindberg, 1964). Genetically determined absences of the eye and optic nerve in mice lead to a reduction in volume of the optic nerve and a slightly reduced volume of the dorsal nucleus. In the superior colliculus there is a reduction in stratum griseum. The visual cortex has a cellular reduction in Layers II, III, and VI (Chase, 1945).

In a case of complete congenital absence of the eye in a human infant surviving two months, there were no optic nerves, tracts, or lateral geniculate nucleus (LGN). On the other hand, the superior colliculus and the striate cortex were normal (Recordon & Griffitsh, 1938). However, no measurements nor comparison with controls were reported.

D. Results of Reduced Sensory Input

1. Disruption of Organization or Overall Dimensions

With one significant exception early morphological studies on animals undergoing sensory deprivation showed little or no effect (Berger, 1900). Superficially, it seemed that the methods were not sensitive enough. On closer examination, most often the controls were inadequate and/or no measurements were taken. Positive results followed measurements with the same methods. Berger measured and came up with positive results in 1900. Sensory deprivation studied in the visual system almost always yielded positive results routinely in controlled studies using quantitative techniques. Many studies to the present have not been performed with blind methodology and therefore must be replicated.

Eyelid suture or dark environment in pigeons for 1–5 days showed no effect on retinal ganglion cells (Schüpbach, 1905). No measurements were reported. Eyelid suture in mice performed at birth showed no effect in protein stained material in the structures from the optic nerve to the visual cortex (Terry, Roland, & Race, 1962).

Goodman (1932) reported no change in Golgi and Nissl preparations of the entire visual system, including the pulvinar, following visual deprivation from birth to 6 months in rabbits. The absence of findings was probably due to the lack of (1) littermate control, (2) standard values from the experimental animal, and (3) quantitative criteria for study. As early as 1900, basing his conclusions on cats and dogs with eyelid suture from birth, Berger suggested that stimulation from the environment is necesary to effect full development of the brain. A variety of measurements of the cortical areas was taken. Often the measurements were at very low magnifications. Nevertheless, the results seem indisputable and, furthermore, have since been replicated. In cats maintained in total darkness from 7 days to 17 weeks, the retina was significantly thinner than it was in the controls (Weiskrantz, 1958). The author believes this may be due to a loss of dendrites or branches within the inner plexiform layer.

2. *Cellular Loss*

Although there have been repeated reports of reduction in volume due to sensory deprivation, particularly due to maturation in the dark, reports of cell loss are not frequent except in the retina of chimpanzee. Thus, so far, sensory deprivation results in a reduction in volume, but apparently results in little or no loss in the numbers of neurons.

Eyelid suture in young rabbits and cats was reported to show a reduction in cells of Layer V of the visual cortex. In rabbits this effect was limited to the rostral binocular portion of the visual area (Umrath, 1955).

Deprivation by eyelid suture in kittens, studied electrophysiologically in the lateral geniculate nucleus, seems to result in a selective loss of a group of neurons defined functionally. Neurons in the lateral geniculate nucleus seem to fall into two classes: fast conducting with phasic responses and slow conducting with tonic responses. A group of large neurons disappears in the lateral geniculate nucleus as a result of deprivation. Perhaps these are the fast-conducting neurons with a phasic response (Sherman, Hoffman, & Stone, 1972; Sherman & Sanderson, 1972). These are reduced in number in Layer A of the lateral geniculate nucleus contralateral to the deprived eye. In this layer, large cells are lacking. Sherman *et al.* therefore conclude that this cell is selectively lost or nonfunctional. He suggests early findings of an across the board reduction of cell size in monocular deprivation is more likely due to loss in the larger Y cells or transient cells. This is an interesting conclusion but must be considered hypothetical. However, these results do indicate the need for histograms to determine the composition of cellular population before assuming that an averaged change in cell volume is an index of somal atrophy rather than a selective loss of a certain cellular population.

In the dark-reared chimpanzee, retinal ganglion cells are reduced to 10% of the normal number. One and one-half hours of diffuse light daily blocks this effect (Riesen, 1965b). Cell loss in the retina of dark reared chimpanzees is striking. This is not the case with cats or rats. Cats and rats showed RNA changes and cell atrophy, but no cell loss (Riesen, 1960). In chimpanzee some of the atrophy of the ganglion cell layer was reversible if normal lighting was restored before 3 months of age. Studying the retinas of rats, cats, and chimpanzees under conditions of dark rearing, Rasch *et al.* (1961) report decreased RNA content, cell cross-sectional area, protein content, and nucleolar volume. In the chimpanzee only, there is striking loss of ganglion cells (90%). In both man and chimpanzee the ganglion cell layer is 8–10 rows deep adjacent of the parafovea. In the cat and rat, there are only 2 rows. The ratio of $\frac{1}{2}$ to $\frac{1}{8}$ receptor cell to ganglion cell is higher in cat and rat ($\frac{1}{2}$) than in chimpanzee ($\frac{1}{8}$). The ability of the receptor cells to activate each ganglion cell is perhaps less in chimpanzee than in cat. Thus minimal activity under conditions of dark adaptation might be less effective in maintaining the ganglion cells. Questions of the number of centrifugal fibers and the possible or even likely difference in the number of synapses per fiber between species are not considered by the authors.

3. Changes in the Soma

Reduced sensory input affects somal and nuclear volume in the relevant system. In the visual system these effects are more pronounced the higher the animal's position in the phylogenetic scale. Adult animals are much less affected than young animals. A few hours of light, or perhaps even less, prevent changes if light exposure is early in life. Extensive exposure to light and even intensified visual experience including training procedures begun after prolonged early deprivation seems to have little or no saving morphological effect. This clinically important facet of visual deprivation needs much more experimentation, particularly in regard to changes in the parameters of the visual experience. The interaction of the utilization of vision in behavior and position on the phylogenetic scale has not been investigated.

In light-deprived mice the supragranular layers of the visual cortex show a reduction in nuclear volume in glia and neurons, as well as a reduction in internuclear material at 30 days. There were no such effects in the pyriform area (Gyllensten, 1959). After prolonged exposure to dark rearing, the percentage differences between control and experimental fall. Gyllensten calls this process "normalization." Also, there are interesting findings in the auditory area that will be reviewed in the discussion section.

In rats, monocularly deprived by eyelid suture from 14–244 days, there is a parallel decrease in leucine uptake and cellular surface (Maraini, Carta, Franguelli, & Santori, 1967). This enzymatic effect may be due to cell size reduction.

Studying the retina of light-deprived rabbits from birth to 60–120 days, no changes in the retina were observed with the usual histological techniques (Schimke, 1959). Changes in a variety of enzymes were observed. Brattgård (1952) suggests that the onset of stimulation induces a "third growth period for nucleoprotein" in the retinal ganglion cells of rabbits.

Prior to stimulation in light deprived rabbits there is no nucleoprotein at all. If an adult animal is deprived of light stimulation for just 3 hr, the nucleoprotein drops to one tenth the control value. He sums up: "The lack of adequate stimulation during the early postnatal period leads not only to incomplete development of the nerve cells, but also to disturbances in their metabolism and chemical composition [Brattgård, 1952, p. 68]."

In cats raised in darkness from birth for 3–36 months, Rasch, Riesen, and Chow (1959) showed a reduction of cytoplasmic RNA not only in rods and cones, but also in bipolar cells and multipolar ganglion cells (40–45%). In addition, mean cytoplasmic volume was reduced, as well as irregular dispersion of filiform Nissl substance.

In the lateral geniculate nucleus of kittens, cell size was decreased 30–40% by eyelid suture and 40% by enucleation (Kupfer & Palmer, 1964). A much smaller but similar effect occurs in adults. Monkeys show a much more severe effect than cats. This author suggests that visual deprivation slows the normal rate of growth without effecting the metabolic activity. He draws this conclusion from the fact that enzymatic activity was similar in the smaller experimental neurons as compared to normal neurons if corrected for size. Monocular and binocular eyelid suture in kittens results in loss of cell, nuclei, and nucleolar volume in the affected layers of the lateral geniculate nucleus (Wiesel & Hubel, 1965a). Casual inspection of the binocularly deprived animals showed little anatomical change. This may explain negative findings where measurements were not taken. Measurements showed a 40% reduction as compared to normal animals. These authors, utilizing physiologic methods in the visual cortex, found more pronounced effects in monocularly deprived animals. Thus, this effect may be in the lack of physiological informational congruence of the two pathways to the cortex. Naturally, the lateral geniculate nucleus is spared, as there are few neurons that have binocular afferents.

In cats monocularly deprived from birth to 16–24 months by eyelid suture, prolonged exposure to light did not reverse the 35% reduction in somal size in the lateral geniculate. If the cats were trained in a visual task 7–12 months, some of these effects were reversed, but this varied from animal to animal (Chow & Stewart, 1972). Under conditions of eyelid suture in kittens from 6–18 days to 3 months, with subsequent exposure to normal lighting up to one year, there is no anatomical recovery in the lateral geniculate nucleus, as well as no or little physiological behavioral recovery (Wiesel & Hubel, 1965b). Hubel and Wiesel (1970) have shown that lid suture in cats between 4 and 6 weeks of age of short duration (as little as 3 days) produces cellular atrophy in the lateral geniculate (see Fig. 4). Even after prolonged exposure to normal lighting and partial behavorial recovery, the neurons of the lateral geniculate nucleus are still atrophic and hypochromic. Prolonged deprivation begun after 3 months

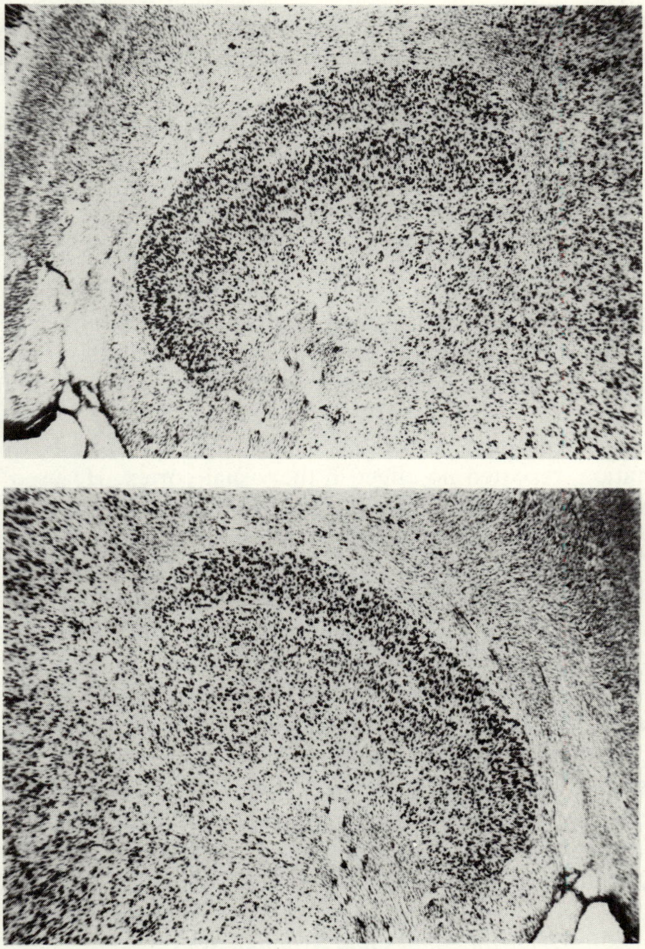

A

B

Fig. 4. Coronal section through (A) left and (B) right lateral geniculate bodies of a kitten whose right eye was closed from days 23–29: "During the most critical period for physiological changes in the cortex even a few days of deprivation gave a distinct difference between geniculate layers [Hubel & Wiesel, 1970, p. 433]."

of age has shown no significant degeneration in the lateral geniculate nucleus (Burke & Hayhow, 1968).

Few studies of limited exposure to a particular type of light have been performed. Le Gros Clark (1943), in a brilliant discursive paper, reported the exposure of three monkeys to red light for one month. Neurons of lamina one in the area of macular projection in two of the monkeys showed "laminar atrophy." The other monkey had a "normal" geniculate nucleus. No measurements were reported and no controls were described.

Chow (1955) studied adult monkeys exposed to red and blue light. He showed no changes in the retina, superior colliculus, lateral geniculate, or striate cortex.

In a man with blindness aparently due to corneal opacities, changes in cell size in the lateral geniculate body were evident. Changes in the visual cortex were reported as absent after 62 years. No control or quantitative data were reported (Hechst, 1933).

4. Changes in Dendrites

Although there are many papers dealing with the effect of reduced sensory input on dendritic spines and synapses, only a few deal with dendritic length and branching. They report a reduction and are in animals deprived from birth.

Goodman (1932) studying rabbits deprived of light from birth but using no quantitation, reported no effect in the visual cortex. He used the Golgi method which stains the entire soma–dendritic complex. This extensive study utilizing meticulous control of the dark environment, and many non-quantitative histological techniques, yielded no positive findings at all.

Reduction in dendritic length and branching of stellate neurons was reported in the striate cortex of cats raised in the dark from birth to 100 days in two of the three littermate pairs. Basal dendrites of pyramids in the cingulate cortex were similarly affected, whereas pyramids of Layer V of the striate cortex were not affected (Coleman & Riesen, 1968). These important results deserve replication.

In dogs deprived of light from birth, Fox, Inman, and Glisson (1968) reported decreased dendritic branching and reduced perikaryal size. Dogs deprived for 5 weeks at 5 weeks of age and in maturity did not show this finding. Quantitative data were not reported.

5. Changes in Dendritic Spines and Synaptic Sites

Reduction in the number of spines observable in Golgi preparations following dark rearing from birth have been repeatedly reported. Whether this a real reduction or a reduction in staining is as yet unanswered. Reduction in synaptic size has also been reported as a consequence of visual deprivation. Unfortunately, few animals higher on the phylogenetic scale than the rabbit have been studied in this manner.

Working with spine counting in visual cortex in mice which are dark-raised from birth, Valverde (1971) concluded that spines will not develop without light, and that some spine development in some pyramidal neurons follows exposure to light even when light exposure is delayed more than 20 days after birth (see Fig. 5). It is difficult to see how the later part

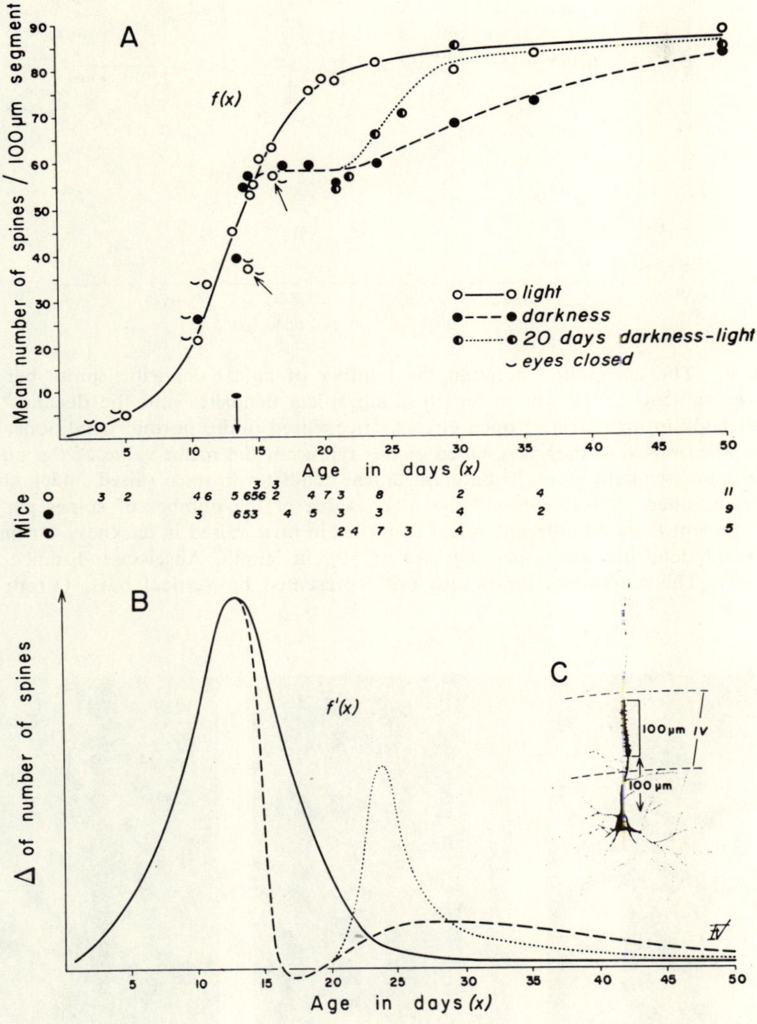

Fig. 5. (A) Mean number of dendritic spines per segment in apical dendrites of Layer V pyramidal cells of the visual cortex as a function of age. The number of animals from which the mean values were obtained for each age group is indicated below the horizontal axis. (B) First-deriviative function indicating the rate of increase of the number of spines in an arbitrary scale as a function of age. Geometrical reconstructions from fitted curves of A. (C) The location of the standard segment in which the number of spines has been counted on each apical dendrite. (From Valverde, 1971.)

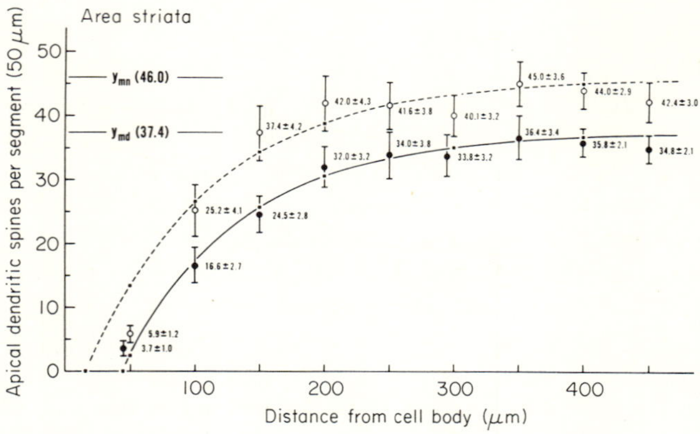

Fig. 6. The correlation between the number of apical dendritic spines per consecutive segments of 50 μm in length along apical dendrites and the distance from the cell body in area striata: open circles, mice raised under normal conditions; filled circles, mice raised in darkness. Open circles represent the mean value of the number of spines per segment from 30 different apical dendrites in mice raised under normal conditions; filled circles represent the mean value of the number of spines per dendritic segment from 30 different apical dendrites in mice raised in darkness. Ordinates: number of dendritic spines per segment of 50μ in length. Abscissas: distance from cell body. The confidence limits also are represented by vertical bars. (From Val-

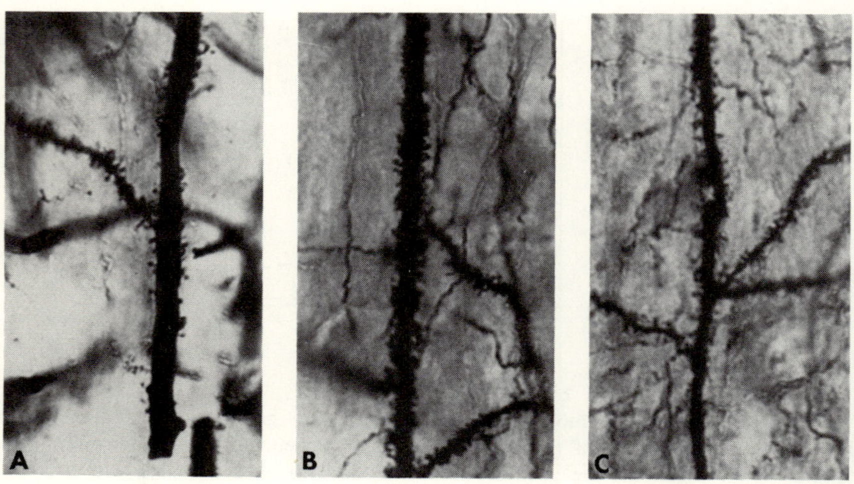

Fig. 7. Photomicrographs of apical dendrites of pyramids in the visual cortex in rabbits: (A) lateral geniculate lesion; (B) control; (C) left eye blinded. Vertical dendrites are apical. Oblique or horizontal ones are branches of the apical dendrite. Thinner fibers in the background are axons. Left: lateral geniculate lesion. Middle: control. Right: left eye blinded. X400. [From Globus & Scheibel, 1967c.]

of his conclusions is supported by the data reported. Further evaluation of Valverde's experiments (Valverde, 1967, 1968; Valverde & Estéban, 1968) in dark-reared mice gave rise to a formula which describes the distribution of spines on apical dendrites as a function of age and distance from the soma. Although there is a reported reduction in total spines, the shape of the curve of their distribution in relation to age and distance from the soma remains the same. He suggests a "soma–dendritic factor" which is responsible for the distribution of spines and is unaffected by visual deprivation. He reports no "normalization" of spines, as might be predicted from the findings of Gyllensten *et al.* (1966) relative to somal sizes (see Fig. 6). The morphological integrity of the dendritic spines is dependent on the structural integrity of the afferent system (Globus & Scheibel, 1967a) as well as on its functional integrity (Globus & Scheibel, 1967c; Valverde, 1967). Globus, using rabbits, reports abnormally formed spines under conditions of visual deprivation rather than a reduction in numbers. In both studies, counts were performed under the same magnification.

In rabbits, light deprived from birth to 30 days, spines were deformed along the apical dendrite. Apparently they were not reduced in number. The stellate cell dendrites and the frequency of cell types are not affected (see Fig. 7). Globus and Scheibel report a greater variance in dendrite length of stellates in the experimental animals. Recalculation of Coleman's and Riesen's data (1968) seemed to show a similar increase in variance. A similar study in pattern deprived monkeys (Globus & Berger, unpublished data) did not show this greater variance in dendrite length of stellates.

In the visual cortex of rats, unilateral lid suture reduced synaptic sites by 20%, but increased synaptic size by 7.5% (Fifková, 1970b). Mentioned by Aghajanian and Bloom (1967) were the then unpublished data showing that there is reduction (30–40%) in E-PTA stained synaptic junctions per unit volume in animals maintained in complete darkness for the first 6 weeks of life.

Cragg (1969) studied the visual cortex of light-deprived rats for the first 3 weeks and then exposed the rats to light for a few hours in the next 10 weeks. Utilizing the electron microscope, he measured synaptic profiles. They were increased in the superficial half of the cortex, but decreased in the deeper half. The density of synapses was reduced in the deeper half of the cortex. In this type of electron microscopic study, it is difficult to identify the postsynaptic neuron. In the visual cortex, axosomatic synapses in rats undergoing monocular eyelid suture at 14 days were found to be smaller. Synapses with round vesicles were more affected than those with flattened vesicles. In rats with eyelid suture, axosomatic synapses having round vesicles in the visual cortex showed a greater reduction in Layer II than in Layer IV. Synapses with flattened vesicles did not show this difference (Fifková, 1970a). As round vesicles may be associated with excitation, and as the synapses with round vesicles show a more pronounced effect relative to layers and magnitude, it may be supposed that eyelid suture has a more pronounced effect on excitation than on inhibition.

6. *Changes in Axons and Glia*

Little or no work has been done in this area.

Summaries of the reduced sensory input studies are given in Table IV, pp. 50–59.

E. Results of Increased Sensory Input

Most experiments dealing with increased sensory input are one of two types. The first paradigm is that of increased electrical stimulation or forced activity (see Table V, p. 64). This paradigm is probably one of stress as well as increased sensory input. The second is the paradigm developed principally by Krech *et al.* (1966). It consists of a very complex environment consisting of toys, other animals, and learning experiences, which is here assumed to be increased sensory input (ECT). This experimental condition is compared to an environment devoid of these things (IC) (see Table VI, p. 66). Which environment is considered the experimental condition is arbitary. I have chosen to consider the enriched environment as the experimental condition.

1. *Disruption of Organization or Overall Dimensions*

Enriched environments (ECT) result in an increase in brain size particularly in the cortex when compared to impoverished environments (IC). ECT rats show greater depth of the visual cortex (Bennett *et al.,* 1964a). Many replications and stringent controls ruled out the possibility that this effect was due to differential handling, differences in locomotion, or the degree of contact with other animals. In young animals it seems to be an effect of the enrichment. Surprisingly, the effect is similar in adult animals (Krech *et al.*, 1966).

Still other conditions were studied. They include social controls, where there are three rats to a cage; extreme impoverishment, where rats are housed individually in an enclosed, temperature controlled, and sound muffled space; and paired isolates, where the animals are housed as in the extreme impoverished environment, but in pairs. These experiments suggest that a social environment (paired) does not significantly prevent the reduction in cortical volume when compared to the enriched environment (Krech *et al.,* 1966). Krech *et al.* (1963) subjected blinded rats to environmentally enriched and impoverished conditions until 80 days of age. Enriched but blinded animals not only showed increased weight of visual cortex over impoverished animals, but total body weights were lower than sighted, enriched animals.

ECT rats show increased weight and depth of occipital cortex over IC rats blinded or raised in the dark and subjected to these experimental conditions from 20 days or birth. Although enriched environment has a generalized effect on brain weight, the most pronounced effect in rats is in the occipital cortex (Bennett *et al.,* 1964a). The generality of this result is difficult to dispute. These authors have approached their results cautiously and thoroughly. There is little doubt that differential experience plays a small but significant effect in overall size of the brain and, in particular, in the occipital cortex of the rat (Rosenzweig *et al.,* 1969).

2. *Cellular Changes*

Few studies have concentrated on changes in cellular types. Apparently, enriched environments do affect the glia/neuronal ratio and, perhaps, the number of short axon cells in the cerebellum.

In rats exposed to ECT–IC environments, the glia/neuron ratio is greater in ECT than IC animals. Both astrocytes and oligodendrocytes account for this increase (Diamond *et al.,* 1966). In rats placed in an enriched environment, there is an increased proliferation of glial cells, particularly in the fibrous portions of the neocortex over isolated animals (Altman & Das, 1964). In rats handled from 3–11 days, the number of interneurons in the cerebellum and hypocampus are increased (Altman *et al.,* 1968).

3. *Changes in the Soma*

Increased stimulation, particularly electrical, results in a variety of somal changes. Changes in nucleoprotein content are reflected by most aniline staining methods. Thus, there is some early literature in this area. Positive results were the reward of those who measured carefully.

A variety of animals were subjected to a variety of severe behavioral tasks. Neurons in the cerebrum, cerebellum, and spinal cord were studied by stains of cellular protein. No effect was noted although some quantitative measures were taken (Kocher, 1916).

Repetitive electrical stimulation of peripheral nerves and twelfth cranial nerve in guinea pig produced minimal or no detectable changes utilizing a thionin histological technique in the postsynaptic neurons. No quantitative measures were taken (Liu *et al.,* 1950). Changes in nucleoproteins within mitochondria, nucleolus, and "tigroid" substances, that is changes of Nissl substance, were reported by Shabadash (1964) as a result of "activity."

TABLE IV

EFFECTS OF ALTERED PRESYNAPTIC ACTIVITY: DECREASED SENSORY INPUT

Procedure	Species	Began	Ended	Structure studied and/or affected	Reference
Eyelid suture, monocular	Chicken	Hatching	17 days	Dark maintained: no change. Light maintained: cerebral hemisphere weighed less. Less acetylcholinesterase activity. Reduced RNA synthesis.	Bondy and Margolis (1971)
Eyelid suture	Pigeon Raven Cookoo	Adult	1–4 days	No change in aniline stains of the retina.	Schüpbach (1905)
Total binocular visual deprivation	Mice	Birth	1–50 days. One group exposed to light after 20 days in darkness	Spines on the apical dendrite in the cerebral cortex studied. Visual cortex affected. Other cortical areas not affected. Some neurons were unaffected within the visual cortex. One-third showed a normal number of spines when exposed to light after 20 days of dark rearing (see Fig. 6).	Valverde (1971)
Total binocular visual deprivation	Mice	Birth	22–25 days	Area striata: approximately 35% decrease in spines of apical dendrites of pyramids from Layer V. No change in area temporalis (see Fig. 5).	Valverde (1967)
Total binocular visual deprivation	Mice	Birth	2, 3, 4 months	Auditory cortex: decrease nuclear size and internuclear volume at 2 months (6%). Increase at 4 months. Both effects more pronounced in supra- than infragranular layers.	Gyllensten *et al.* (1966)
		Adult	To 7 months	Auditory cortex: increase in nuclear size and internuclear material (see Figs. 9 and 10).	

Total binocular visual deprivation	Mice	Birth	2, 3, 4 months	Visual cortex: reduction in thickness (4.47%). Geniculate body: reduction in internuclear material (20%). Superior colliculus: same measure (9.5%).	Gyllensten *et al.* (1965)
		4 months	7 months	Visual cortex: no change in thickness. Geniculate body: reduction in internuclear material (18.2%). Superior colliculus: same measure (8.8%). (See Figs 7 and 8.)	
Eyelid suture	Mice	Birth (4–6 days)	3–11 weeks later	No findings in the entire visual system: optic nerve, optic tract, striate cortex, LGN, and visual cortex.	Terry *et al.* (1962)
Total binocular visual deprivation	Mice	Birth	20–30 days	Visual cortex: reduction in diameter of cell nuclei of Layers II–IV and glia (5–6%). Reduction of quantity of internuclear material in Layers II–IV (7–8%). No absolute change in degree of vascularity. None of these findings occurred in pyriform area.	Gyllensten (1959)
Monocular eyelid suture	Rat	14 days	2 months with 8, 11, or 16 hr illumination daily	Retina: Opened eye, damage to receptors, decreased synaptic density in inner plexiform layer (24%). Closed eye, synaptic density of inner plexiform layer increased (28%) as compared to controls.	Fifková (1972)
Monocular eyelid suture	Rat	6 weeks	3 months	LGB (dorsal part), (10%), and nucleus (8%) lateralis pars posterior volumes reduced. Visual cortex: Layers II–IV thickness decreased (8%). Layers V and VI, no change. Increase in cell density in Layers III and IV (11%).	Fifková (1970c)

TABLE IV *(continued)*

Procedure	Species	Began	Ended	Structure studied and/or effected	Reference
Monocular eyelid suture (continued)	Rat	14 days	3 days	LGB (dorsal part): no change. Visual cortex: thickness, no change.	Fifková (1970c)
			10 days	LGB (dorsal part): No change. Visual cortex: Layers II–IV decreased thickness (5%). Layers III and IV, increased cell density (7%). Reduction in spine density (17%) in Layer IV on the apical dendrite of pyramids from Layer V.	
			30 days	LGB (dorsal part): volume decrease (15%). Visual cortex: layers II–IV, decreased thickness (9%). Layers III and IV, increased cell density (13%). Reduction in spine density (28%) in Layer IV on the apical dendrite of pyramids from Layer V.	
		14 days	2 months sutured, 10 days light-exposed	LGB (dorsal part): volume decreased (10%). Visual cortex: layers II–IV, decreased thickness (10%). Layers III and IV, increased cell density (11%).	
			2 months sutured, 30 days light-exposed	LGB (dorsal part): Volume decreased (7%). Visual cortex: layers II–IV, decreased (6%). Layers III and IV, increased cell density (10%).	
Monocular eyelid suture	Rat	14–15 days	8 weeks	Visual cortex: layers II–V, reduction in synaptic activity (20%). Mean size of synaptic contacts, in upper levels of cortex, increased (7.5%). Only axodendritic synapses studied.	Fifková (1970b)

Monocular eyelid suture	Rat	14–15 days	8 weeks	Visual cortex: size of axosomatic synapses decreased (23%) in Layers II–V. Synapses with round vesicles more affected than those with flattened.	Fifková (1970a)
Total binocular visual deprivation	Rat	Birth	After weaning (3 weeks), 4–5 weeks of light exposure	Light exposed rats: lateral geniculate, average diameter of axon terminals decreased (15%), but density was increased (34%). Thalamus and ventro-basal complex: no change.	Cragg (1969)
		3 weeks	3 months	Dark exposed rats; axon terminals (11%), density decreased (29%).	
Monocular eyelid suture	Rat	14–15 days	8–9 weeks	Optic tract and superior colliculus: no change. LGB (dorsal part) decreased volume (5.07%). Primary visual area decreased volume (16%). Decreased cell numbers in pulvinar (7%), and LGB (dorsal part) (13.5%). Cells of Layer IV increased (11.5%).	Fifková and Hassler (1969)
Monocular eyelid suture	Rat	14–15 days	8–9 weeks	Visual cortex: decreased cell density. Decreased spine density in Layer IV (25–30%).	Fifková (1968)
Total binocular visual deprivation	Rat	Birth	After weaning (3 weeks), 10 weeks of light exposure	Light exposed rats: visual cortex, superficial half, increased size of synaptic profiles. Deeper half, decreased.	Cragg (1967)
		Birth	13 weeks	Dark-reared rats: visual cortex, synaptic density lower.	
Total binocular visual deprivation	Rat	Birth	21 days	Decreased acetylcholinesterase activity in superior colliculus and LGB, not in visual cortex.	Maletta and Timiras (1967)
		Adult	21 days	No histological or enzyme changes seen.	

TABLE IV *(continued)*

Procedure	Species	Began	Ended	Structure studied and/or affected	Reference
Monocular eyelid suture	Rat	14 days	4–7 months	No changes in gross morphology and leucine-H^3 uptake in retina and visual cortex. Decreased leucine-H^3 uptake in LGN neurons (20%) and of cellular surface (20%).	Maraini *et al.* (1967)
Total binocular visual deprivation	Rat	Birth	90 days	Decrease RNA concentration in ganglion cells of retina (30%).	Riesen (1965a, b)
		Birth	90 days deprivation, followed by 60 days normal light	As above, but only 15% decrease.	
Total binocular visual deprivation	Rabbit	Birth	30 days	Deformity of spines along apical dendrites of pyramids in visual cortex. Stellate dendrites and frequency of cell types unchanged.	Globus and Schiebel (1967a)
Eyelid suture	Rabbit	8 days	10–26 days	Decreased binocular part of Layer IV. Monocular parts not effected in visual areas I and II. Superior colliculus: decreased cell process.	Umrath (1965)
		Adult		No change.	
Eyelid suture	Rabbit	8–9 days	30 days	Visual cortex: no change.	Dzidzishvili (1963)

Total binocular visual deprivation	Rabbit	Adult	3 hr	Retinal ganglion cells: decreased dry mass (74%). Visual cortical cells: no change.	Gomirato and Baggio (1962)
Total binocular visual deprivation	Rabbit	Birth	26, 60, 120 days	Histology of retina unaffected. Decreased malic dehydrogenase, lactic dehydrogenase, acid phosphatase activities. Increased glucose 6-phosphate dehydrogenase activity.	Schimke (1959)
Monocular eyelid suture	Rabbit	Adult	Few days to a month	No change in 17, 18 binocular areas, or in visual areas I and II cell counts.	Lindner and Umrath (1955)
Total binocular visual deprivation	Rabbit	Birth	10 weeks	Retinal ganglion cells: protein fraction decreased (50%) of controls, absence of nucleoprotein.	Brattgärd (1952)
		Adult	3 hr	Nucleoprotein decreased (10%) of control retinal ganglion cells.	
Total binocular visual deprivation	Rabbit	Birth	6 months	No change in: retina, optic nerve, superior colliculus, LGB, pulvinar, and striate cortex.	Goodman (1932)
Monocular or binocular eyelid suture	Cat	Birth	16–24 months	Monocular: decreased somal size (35%) in LGB, reversed by forced usage. Binocular: no systematic change in somal size.	Chow and Stewart (1972)
Monocular or binocular eyelid suture	Cat	8–10 days	8–12 months	LGN: 2 cell types, X cells (sustained response cells) and Y cells (transient response cells). Loss of Y cells to electrophysiological recording. Layer A: cells shrunken. Loss of large cells.	Sherman and Sanderson (1972)

TABLE IV *(continued)*

Procedure	Species	Began	Ended	Structure studied and/or affected	Reference
Monocular eyelid suture	Cat	4–5 weeks	3–6 days	LGN: cells smaller, paler to Nissl stain. (See Fig. 4.)	Hubel and Wiesel (1970)
		Birth	3 months deprivation, then 5 years light exposure	LGN: no obvious recovery in cellular atrophy.	
		4 months	3 months	LGN: no appreciable atrophy of cells.	
Total binocular visual deprivation	Cat	Birth	6 months	Striate cortex: layer IV, no difference in length of 1 and 2 order dendrites of stellate cells. Over 12% reduction in third-order dendritic length. Also reduction in branching. No effect on pyramids of Layer V. Decrease in pyramidal dendritic branching of cingulate cortex.	Coleman and Riesen (1968)
Total binocular visual deprivation	Cat	Birth	4–39 months	50% reduction in RNA in ganglion cells.	Riesen (1965a, b)
		Birth, with 1 hr normal light/day	4–39 months	25% reduction in RNA ganglion cells.	
Eyelid suture	Cat	Young		No change except decreased in anterior part of visual areas in Layer IV.	Umrath (1965)
		Adult		Decreased cell density contralateral throughout visual system.	

Monocular and binocular eyelid suture	Cat	6–18 days	2.5–4.5 months	No obvious changes in retina or cortex. Monocular: LGN change in staining characteristics in relevant layers, decrease in cell volume (30–40%) and nuclei. Binocular: LGN little to see on casual inspection. Comparison with normal animals showed changes. Cell volume shrinkage (40%). Similar effects in nucleus and nucleolus.	Wiesel and Hubel (1965a)
Monocular and binocular eyelid suture	Cat	6–18 days	3 months deprivation, followed by 3–14 months light exposure	LGN atrophy: no recovery as above.	Wiesel and Hubel (1965b)
Monocular eyelid suture	Cat	4 days	5–28 days	LGN: decrease in cell size (30–40%) in kittens only. Enzyme activity the same in affected cells as opposed to unaffected cells.	Kupfer (1964)
		5 weeks	8 weeks	LGN: cells slightly smaller when compared to a normal kitten.	
Visual deprivation—opaque ocular	Cat	Birth	2–2½ months	LGB: 40% reduction in mean cross-sectional volume. No cortical change.	Hubel and Wiesel (1963)
Visual deprivation—translucent ocular		Birth	2–2½ months	LGB: 10–15% reduction in mean cross-sectional volume.	
Monocular eyelid suture or translucent contact ocular	Cat	Birth	3 months	Decreased cell areas (40–25%). Nuclei and nucleoli shrunken. No change in retina, optic nerve, striate cortex, superior colliculus.	Wiesel and Hubel (1963)
Eyelid suture		2 months Adult	5 months 3 months	Similar to above but less severe. No change.	

TABLE IV *(continued)*

Procedure	Species	Began	Ended	Structure studied and/or affected	Reference
Total binocular visual deprivation	Cat	Birth	3–36 months	Decreased cytoplasmic and nucleolar RNA levels in neurons from multipolar, bipolar, receptor cell layers (40–50%). Decreased protein levels. Mean cytoplasmic volume reduced. Irregular dispersion of filiform Nissl substance in ganglion cells. Reduced mean nucleolar volume.	Rasch *et al.* (1961)
Total monocular and binocular visual deprivation	Cat	Adult	Up to 966 days	Retina and LGB. no change.	Burke and Hayhow (1960)
Total binocular visual deprivation	Cat	7 days	17 weeks	Inner plexiform layer: decreased fibers (20%), decreased thickness (15%). Optic tract: decreased fibers (6%).	Weiskrantz (1958)
Binocular eyelid suture	Dog	1 day	130 days	Retina, optic nerve, lateral geniculate: no change. Golgi of cortex showed reduced cell size. Reduced gyri and cortical thickness.	Berger (1900)
	Cat	5 days	95 days	Optic nerve, lateral geniculate: reduced volume.	
Binocular occlusion	Dog	Birth	5 weeks	Decreased dendritic branching in Layer V. Decreased thickness of apical dendrites.	Fox, Inman, and Glisson (1968)
		Adult	5–10 weeks	No findings in adult.	
Eyelid suture	Dog	Young		Decreased Layer IV in visual area. Increased cell density in anterior part of contralateral visual area.	Umrath (1965)

Patterned deprivation—ocular	Monkey	Birth	18 months	Cortex 17, 18, associate, motor, sensory, and frontal: no change. Golgi study.	Berger and Globus (unpublished data)
Total binocular visual deprivation or exposure to blue, red light	Monkey (*Macaca mulatta*)	Immature	8 months	Retina, superior colliculus, lateral geniculate, and striate cortex: no change.	Chow (1955)
Total red light exposure	Monkey	Adult	1 month	Two animals. LGN selective laminar atrophy in the region of macular projection. Limited to Layer I. One animal, no effect.	Le Gros Clark (1943)
Total binocular visual deprivation	Chimpanzee	Birth	6 months	Disc pallor.	Riesen (1965a, b)
			7 months	Retina: 90% of ganglion cells disappear. No change in receptors or bipolars.	
			18 months	Ganglion cells reduced cytoplasmic volume.	
			23 months	Ganglion cells, receptors, and bipolar cells disappear.	
Total binocular visual deprivation	Chimpanzee	Birth	Adult	Less retinal ganglion cells and optic fibers. No change in receptor or bipolar cells. Decreased nucleolar volume. Decreased RNA content. Recovery of RNA if light instituted at 3 months.	Riesen (1960)
Total binocular visual deprivation	Chimpanzee	Birth	7 months with 1.5 hr diffuse light daily	Retina normal.	Chow *et al.* (1957)
		Birth	33 months	Disappearance of ganglion cells in retina.	
		8 months	24 months	Intact receptive and bipolar cell layers.	

Unfortunately, experimental details were not reported. In rats, perikarya within the outer third of the cortex above the posterior commissure were considerably larger in ECT animals (17.7%) than in IC controls. The middle third and lower third also showed effects, but they were less pronounced (Diamond, 1967).

Hamberger and Hydén (1949) showed changes in the nucleus and Nissl substance in neurons of the Deiters' and vestibular nuclei. Different levels of stimulation show a graded change from increased nucleoprotein for mild to moderate stimulation, to a striking decrease of nucleoprotein content following hyperstimulation (see Fig. 8). In adult rabbits, vestibular

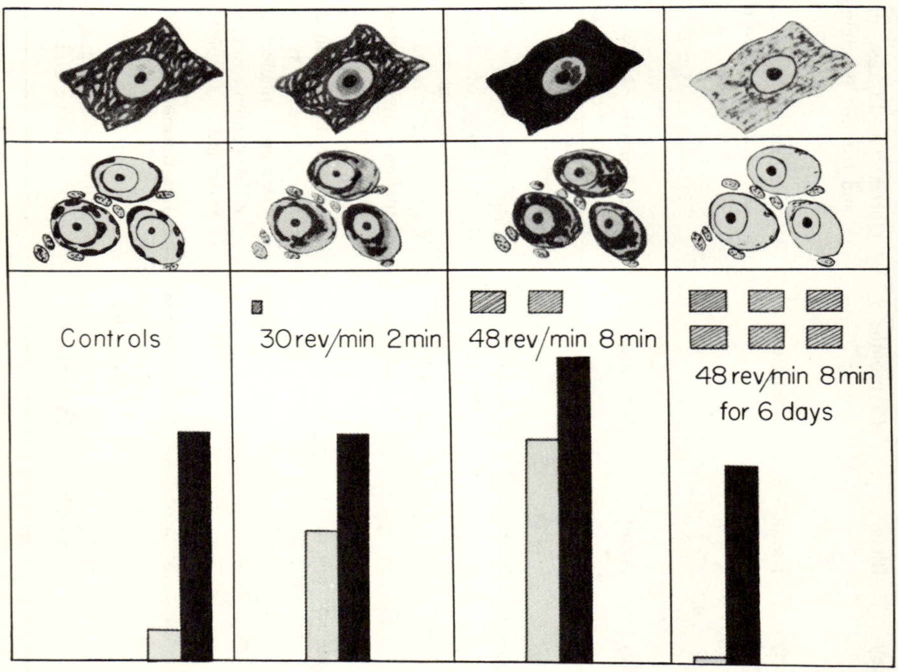

Fig. 8. Diagram illustrating the correlation between the cytochemical changes in the rabbit nerve cells of the vestibular ganglion and those of Deiters' nucleus in connection with vestibular stimulation. The degree of density demonstrates the difference in the nucleoprotein content of the nerve cells. The size and number of the shaded rectangles show the amount of vestibular stimulation given. The reaction capacity of the cells, judged by the increase in their nucleoprotein content, is seen from the columns. The white columns designate the controls and the black, the cells of the stimulated animals. The nerve cells of the vestibular ganglion react quantitatively with greater changes. The reaction in Deiters' nucleus takes place in the same period of time, but is less extensive. (From Hamberger & Hydén, 1949.)

stimulation by centrifugation results in changed RNA and protein content in Deiters' nucleus. In neurons, they are increased; in oligodendroglial cells, decreased (Hydén & Pigon, 1960). These authors concluded: "The nerve cell plus the surrounding glial cells seem to constitute a functional unit in the central nervous system [p. 71]." In adult rabbits using microroentgen radiographic technique, intense illumination results in a decrease in nuclear protein mass of retinal cells, but not cortical cells; darkness causes a slight reduction in both (Gomirato & Baggio, 1962). Changes in ganglion cells of the superior cervical ganglion as the result of stimulation have been reported as early as 1894 by Mann.

In cats continuous stimulation (50 pulses/sec) of the hypoglossal nerve depletes the Nissl substance for the first 3 days, then it recovers. During recovery the nuclear membrane becomes prominent. There is no sign of degeneration for up to 38 hr (Bertram & Barr, 1949).

In mature female cats, motor neurons have a nuclear satellite. This structure is stained in Cresyl Violet and Thionin methods. In the hypoglossal nucleus, during intense stimulation, the nucleolar sattelite moves further away from the nucleolus. This corresponds to the period of synthesis of ribose nucleoprotein (Barr & Bertram, 1949).

4. *Changes in Dendrites*

The effect of intense stimulation on dendritic growth has not been studied; however, enriched environments result in increased dendritic length and branching.

In rats subjected to ECT–IC environments, Holloway (1966) reports increased dendrite branching (ECT) in littermate pairs. Considerable variations in results were reported (11 out of 15 cases). In rats, higher-order dendrite branching was increased under ECT conditions in stellates and pyramid cells in Layers II, III, and IV. Basilar dendrites were counted in pyramid cells (Volkmar & Greenough, 1972). The authors believe that this effect is due to the degree of stimulation involved in the environmental situation in which the animal is reared.

5. *Changes in Dendritic Spines and Synapses*

Increased environmental stimulation seems to increase the number of dendritic spines, or at least to accelerate their development. On the EM level, complex changes take place. This area of research is just being launched. This type of study specifies those morphological features involved in changing the parameters of synaptic function and thus may be of service to the neurochemist in designing experiments and techniques preliminary to the study of the synaptic changes involved in learning.

In rats reared under ECT or IC conditions for 30 days after weaning, the spine density was increased along the basal, oblique, and terminal dendrites. These spines are thought to be the site of intracortical afferents (Globus, Rosenzweig, Bennett, & Diamond, 1973). The authors believe this change to be a consequence of increased "demand of integration of complex multisensory information [p. 179]." In rats from birth to 8 days, there were more pyramidal cells impregnated by the rapid Golgi method and an increased spine density in those cells that were impregnated (Schapiro & Vukovich, 1970). This stimulation included handling, stroking, shaking, immersing in warm and cold water, loud noises, flashing lights, and electric shock for 3–5 times daily for 20–30 min. These conditions might be considered hyperstimulation and/or stressful. Synapses in the occipital cortex, Layer III, are larger in ECT (roughly 10%) than in IC animals. The measures were taken on the postsynaptic thickening (West & Greenough, 1972).

In an EM study in adult dogs and cats following cortical lesions and stimulation, Mikeladze (1969) reported great variability in spine shape, postsynaptic membrane thickness, and synapses. Unfortunately he did not make clear which finding belongs to which experimental condition. Nevertheless, he states that functional states affect these structures.

6. *Changes in the Axons and Glia*

No studies have been reported. However, one might expect a change in diameter of presynaptic terminals to match changes reported in the postsynaptic thickening.

The effects of altered presynaptic activity are given in Table V, and the effects of altered innervation are summarized in Table VI.

III. Discussion

A. Some Problems Related to Individual Variation

Experiments purporting to elucidate factors influencing growth secondary to changes in afferent integrity and function should control for individual variation. Other significant factors contributing to individual variation are genetic, hormonal, nutritional, and, perhaps, behavioral.

Genetic control is harder to achieve the higher the position on the phylogenetic scale. Visual deprivation in rabbits of the same litter produces changes in the dendritic spines (Globus & Scheibel, 1967a). Pattern deprivation from birth to 18 months in monkeys yielded no significant changes in the number and distribution of spines in pyramids in the visual cortex (Berger & Globus, unpublished data). There were changes thought to be due to the treatment, but individual variation, indicated by variance within the controls, was apparently so large as to vitiate the effects of treatment. In a number of studies of visual deprivation from birth, the results could be interpreted to mean that a loss of sensory input leads to greater variation in dendritic length in experimental animals than controls. Coleman and Riesen (1968) showed reduced dendritic branching in stellates of the striate cortex in only 2 of 3 littermate pairs of cats. Recalculation of Coleman and Riesen's data in cats and Globus and Scheibel's data in rabbits indicates greater variation in dendritic length in stellate cells in the visual deprived group as opposed to the controls. Berger and Globus (unpublished data) did not find this in stellates of monkeys which were pattern deprived. Aberrant results in occasional littermate pairs have been observed by others. Globus and Scheibel (1967a) have ascribed this effect to a loss of functional factors regulating growth of dendrites: in one animal leading to excessively long, and, in the other, excessively short dendrites. This postulates that normal function exercises control of dendritic growth. The evidence for this interesting hypothesis is still scant.

Torvik (1956), studying kittens' inferior olive and pontine nuclei, noted that the same lesion in the same species at the same time produces different effects. He ascribes this to individual variability in development.

To summarize: Increased variance can not be considered the result of reduced sensory input until all genetic, nutritional, hormonal, and, perhaps, even behavioral factors are adequately controlled.

B. Problems Related to Experimental Methods

Conclusions are only as sound as the knowledge of what happens as a result of the experimental procedure. Many experiments designed to reduce sensory input may increase neuronal activity. On the other hand, seemingly innocuous procedures such as dilating the pupil or increasing its exposure to light may effect changes that reduce a study of decreased function to a study of degenerative effects. Only a few examples have been selected.

Does reducing the amount of adequate stimuli also reduce neuronal activity? "The spontaneous activity, so lively in the mammalian retina, is thus the background against which effects of stimulation are displayed [Granit, 1955, p. 85]." The "spontaneous" activity referred to is in dark adapted animals. Slow rhythms in the dark adapted retina are disturbed by light (Rodieck & Smith, 1966). This can be taken as evidence of reduced activity under light stimulation. Retinal ganglion cells respond to changes of illumination, not to steady illumination or darkness (Granit, 1947). Steady illumination or dark adapted, unopened eyes produces maintained

TABLE V

EFFECTS OF ALTERED PRESYNAPTIC ACTIVITY: INCREASED SENSORY INPUT

Procedure	Species	Began	Ended	Structure studied and/or affected	Reference
Variety of relatively stressful stimulation	Rat	Birth	8 days	Increased spine density in neurons of cortex. Increased Golgi impregnation.	Schapiro and Vukovich (1970)
Electrical stimulation	Guinea pig	Adult	24 hr and 1–7 days later	Spinal ganglia and spinal cord: no change in Nissl pattern of post-synaptic neurons.	Liu *et al.* (1950)
Intense white light	Rabbit	Adult	3 hr	Reduction in nuclear protein mass in retinal cells (43%–100%). No effect on cortical cells.	Gomirato and Baggio (1962)
Vestibular stimulation 25 min/day	Rabbit	Adult	1–7 days	Deiters' nucleus: increased RNA, increased protein per nerve cell. Oligodendroglia: RNA and respiratory enzymes decreased.	Hydén and Pigon (1960)
Rotary stimulation (2–16 min)	Rabbit	Adult	1–6 days	Increase of chromocentric areas in nucleus. Increase nucleoprotein content in cells of Deiters' nucleus. Fatigue results in decrease of RNA and protein content. (See Fig. 11.)	Hamberger and Hydén (1949)
Stimulation of superior cervical ganglion	Rabbit	Adult	2–177 days	Swollen cells, reduction in Nissl substances, nucleus eccentric.	Sternschein (1921)

Stimulation	Rabbit	Adult	15 min–9 hr	Sympathetic ganglion cell and nucleus increase in size. Nucleolus increases in size. Longer periods of stimulation darkens.	Mann (1894–1895)
Electrical stimulation of hypoglossal nerve	Cat	Adult	?	Nucleolar satellite moves more distant to the nucleolus.	Barr and Bertram (1949)
Electrical stimulation of hypoglossal nerve	Cat	Adult	½ day–15 days	Nucleus of hypoglossal nerve: Nissl substance depleted after 12–60 hr. Recovery to 384th hr. Nucleolus enlarged. Nuclear membrane becomes prominent. No nuclear eccentricity.	Bertram and Barr (1949)
Electrical stimulation of cortex	Cat Dog	Adult	Few min	Dendritic spines sometimes were swollen 10–20 μm. No change in axonal terminals.	Mikeladze (1969)
Electrical stimulation, forced behavior, strychnine, blood loss	Dog Cat Pigeon Sparrow Frog Rat	Adult	1–10 hr	Neurons studied by cell body stains in cruciate gyrus, cerebellum, motoneuron in spinal cord, and dorsal ganglia: no change found over resting controls.	Kocher (1916)
Stimulation	Dog	Adult	12 hr eye covered	Retina, lateral geniculate, visual cortex: nuclei darker in neurons of covered eye.	Mann (1894–1895)

TABLE VI

Effects of Altered Innervation: Enriched Environments

Procedure	Species	Began	Ended	Structure studied and/or affected	Reference
Environmentally enriched, impoverished (ECT vs. IC)	Mice Gerbils	?	?	Significant brain difference, but occipital effect does not dominate.	Rosenzweig *et al.* (1969)
ECT vs. IC	Rat	25 days	55 days	Visual cortex: ECT > IC spines on basal 9.7%, oblique 3.6%, and terminal dendrites, 0.05%.	Globus *et al.* (1973)
Environmentally enriched vs. normal colony	Rat	25 days	Newborns–650 days	Frontal, somesthetic, and occipital cortex: increase in depth until 26 days of age, then slow decrease (6%) until 650 days. Greatest difference in cell counts between 25–41 days (30%).	Diamond *et al.* (1973)
ECT vs. IC and social control (SC)	Rat	22–25 days	29–31 days	Occipital cortex: increased higher order dendritic branching in Layer IV stellates, pyramids from Layers II, IV, and V–ECT > SC > IC.	Volkmar and Greenough (1972)
ECT vs. IC	Rat	Young, adult	30, 80 days	Increased brain weight, cortical depth, AChE and ChE activities—especially in occipital cortex.	Rosenzweig *et al.* (1969)
Total unilateral visual deprivation ECT vs. IC	Rat	20 days Birth	100 days 65 days	Less affected but still present. Dark raised occipital cortex 8.2%. Light-raised occipital cortex 7.2%.	
Enucleated ECT vs. IC	Rat	25 days	105 days	ECT > IC blinded 3.6%, weight of cortex and occipital cortex.	
Handled 15 min. daily, thymidine-H^3 injected IP	Rat	2–11 days	6 hr. 3 days, 30 days	Brain weight and areal measurements decreased. Increased cell proliferation. Formation of interneurons in cerebellum.	Altman *et al.* (1968)

Total unilateral visual deprivation ECT vs. IC	Rat	22 days	80 days	No effect in sensory cortex. IC: lighter somesthetic and auditory cortex.	MacNeill and Zubeck (1967)
ECT vs. IC	Rat	25 days	46–105 days	Increased cortical depth.	Diamond (1967)
ECT vs. IC, social controls (SC), extreme impoverishment (IEI), paired extreme impoverishment (PEI)	Rat	22 days	80 days	Effect on cortical volume: ECT (4%) > SC > PEI ≅ IEI (9%).	Krech *et al.* (1966)
ECT vs. IC	Rat	25 days	85 days	Increased dendritic branching of stellate cells in ECT.	Holloway (1966)
ECT vs. IC	Rat	25 days	85 days	Increased visual cortical depth ECT > IC by 6.4%. Increased glia ECT > IC by 14%.	Diamond *et al.* (1966)
ECT vs. IC	Rat	25 days	105 days	ECT increases the depth of the neocortex by 6%. Decreased neuronal density by 17%.	Diamond *et al.* (1964)
ECT vs. IC	Rat	25 days	105 days	Visual cortex, ECT > IC by 6.2%; somesthetic cortex, ECT > IC by 2.7%.	Bennett *et al.* (1964b)
ECT vs. IC	Rat	25 days	80 days	Visual cortex, ECT > IC by 7%; somesthetic cortex, ECT > IC by 3%.	Bennett *et al.* (1964a)
ECT vs. IC	Rat	25 days	4–5 months	Cortex and subcortical increased glia, increased volume. Labeled with thymidine-H^3.	Altman and Das (1964)
Enucleated ECT vs. IC	Rat	25 days	80 days	Visual cortex: blinded ECT weights increased over IC.	Krech *et al.* (1963)

activity of ganglion cells of the retina. "Visual stimuli are therefore transmitted by modulating the ever present background activity [Kuffler, FitzHugh, & Barlow, 1957]." Further transient changes occur even 5 min after changing illumination.

In anesthetized cat recording from the optic chiasm, tonic activity increased in 85% of the implants as a result of an increase in the level of steady illumination; 15% of the implants showed a reversed effect. The same results were obtained in unanesthetized precollicular decerebrate preparations. This study, unlike a number of others, indicates that decreased illumination, such as in visual deprivation, may result in decreased activity (Arduini & Pinneo, 1962).

In cats maintained in darkness up to 1000 days, the lateral geniculate electrophysiological response showed little or no change. Burke and Hayhow (1968) believe this is evidence that the ganglion cells continue to discharge in total darkness for long periods. In anesthetized adult cats unit firing in the lateral geniculate nerve persists after prolonged dark adaption. Rates between 4 and 6 Hz were seen in stable units. Often units changed firing patterns. This dark firing was dependent on a functional retina and was not blocked by lesions at the intercollicular level of the brain stem. It was not affected by minor fluctuations of body temperature, ventilation rate, or rate of infusion of anesthetic or relaxant (Levick & Williams, 1964).

"Dark discharge (in retina) exerts a constraining influence on the excitability of the geniculate neurons, although this influence is not evenly distributed within the geniculate nucleus [Arduini, 1961]." Constant illumination with stimulation of the lateral geniculate body potentiates the visual cortical response, defined as lowering the threshold and increasing the magnitude of the response. Thus the constant influence of afferent impulses modifies the excitatory state of the central neurons and increases the efficiency of their activities (Chang, 1952). In terms of these complex physiological activities, it is difficult to feel safe in assuming that diminished light or noise results in reduced neuronal activity. Nevertheless, for the purposes of clarity, this simplistic view has been assumed: Increased stimulation produces increased neuronal activity in the aggregate, and vice versa.

What is the effect of deafferentation? For purposes of this paper we have assumed reduced postsynaptic activity; however, there is at least some doubt. Furthermore, are the long term effects the same as the short-term effects? According to Drake and Stavraky (1948): "In conclusion, it may be emphasized once again that the present investigation shows the principle of sensitization by denervation within the central nervous system holds true not only in the case of decentralization but in deafferentation as well [p. 237]." Deafferentation disturbs the behavior of the postsynaptic neuron.

What is the anatomical basis for the "law of denervation?" Loeser (1967) showed higher activity in neurons of the dorsal horn at 4 weeks following dorsal rhizotomy.

Is a total reduction of sensory input the end result of reducing light? Crozier and Pincus (1937) reported eyelid suturing in rats enhances relative stimulating efficiency of red light. Thus, it may be concluded that eyelid suture experiments may be studies of reduced light intensity of most wavelengths or more likely studies of the effect of predominance of red light on the retina as well as the reduction of patterned light.

The effect of binocular visual deprivation is certainly different than that of monocular even in regard to the individual cells within the cortex. This is particularly true if the neuron studied receives binocular input. The deranged behavior of individual neurons would then pass that effect onto the next postsynaptic neuron. Furthermore, if the postsynaptic neuron receives input from two sources, and if these sources are out of phase, then they yield contradictory information. The postsynaptic neuron is "jammed." Presumably, it receives no coherent information, although the number of action potentials which are "seen" are identical to that received prior to the disruption of one of the afferent systems. Thus, there would be no interference with postulated anatomical or physiologic dependence, but significant interference with informational dependence. An experimental example: Extracellular recording of monocularly and binocularly visually deprived cats shows drastic changes in the receptive fields, firing patterns, and fatigability of visual cortical neurons (Ganz *et al.*, 1968).

Another method of "jamming" is hyperstimulation over certain, but as yet unknown, levels of activity. As the level of stimulation is increased, more and more afferent volleys would theoretically take on "jamming" qualities. In this case, however, there is also an effect on physiologic dependence as, presumably, the amount of transmitter released is proportional to the number of action potentials arriving at the synaptic site. These statements may be broken down into two hypotheses as illustrated in Figures 9 and 10.

In some cases experiments purporting to show one effect may be examples of either deafferentation or reduced afferent activity. An example of this experimental problem is the study of dendritic morphology by Grant and Aldskogius (1967) and Grant (1968). They reported an interesting finding utilizing the Nauta stain in neurons whose axons have been transected. The dendrites of these neurons undergo a chemical change that results in a dark metallic deposit within them. They are thus seen beaded and apparently undergoing degeneration. These authors concluded that this was a consequence of axon transection and Wallerian degeneration. Another possibility is a transneuronal effect mediated through axon collaterals. Cortical undercutting and slab procedures resulted in interruption of both

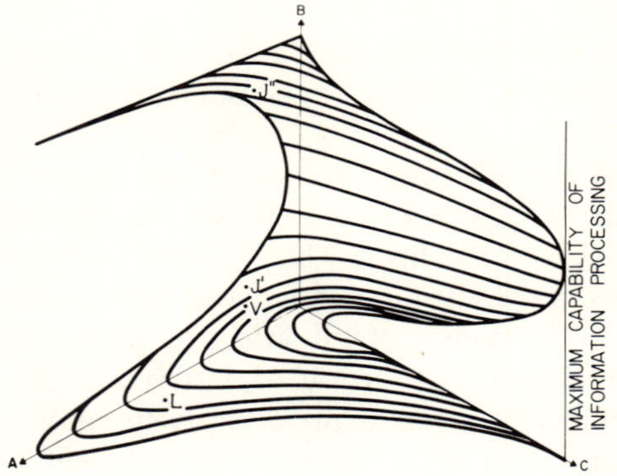

Fig. 9. Three-dimensional graphic illustration of the hypothesis: Morphological feature is dependent on a normal amount of information processing. Diagram of the relation between the amount of information on a presynaptic input system, B; the information processing capability of a hypothetical neuronal structure, C; and the degree of morphological change, A. If the eyelids are sutured, B is small, C is small, and A is large in the lateral geniculate neurons (point L). In the same experimental treatment, but in case of the visual association cortex, B is relatively larger because of continuing input from the other cortical areas, C is larger for the same reason, and, thus, the morphological change is also less (point V). With this hypothesis, "jamming" of the input system and/or similar overload (J″) should produce the same morphological effects as deprivation (J′) because both reduce the information available.

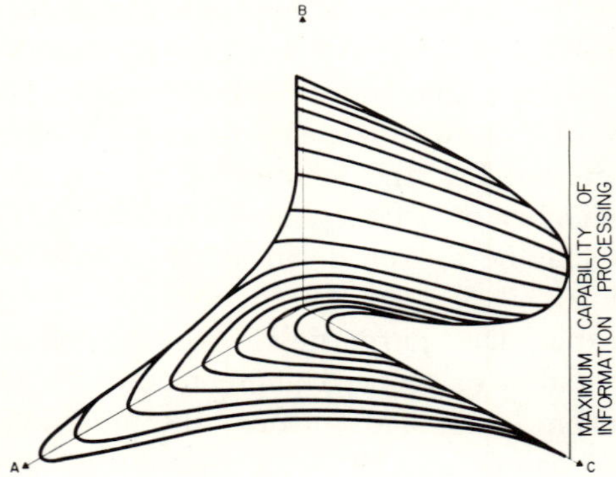

Fig. 10. Three-dimensional illustration of the hypothesis: Morphological feature is dependent on the presence of a normal number of synapses and the proper amount of released transmitter but independent of the order of action potentials within the afferent volley. In this case the morphological feature would not respond to overload by structural change. Note that the two hypotheses cannot be distinguished on the lower part of the graph by experiments involving overload or hyperstimulation.

efferent and afferent axons as well as many afferent axons to the slab from short axon cells just outside the slab. The effects of efferent interruption were retrograde degeneration; those of afferent interruption were transneuronal (Benhamida & Ruiz de Pereda, 1969). Thus, one must study the effects of retrograde degeneration, effect the slab, and then deduct the effects due to transneuronal degeneration. Therefore, these methods may be pertinent but are of limited usefulness to the investigative areas covered by this review.

Timing of sacrifice may also be an important factor. In the somatosensory cortex, Jones and Powell (1970a, b, c), and in the visual cortex, Garey and Powell (1971), did not find evidence that dendritic spines were detached from the postsynaptic dendrite following lesions of the respective nuclei of the thalamus. These studies were performed at 5 and 6 days. Ghetti and Wiśniewski (1972) did not show detachment and glial engulfment in cat striate cortex after lesions of lateral geniculate body; however, they utilized longer survival times. Thus, the timing following the lesion is often critical to the definition of the effect of presynaptic manipulation.

Constant awareness of untoward pathological conditions affecting the outcome is well illustrated in a paper by Matthews and Powell (1962). In an experiment utilizing surgical excision of one olfactory mucosa, several of the rabbits contracted atrophic rhinitis on the control side. These authors were astute enough to discover this and utilize it in their study.

Often controls within the same animal are accepted. Fifková reports a dramatic example of this type of error in experimental design. Moderate damage is sustained by the receptors of the retina in the open eye of monocularly deprived rats, apparently due to increased duration of eye opening (Fivková, 1972). This finding throws doubt on the claim that this eye and its visual system can be used as a sole control in monocular deprivation or surgical experimental procedures.

Experimental variation in measures is affected by the procedure chosen: For instance, total visual deprivation produced a larger reduction (39%) in spines on pyramids in the visual cortex of mice (Valverde, 1967) than unilateral lid suture in rats (25–30%) (Fifková, 1968). Apparently total visual deprivation is an experimental manipulation that affects a number of modalities that remain unaffected by unilateral lid suture.

C. Problems Related to Species Differences

Species selection is dependent on the experimental procedure and the time of initiation of experimental treatment. Examples abound in the results section, but a few are used as illustrations here. The goals of the experiment dictate the species utilized. Rodents show changes in superior colliculus on optic nerve section, but primates and carnivores do not. In rats, 60 days of visual experience does not diminish the effect of unilateral eyelid suture on the volume of the lateral geniculate, the cell densities in Layers II–IV in the visual cortex, or the density of spines on the apical dendrite. Eyelid suture at 11 days produces similar effects. Thus, previous light experience does not safeguard the pertinent structures against the effects of visual deprivation. Also, there seems to be little or no recovery in these structures even after 30 days following eye reopening. Furthermore, in the rat a 3-day period of deprivation produces no effect, 10 days deprivation a more pronounced effect, and 30 days a maximal effect. In regard to the decrease in spines, the effect of 30 days of deprivation is almost twice as great as that of 10 days of deprivation (Fifková, 1970c). Rats have few uncrossed optic fibers; cats have many. Rats have an unstratified lateral geniculate body, cats a stratified lateral geniculate body. Experimental designs may take advantage of these differences. Other anatomical differences are of importance: for instance, the eyelids of rats are thinner than the nictitating membrane of cats. When these structures are sutured, more light is admitted to the retina in rats than cats, although patterned light is blocked in both. Perhaps the experiments with semiopaque occluders in cats are therefore more comparable to lid suture in rat than suture of the nictitating membrane in cats. When the treatment is applied at birth, maturity at birth is an important consideration. For instance, mice at birth are considered very immature, roughly equivalent to a 5-month human fetus. Rabbits are also relatively immature. Cats and monkeys are more mature at birth in terms of central nervous system development than these species.

D. Problems Related to Data Collection

It is difficult to make generalizations about these often after the fact, and startling problems. The only generalizations that I can think of are: (1) the disclosure of the these problems stems most often from your colleagues; (2) they are often dismaying; (3) your consolation is based on the hope and high probability that you will be able to return the favor.

Often it is preferable not only to compare changes in an affected structure, but also in an area thought not to be affected. For example, in mice raised in the dark from birth, there is no change in spine densities along the apical dendrites in pyramids of the area temporalis, while there is a 35% reduction in the spine counts in the area striata (Valverde, 1967). Thus, the use of this technique in data collection helps rule out trophic effects as opposed to specific effects of sensory deprivation. In selecting the area involved, care must be exercised to avoid structures undergoing indirect changes such as "normalization." For example, taking a clue from physiological studies which showed evoked potentials in the cingulate cortex after photic stimulation, Coleman and Riesen (1968) studied dendritic branching under conditions of long term total visual deprivation. Reduction in basal dendritic length and branching was demonstrated in this cortical area. Obviously this cortical area would not be a good standard or control for a visual deprivation or hyperstimulation study.

Effects may decrease with the prolongation of the treatment. Enucleated mice at birth show less effect at 48 days than at 24 days, both in spine counts in the Layer IV and on dendritic orientation (Valverde, 1968). Whether this is a "compensatory" mechanism as the author suggests, a slight change in the method of gathering the data, or an artifact of timing related to the developmental stage, is difficult if not impossible to assess.

The anatomical facts often affect the data base. In rat visual cortex, 85% of axosomatic synapses have flattened vesicles (Fifková, 1970a). Obviously it is more difficult to obtain a suitable sample size of axosomatic synapses having round vesicles. Care should be exercised to vary sample size to assure a reasonable level of significance depending on population. Often changes vary in different parts of a single structure. Thus, findings in the lateral geniculate body of rat differ from the rostral to caudal dimensions, presumably due to cell size, density, and distribution of the afferent system (Fifková & Hassler, 1969).

Suppose that in a given structure there are several cell types. If only one cell type shows an effect of altered presynaptic activity, then it is reasonable to conclude that this is not a trophic, nutritional, or environmental effect. That is, this effect is a result of altered presynaptic function, as the other neurons were unaffected.

Depending on the anatomical level, effects are different. For instance, rats undergoing enucleation (Tsang, 1937) and lid suturing (Fifková, 1968) produce different volume effects at the lateral geniculate body, but similar effects at the cortex.

Within the same species the timing of transneuronal degeneration varies. With deafferentation in rabbits involving the olfactory mucosa, degeneration occurs within one month. With enucleation, no changes occur until 5–6 months (Cook *et al.*, 1951).

A criterion often used to distinguish neurons from glia is the presence of a distinct nucleolus. However, with very small cells such as stellates of Layer IV of the visual cortex, additional criteria are necessary, such as a cytoplasmic fringe surrounding the nucleus (Fifková & Hassler, 1969).

E. Problems of Developmental Stage

The timing of the experimental treatment is crucial. Critical developmental events to be considered are:

1. cessation of cell division;
2. organ formation;
3. arrival of afferent systems;
4. early synaptic function;
5. mature synaptic function;
6. maximum growth.

Naturally, the onset of receptor function, opening of eyes, etc., are also critical to experimental design. Thomas and Schaefer (1961), in a review article on the effects of early experience and stimulation on behavior, set forth these postulates (see Fig. 11). These effects apply equally to ana-

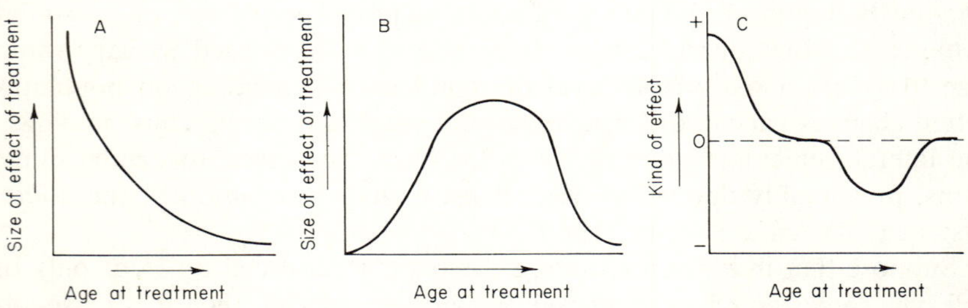

Fig. 11. Hypothetical relationships between age at treatment and size or type of effect produced. (A) The hypothesis states simply that the effect of stimulation is inversely proportional to age. (B) The hypothesis of the critical period type, stating that there is a specific time during which certain kinds of stimulation will have maximal effect. (C) The hypothesis that stimulation at the earliest stage of development has an effect which is opposite to the effect of the same stimulation at a later stage of development. (From Thompson & Schaefer, 1961.)

tomical results. Further postulates may be formulated. A few experimental facts are cited as illustrations.

In the pontine nucleus and inferior olive, processes responsible for mild transneuronal effects in adult cats cause severe cell loss in young animals (Torvik, 1956). In kittens, the degree of damage depends on the period of deprivation, being most damaging between 1–3 months of life (Wiesel & Hubel, 1956b). Using lesions of the thalamus and cerebral cortex, dendritic spines of stellate neurons in the caudate were studied in cats from 13–56 weeks of age. The effects of the lesion at these various ages was the same (Kemp & Powell, 1971). The afferent systems to the caudate are mature long before the placement of these lesions. In order to study the relation between development and spine formation, the events of afferent system arrival, early, and mature functioning must be accounted for in the experimental design.

F. Problems Related to Interpretation of Results

There are several major problems in the interpretation of results. Embedded in the matrix of these unsolved problems are the alternative conclusions that will lend significance or its lack to this investigative area. Some of these problems are:

1. Does deafferentation and/or disuse result in degeneration or developmental failure of the dendritic spine and/or the synaptic site?
2. Are changes observed following reduced stimulation a result of changes in anatomical, physiological, and/or informational processes?
3. Once a morphological change has been effected, can it be reversed?
4. Does environment and thus behavior control brain growth or neuronal connectivity?

Question 1. *Does deafferentation and/or disuse result in a degeneration or developmental failure of the dendritic spine and/or of the synaptic site?*

This question is complex and involves a number of technical problems that are better left to the original scientific papers. Nevertheless, I will briefly discuss the case for and against the loss of spines as a consequence of deafferentation, as well as mention some technical problems.

Spine densities vary from animal to animal in the normal population, resulting in high statistical variance and, therefore, requiring special statistical methods of analysis. Further difficulties are encountered as the density of spines varies at different distances from the soma (Globus & Scheibel, 1966; Kemp & Powell, 1971; Valverde, 1967; Valverde, 1968; Valverde & Esteban, 1968). This means that comparison must be made at standard distances from the soma.

The remaining synapses may serve to maintain intact the morphology of the dendritic spine, although another afferent system has degenerated. It may also be that a spine may have more than one synapse. Presumably the loss of one afferent would not cause the loss of the spine.

Furthermore, there have been reports that neurons which are undergoing loss of afferent systems may fail to impregnate with the Golgi method (Cowan, 1970; Matthews & Powell, 1962; Powell, 1967). If true, this effect would eliminate from quantitation exactly those neurons most affected by the loss of the afferent system. There are at least two reports of neurons not taking on the impregnation in the Golgi technique: in rats (Schapiro

& Vukovich, 1970) under conditions of isolated or nonstimulating environments, and in rabbits under conditions of deafferentation (Matthews & Powell, 1962). The latter authors suggest that activity in the principal dendrites is necessary to maintain the integrity of the whole of the neuron.

Colonnier (1964), in an EM study of rat cerebral cortex following slab production, reported the phagocytosis of not only the deafferentated synapses, but also of the still attached dendritic spine. Westrum (1966) reported changes following deafferentation in the postsynaptic surfaces of neurons in the prepyriform cortex. They consisted of postsynaptic structures in contact with glycogen containing glial processes. He concludes that the postsynaptic elements may maintain their morphological integrity up to several weeks. Although there are some confusing aspects in the statement of findings, Szentágothai (1965) seems to suggest that there is a loss of spines in pyramidal cells following slab production. This author does not specify directly whether the spine loss is secondary to transneuronal or retrograde degeneration. However, interpretations made elsewhere in the paper lead me to believe that he assumes a transneuronal effect. Studying the lateral geniculate body of rats (25–150 days) with enucleation or optic nerve transection, McMahan (1967) observed synaptic organelles extending deeply into the dendritic cytoplasm. This author reported both normal and thickened synapses at the site of phagocytized boutons.

Age of the animal following deafferentation seems to be critical in differentiating failure of spine development, actual spine loss, and failure to impregnate with the Golgi method. There is insufficient evidence for a definitive answer to this important question. Nevertheless, it is probably true that early deafferentation, or visual deprivation, if instituted prior to establishment of synaptic continuity, results in failure of the spine to develop in the striate cortex. In some structures such as the cerebellum (Mouren-Mathieu & Colonnier, 1969) and the caudate (Kemp & Powell, 1971), deafferentation, even in the adult, effects spine degeneration.

QUESTION 2. *Are changes observed following reduced stimulation a result of changes in anatomical, physiological, and/or informational processes?*

Changes in dendritic branches following transection of afferent systems may be due to a reduction of impulses or a loss of controlling factors maintaining neuronal morphology normally furnished by the afferent systems but not related to impulse conduction. Deafferentation results in a poverty of polarizing input. This may effect the morphological change based on the requisite ionic alterations due to the lack of polarizing input. Altered extracellular and glial space under EM observation tends to support this conception of the mechanism of morphologic alteration. Similarly, lack of spike generation at the initial segment may cause primary changes which, in turn, could affect axonal structures (Pinching & Powell, 1971). Although altered dendrites and spines may be dominated by the polarizing influence of dendrites with normal synaptic input it could effect a changed firing pattern and, in turn, affect the postsynaptic neuron. In any case, there is little data base for a hypothesis about the mechanism of the variety of well established changes. A unique hypothesis for a mechanism is suggested by the basic work of Scheibel and Scheibel (1955) showing that axons may terminate on neuroglia. The possibility must be at least considered that transneuronal effects may be mediated by glia.

QUESTION 3. *Once a morphological change has been effected, can it be reversed?*

Studies in immature *Macaca mulatta* utilizing total visual deprivation showed no histological effects throughout the visual system (Chow, 1955). The author rightfully warns that too much emphasis should not be placed on these negative results since the animals were exposed to 2–3 min of normal lighting per day. It is probable that such a minimal exposure is sufficient to safeguard the animal, especially as the treatment was not instituted at birth. In monocularly deprived cats, forced visual stimulation and learning seems to reverse the reduction in somal size (Chow & Stewart, 1972). Using electrophysiological and behavioral data these authors conclude, "One might propose that as a change is produced by an inequality in stimulus directed growth, it may be necessary to initiate a stimulus inequality in the opposite direction in order for compensation to occur [p. 438]." Furthermore, as the binocularly deprived animals show little change in lateral geniculate body somal size, it seems reasonable to conclude that inequality of bilateral excitation has a more dramatic effect on somal size than an equal, bilateral effect. This may be a "jamming" effect.

In a variety of behavioral studies following early deprivation, partial recovery was demonstrated (Hubel & Wiesel, 1970; Wilson & Riesen, 1966). On the other hand, a very short exposure to light apparently has great efficacy in blocking the effect on the morphologic changes resulting from visual deprivation.

QUESTION 4. *Does environment and thus behavior control brain growth or neuronal connectivity?*

In weight and area measurements, handled rats show a retardation of growth: Cell proliferation particularly in the microneurons of the cerebellum and hippocampal dentate gyrus is increased. Altman *et al.* (1968) conclude that the "brains of the handled animals, which mature slower and are exposed longer to modulatory environmental influences, are structurally different from the brains of the unhandled animals [p. 19]." Furthermore, they suggest that the anatomical substrate may be "input-regulated (behavioral) control over the finer aspects of the interconnection of neurons." Globus *et al.* (1973) have shown an increased number of dendritic spines, and, therefore, synapses in pyramidal cell dendrites in rats exposed to environmental complexity as compared to rats maturing in a relatively impoverished environment. Although the experimental design differs from Altman *et al.* (1968), the experiments are similar in that the behavioral

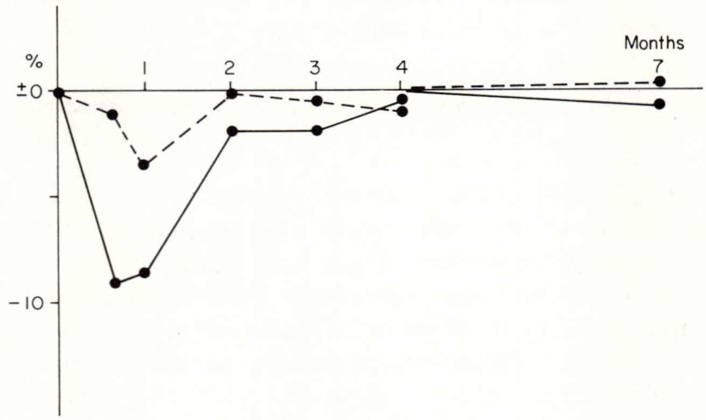

Fig. 12. Nuclear diameter: change in visually deprived mice. The solid line represents Layers II–IV of the visual cortex; the dashed line represents Layers V–VI. (From Gyllensten *et al.*, 1965.)

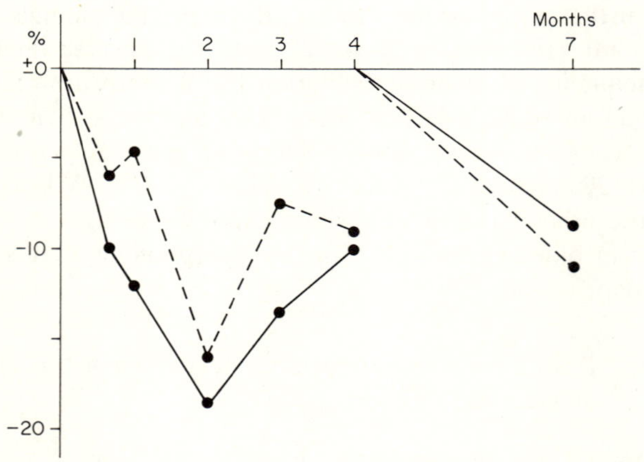

Fig. 13. Internuclear material per nucleus: change in visually deprived mice. The solid line represents II–IV of the visual cortex; the dashed line represents Layers V–VI. Internuclear material per nucleus is taken as a rough measure of the volume of cytoplasm. (From Gyllensten *et al.*, 1965.)

treatment begins at weaning (21 days) and lasts for 30 days. The increase in spines may be the anatomical substrate of the behavioral control of the interconnection of neurons postulated by Altman and co-workers

"Normalization" is described by Gyllensten, Malmfors, and Norrlin (1965), in reference to nuclear diameter and internuclear material per nucleus. These authors apply this term to the fact that these measures tend toward the "normal" value after prolonged periods of total visual deprivation (see Figs. 12 and 13). This phenomenon was seen in the cortex, but not in subcortical structures. These hypotheses are offered to explain normalization:

1. Growth of the visual cortex depends primarily on genetic factors which compensate for the lack of functional stimulation.
2. The retina, even in dark-reared animals, exhibits "spontaneous" activity (Arduini & Pinneo, 1962; Granit, 1955). After some time, tonic discharge may provide functional stimulus for growth.
3. Nonvisual function in the visual cortex increases during visual deprivation. This third explanation is the only one that accounts for the fact that subcortical centers do not show this effect.

In mice reared in the dark, the auditory cortex shows a transient hypotrophy: 6% in the auditory cortex, and 15–20% in the visual cortex. After 2 months of dark rearing, normalization occurs in both cortexes. After 4 months, "normalization" had occurred in the visual cortex and hypertrophy of 5–15% in the auditory cortex. The effect in the auditory cortex was more pronounced in the upper layers (Gyllensten *et al.,* 1966). Hypotheses for the hypotrophy of the auditory cortex are the reduction of associative stimuli, a generalized effect on the entire cerebral cortex, or hormonal effects mediated through the hypothalamus. Hypotheses for the hypertrophy occurring at 4 months include an increased reliance on auditory stimuli for orientation (see Figs. 14 and 15). This hypothesis gains support from the fact that the supragranular layers, where the hypertrophy is most striking, are the layers of greatest changes. Furthermore, adult mice reared in the dark showed a consistent effect. A more complex and less supported hypothesis is that the hypertrophy is due to a lack of "morphogenetic inhibition [De Oliveira Castro, 1963; Röhlich & Török, 1962]." In conclusion, it seems clear that the environment or, perhaps, the behavior induced by that environment, produces a modulating effect on brain growth (Rosenzweig *et al.,* 1969) and connectivity (Cragg, 1968; Globus *et al.,* 1973; Møllgaard, Diamond, & Bennett, 1971). While the total variance in growth and connectivity accounted for by moderate changes in environment within the limits of normal growth is less than 15%, it is difficult to assume the position that this change is insignificant in terms of adaptability.

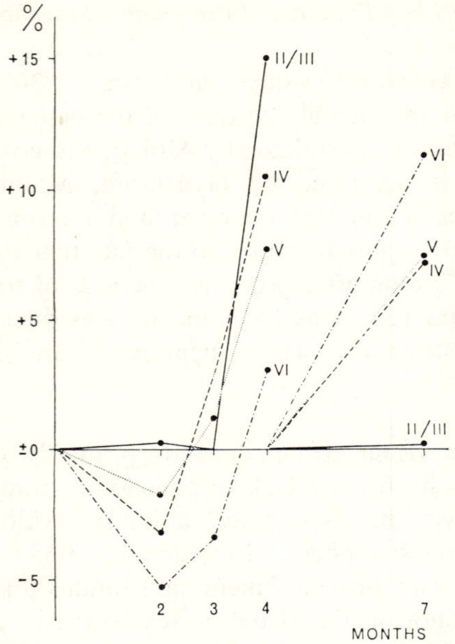

Fig. 14. Internuclear material per nucleus in different layers of the auditory cortex: change in visually deprived mice. The first group of curves refer to growing mice reared in the dark from birth; the second to adult mice reared in darkness from four to seven months of age. II/III, external granular and pyramidal-cell layer; IV, internal granular layer; V, internal pyramidal-cell layer; VI, multiform layer. Control taken as O. (From Gyllensten *et al.*, 1966.)

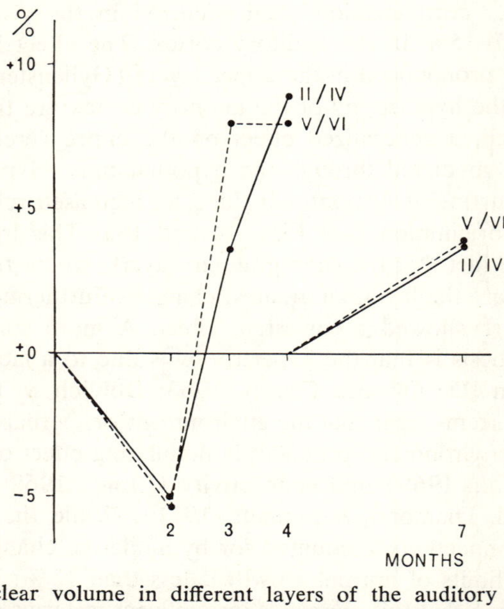

Fig. 15. Nuclear volume in different layers of the auditory cortex of visually deprived mice: change in per cent of corresponding controls. Cortical layers denoted as in Figure 9. (From Gyllensten *et al.*, 1966.)

G. Gaps in Experiments Performed

Unfortunately gaps of knowledge abound in this subject. The following experiments have come to mind. Most of them have never been cited in the literature, at least in regard to their morphological effects:

1. Block of afferent system produced by slow infusion of substance such as Novocaine.
2. Ecological niche as it alters the effects of deafferentation or sensory deprivation (visual deprivation in moles, bats, etc.).
3. Almost any kind of hyperstimulation experiment.
4. Long term effects of sensory deprivation and/or deafferentation, both partial and complete, on glia.
5. Frequency specific light hyper- or hypostimulation.
6. Minimum exposure of patterned light in terms of timing and amount to block effects of visual deprivation.

IV. Summary

Deafferentation affects somal size and postsynaptic structures often leading to dendritic and spine degeneration. Effects seem to hold throughout the phylogenetic scale in regard to synaptic sites and to be more pronounced in primates in regard to size. Effects are more severe if the treatment is initiated before the establishment of synaptic continuity and if the deafferentation is complete rather than partial.

Sensory deprivation results in similar but less profound effects. The same generalization holds true as for deafferentation. Recovery in morphological structures has not been demonstrated. A small amount of exposure to normal stimulation often has the capability of preventing the effect. Furthermore, the conditions of environments affect brain growth, glia, and connectivity within specific limits.

Finally, this investigative field, although now burgeoning, abounds with research possibilities. The filling of these lacunae promise significant clues to the organelles involved in learning and brain development, and will certainly point the way to more relevant and sensitive biochemical studies.

Acknowledgments

Appreciation is expressed for bibliographic help to Edith Askew, Pamela Kaups, Orilla A. Globus, and John Parnavelas and for typing assistance to Penelope Kimbrell.

References

Aghajanian, G. K., & Bloom, F. E. The formation of synaptic junctions in developing rat brain: A quantitative electron microscopic study. *Brain Research,* 1967, **6**, 716–727.

Allison, A. C. The secondary olfactory areas in the human brain. *Journal of Anatomy,* 1954, **88**, 481–488.

Altman, J., & Das, G. D. Autoradiographic examination of the effects of enriched environment on the rate of glial multiplication in the adult rat brain. *Nature,* 1964, **204**, 1161–1163.

Altman, J., Das,, G. D., & Anderson, W. J. Effects of infantile handling on morphological development of the rat brain: An exploratory study. *Developmental Psychobiology,* 1968, **1**, 10–20.

Arduini, A. Influences of visual deafferentation and continuous retinal illumination on the excitability of geniculate neurons. In R. Jung & H. Kornhuber (Eds.), *The visual system. Neurophysiology and psychophysics.* Berlin and New York: Springer-Verlag, 1961.

Arduini, A., & Pinneo, L. R. Properties of the retina in response to steady illumination. *Archives Italiennes de Biologie,* 1962, **100**, 425–448.

Bach, L. von Zur feinen Anatomie und Pathologie der Ganglienzellen der Retina. *International Ophthalmologic Congress, Transactions,* 1894, **8**, 137–138.

Barr, M. L., & Bertram, E. G. A morphological distinction between neurones of the male and female and the behaviour of the nucleolar satellite during accelerated nucleoprotein synthesis. *Nature,* 1949, **163**, 676–677.

Barron, D. H. Structural changes in anterior horn cells following central lesions. *Proceedings of the Society for Experimental Biology and Medicine,* 1933, **30**, 1327–1329.

Benhamida, C., & Ruiz de Pereda, G. Répartition des éspines dendritiques dans le cortex cérebral. *Journal of Neurological Sciences,* 1969, **9**, 1–10.

Benhamida, C., Ruiz de Pereda, G., & Hirsch, J. C. Les éspines dendritiques du cortex de gyrus isolé de chat. *Brain Research,* 1970, **21**, 313–325.

Bennett, E. L., Diamond, M. C., Krech, D., & Rosenzweig, M. R. Chemical and anatomical plasticity of brain. *Science,* 1964, **146**, 610–619. (a)

Bennett, E. L., Krech, D., & Rosenzweig, M. R. Reliability and regional specificity of cerebral effects of environmental complexity and training. *Journal of Comparative and Physiological Psychology,* 1964, **57**, 440–441. (b)

Berger, H. Experimentall-anatomische Studien über die durch den Mangel optischer Reize veranlassten Entwicklungshemmungen im Occipitallappen des Hundes und der Katze. *Archiv für Psychiatrie und Nervenkrankheiten,* 1900, **33**, 521–567.

Bertram, E. G., & Barr, M. L. Cytological changes in motor nerve cells following prolonged electrical stimulation of their axons. *Anatomical Record,* 1949, **103**, 567.

Bloom, F. E. Correlating structure and function of synaptic ultrastructure. In F. O. Schmitt (Ed.), *The neurosciences: Second study program.* New York: Rockefeller Univ. Press, 1970. Pp. 729–747.

Bondy, S. C., & Margolis, F. L. *Sensory deprivation and brain development: The avian visual system as a model.* Jena: Fischer, 1971.

Bowsher, D. Trans-neuronal degeneration in the specific sensory nucleus of the thalamus. *Journal of Anatomy,* 1957, **91**, 611.

Brattgård, S. O. The importance of adequate stimulation or the chemical composition of retinal ganglion cells during early post-natal development. *Acta Radiologica, Supplementum,* 1952, **96**, 1–80.

Burke, W., & Hayhow, W. R. Disuse in the lateral geniculate nucleus of the cat. *Journal of Physiology,* 1968, **194**, 495–519.

Burns, B. D. Some properties of isolated cerebral cortex in the unanaesthetized cat. *Journal of Physiology,* 1951, **112**, 156–175.

Burns, B. D. *The mammalian cerebral cortex.* London: E. Arnold, 1958.

Chang, H. T. Cortical response to stimulation of lateral geniculate body and the potentiation thereof by continuous illumination of retina. *Journal of Neurophysiology,* 1952, **15**, 5–26.

Chase, H. B. Studies on an anophthalmic strain of mice. V. Associated cranial nerves and brain centers. *Journal of Comparative Neurology,* 1945, **83**, 121–139.

Chow, K. L. Failure to demonstrate changes in the visual system of monkeys kept in darkness or in colored lights. *Journal of Comparative Neurology,* 1955, **102**, 597–606.

Chow, K. L., Riesen, A. H., & Newell, F. W. Degeneration of retinal ganglion cells in infant chimpanzees reared in darkness. *Journal of Comparative Neurology,* 1957, **107**, 27–42.

Chow, K. L. & Stewart, D. L. Reversal of structural and functional effects of long-term visual deprivation in cats. *Experimental Neurology,* 1972, **34**, 409–433.

Coleman, P. D., & Riesen, A. H. Environmental effects on cortical dendritic fields. I. Rearing in the dark. *Journal of Anatomy,* 1968, **102**, 363–374.

Colonnier, M. Experimental degeneration in the cerebral cortex. *Journal of Anatomy,* 1964, **98**, 47–53.

Colonnier, M., & Gray, E. G. Degeneration in cerebral cortex. In S. S. Bresse, Jr. (Ed.), *Electron microscopy. Fifth international congress for electron microscopy,* Vol. 2. New York: Academic Press, 1962.

Cook, W. H., Walker, J. H., & Barr, M. L. A cytological study of transneuronal atrophy in the cat and rabbit. *Journal of Comparative Neurology,* 1951, **94**, 267–292.

Cowan, W. M. Anterograde and retrograde transneuronal degeneration in the central and peripheral nervous systems. In W. J. H. Nauta & S. O. E. Ebbesson (Eds.), *Contemporary research methods in neuroanatomy.* New York: Springer Publ., 1970.

Cragg, B. G. Changes in visual cortex on first exposure of rats to light. *Nature,* 1967, **215**, 251–253.

Cragg, B. G. Are there structural alterations in synapses related to functioning? *Proceedings of the Royal Society of London, Series B,* 1968, **171**, 319–323.

Cragg, B. G. The effects of vision and dark-rearing on the size and density of synapses in the lateral geniculate nucleus measured by electron microscopy. *Brain Research,* 1969, **13**, 53–67.

Cragg, B. G. What is the signal for chromatolysis? *Brain Research,* 1970, **23**, 1–21.

Crozier, W. J., & Pincus, G. Photic stimulation of young rats. *Journal of General Psychology,* 1937, **17**, 105–111.

DeLong, G. R., & Sidman, R. L. Effects of eye removal at birth on histogenesis of the mouse superior colliculus: An autoradiographic analysis with tritiated thymidine. *Journal of Comparative Neurology,* 1962, **118**, 205–223.

de Oliviera Castro, G. Effects of reduction of nerve centers on the development of residual ganglia and on nerve patterns in the wing of the chick embryo. *Journal of Experimental Zoology,* 1963, **152**, 279–293.

Diamond, J., Gray, E. G., & Yasargil, G. M. The function of the dendritic spine—an hypothesis. In P. Andersen & J. K. S. Jansen (Eds.), *Excitatory synaptic mechanisms.* Oslo: Universitetsforlaget, 1970. Pp. 213–222.

Diamond, M. C. Extensive cortical depth measurements and neuron size increases in the cortex of environmentally enriched rats. *Journal of Comparative Neurology,* 1967, **131**, 357–364.

Diamond, M. C., Cosenza, C., & Johnson, R. E. An attempt to alter neuron number by environmental stimulation. *Anatomical Record,* 1973, **175**, 306.

Diamond, M. C., Krech, D., & Rosenzweig, M. R. The effects of an enriched environment on the histology of the rat cerebral cortex. *Journal of Comparative Neurology,* 1964, **123**, 111–120.

Diamond, M. C., Law, F., Rhodes, H., Lindner, B., Rosenzweig, M. R., Krech, D., & Bennett, E. L. Increases in cortical depth and glia numbers in rats subjected to enriched environment. *Journal of Comparative Neurology,* 1966, **128**, 117–125.

Dolley, D. H. The morphology of functional depression in nerve cells and its significance for the normal and abnormal physiology of the cell. *Journal of Medical Research,* 1913, **29**, 65–129.

Donaldson, H. H. Anatomical observations on the brain and several sense-organs of the blind deaf-mute, Laura Dewey Bridgman. *American Journal of Psychology,* 1890, **3**, 293–342.

Donaldson, H. H. Anatomical observations on the brain and several sense-organs of the blind deaf-mute, Laura Dewey Bridgman. *American Journal of Psychology,* 1891, **4**, 248–294.

Drake, C. G., & Stavraky, G. W. An extension of the "law of denervation" to afferent neurones. *Journal of Neurophysiology*, 1948, **11**, 229–238.

Dzidzishvili, N. N. Electrocorticographical study after exclusion of sight function. *Gagra Symposium,* 1963, **4**, 203–224.

Fifková, E. Changes in the visual cortex of rats after unilateral deprivation. *Nature,* 1968, **220**, 379–381.

Fifková, E. Changes of axosomatic synapses in the visual cortex of monocularly deprived rats. *Journal of Neurobiology,* 1970, **2**, 61–71. (a)

Fifková, E. The effect of monocular deprivation on the synaptic contacts of the visual cortex. *Journal of Neurobiology,* 1970, **1**, 285–294. (b)

Fifková, E. The effect of unilateral deprivation on visual centers in rats. *Journal of Comparative Neurology*, 1970, **140**, 431–438. (c)

Fifková, E. Effect of light and visual deprivation on the retina. *Experimental Neurology,* 1972, **35**, 450–457.

Fifková, E., & Hassler, R. Quantitative morphological changes in visual centers of rats after unilateral deprivation. *Journal of Comparative Neurology,* 1969, **135**, 167–178.

Foerster, O., & Gagel, O. Die tigrolytische Reaktion der Ganglienzelle. *Zeitschrift für Mikroskopische Anatomische Forschung,* 1934, **36**, 567–575.

Fox, M. W., Inman, O., & Glisson, S. Age differences in central nervous effects of visual deprivation in the dog. *Developmental Psychobiology,* 1968, **1**, 48–54.

Ganz, L., Fitch, M., & Satterberg, J. A. The selective effect of visual deprivation on receptive field shape determined neurophysiologically. *Experimental Neurology,* 1968, **22**, 614–637.

Garey, L. J., & Powell, T. P. S. An experimental study of the termination of the lateral geniculo-cortical pathway in the cat and monkey. *Proceedings of the Royal Society of London, Series B,* 1971, **179,** 41–63.

Ghetti, B., Horoupian, D. S., & Wiśniewski, H. M. Transsynaptic response of the lateral geniculate nucleus and the pattern of degeneration of the nerve terminals in the rhesus monkey after eye enucleation. *Brain Research,* 1972, **45**, 31–48.

Ghetti, B., & Wiśniewski, H. M. On degeneration of terminals in the cat striate cortex. *Brain Research,* 1972, **44**, 630–635.

Gibson, W. C. Degeneration and regeneration of sympathetic synapses. *Journal of Neurophysiology,* 1940, **3**, 237–247.

Glees, P., Hasan, M., & Tischner, K. Ultrastructural features of transneuronal atrophy in monkey geniculate neurons. *Acta Neuropathologica,* 1967, **7**, 361–366.

Globus, A. Neuronal ontogeny: Its use in tracing connectivity. In M. B. Sterman, D. J. McGinty, & A. M. Adinolfi (Eds.), *Brain development and behavior.* New York: Academic Press, 1971. Pp. 253–263.

Globus, A., Rosenzweig, M. R., Bennett, E. L., & Diamond, M. C. Effects of differential experience on dendritic spine counts in rat cerebral cortex. *Journal of Comparative and Physiological Psychology,* 1973, **82**, 175–181.

Globus, A., & Scheibel, A. B. Loss of dendritic spines as an index of presynaptic terminal pathways. *Nature,* 1966, **212**, 463–465.

Globus, A., & Scheibel, A. B. The effect of visual deprivation on cortical neurons: A Golgi study. *Experimental Neurology,* 1967, **19**, 331–345. (a)

Globus, A., & Scheibel, A. B. Synaptic loci on parietal cortical neurons: terminations of corpus callosum fibers. *Science,* 1967, **156**, 1127–1129. (b)

Globus, A., & Scheibel, A. B. Synaptic loci on visual cortical neurons of the rabbit: The specific afferent radiation. *Experimental Neurology,* 1967, **18**, 116–131. (c)

Goldby, F. A note on transneuronal atrophy in the human lateral geniculate body. *Journal of Neurology and Neurosurgery and Psychiatry,* 1957, **20**, 202–207.

Gomirato, G., & Baggio, G. Metabolic relations between the neurons of the optic pathway in various functional conditions. *Journal of Neuropathology and Experimental Neurology,* 1962, **21**, 634–644.

Goodman, L. Effect of total absence of function on the optic system of rabbits. *American Journal of Physiology,* 1932, **100**, 46–63.

Granit, R. Visual cells of guinea pig. *Nature,* 1947, **160**, 838.

Granit, R. *Receptors and sensory perception: A discussion of aims, means and results of electrophysiological research into the process of reception.* New Haven: Yale University Press, 1955.

Grant, G. Silver impregnation of degenerating dendrites, cells and axons central to axonal transection II. A Nauta study on spinal motor neurones in kittens. *Experimental Brain Research,* 1968, **6**, 284–293.

Grant, G., & Aldsoguis, H. Silver impregnation of degenerating dendrites, cells, and axons central to axonal transection. Part I: A Nauta study on the hypoglossal nerve in kittens. *Experimental Brain Research,* 1967, **3**, 150–162.

Gray, E. G. Axo-somatic and axo-dendritic synapses of the cerebral cortex: an electron microscope study. *Journal of Anatomy,* 1959, **93**, 420–433.

Gray, E. G., & Hamlyn, L. H. Electron microscopy of experimental degeneration in the avian optic tectum. *Journal of Anatomy,* 1962, **96**, 309–316.

Gyllensten, L. Postnatal development of the visual cortex in darkness (mice). *Acta Morphologica Neerlando-Scandinavica,* 1959, **2**, 331–345.

Gyllensten, L., & Lindberg, J. Development of the visual cortex in mice with inherited retinal distrophy. *Journal of Comparative Neurology,* 1964, **122**, 79–90.

Gyllensten, L., Malmfors, T., & Norrlin, M. L. Effect of visual deprivation on the optic centers of growing and adult mice. *Journal of Comparative Neurology,* 1965, **124**, 149–160.

Gyllensten, L., Malmfors, T., & Norrlin, M. L. Growth alteration in the auditory cortex of visually deprived mice. *Journal of Comparative Neurology,* 1966, **126,** 463–469.

Haddara, M. A. H. Studies in the postnatal development of the visual cortex of the mouse. Unpublished doctoral dissertation, University of London, 1955.

Hamberger, C. A., & Hydén, H. Transneuronal chemical changes in Deiters' nucleus. *Acta Otolaryngologica Supplementum,* 1949, **75**, 82–113.

Hamlyn, L. H. The effect of preganglionic section on the neurons of the superior cervical ganglion in rabbits. *Journal of Anatomy (London),* 1954, **88,** 184–191.

Hamori, J. Presynaptic-to-presynaptic axon contacts under experimental conditions giving rise to rearrangements of synaptic structures. In C. van Euler, S. Skoglund, & U. Söderberg (Eds.), *Structure and function of inhibitory neuronal mechanisms.* London: Pergamon, 1968. Pp. 71–80.

Hechst, B. Über das Verhalten der aüsseren Kniehöcker und der Sehrinde bei einseitiger peripherer Blindhert. *Archiv für Psychiatrie,* 1933, **100**, 19–31.

Hess, A. Optic centers and pathways after eye removal in fetal guinea pigs. *Journal of Comparative Neurology,* 1958, **109**, 91–115.

Holloway, R. L., Jr. Dendritic branching: Some preliminary results of training and complexity in rat visual cortex. *Brain Research*, 1966, **2**, 393–396.

Hubel, D. H., & Wiesel, T. N. The period of susceptibility to the physiological effects of unilateral eye closure in kittens. *Journal of Physiology*, 1970, **206**, 419–436.

Hydén, H., & Pigon, A. A cytophysiological study of the functional relationship between oligodendroglial cells and nerve cells of Deiters' nucleus. *Journal of Neuro-chemistry*, 1960, **6**, 57–72.

Illera, A. J. The effects of cerebellar lesions on Purkinje cell structure. *Anatomical Record,* 1968, **160**, 369.

Jones, E. G., & Powell, T. P. S. Electron microscopy of the somatic sensory cortex of the cat. I. Cell types and synaptic organization. *Philosophical Transactions of the Royal Society of London, Series B,* 1970, **257**, 1–11. (a)

Jones, E. G. & Powell, T. P. S. An electron microscopic study of terminal degeneration in the neocortex of the cat. *Philosophical Transactions of the Royal Society of London, Series B,* 1970, **257**, 29–43. (b)

Jones, E. G., & Powell, T. P. S. An electron microscopic study of the laminar pattern and mode of termination of afferent fibre pathways in the somatic sensory cortex of the cat. *Philosophical Transactions of the Royal Society of London, Series B,* 1970, **257**, 45–62. (c)

Jones, W. H., & Thomas, D. B. Transsynaptic atrophy in the cerebral cortex. *Nature,* 1956, **178**, 47–48.

Jones, W. H., & Thomas, D. B. Changes in the dendritic organization of neurons in the cerebral cortex following deafferentation. *Journal of Anatomy,* 1962, **96,** 375–381.

Kemp, J. M., & Powell, T. P. S. The termination of fibers from the cerebral cortex and thalamus upon dendritic spines in the caudate nucleus: a study with the Golgi method. *Philosophical Transactions of the Royal Society of London, Series B*, 1971, **262**, 429–439.

Kocher, R. A. The effect of activity on the histological structure of nerve cells. *Journal of Comparative Neurology*, 1916, **26**, 341–357.

Krech, D., Rosenzweig, M. R., & Bennett, E. L. Effects of complex environment and blindness on rat brain. *Archives of Neurology,* 1963, **8**, 403–412

Krech, D., Rosenzweig, M. R., & Bennett, E. L. Environmental impoverishment, social isolation and changes in brain chemistry and anatomy. *Physiology and Behavior*, 1966, **1**, 99–104.

Kruger, L., & Hamori, J. An electron microscopic study of dendritic degeneration in the cerebral cortex resulting from laminar lesions. *Experimental Brain Research,* 1970, **10**, 1–16.

Kuffler, S. W., FitzHugh, R., & Barlow, H. B. Maintained activity in the cat's retina in light and darkness. *Journal of General Physiology*, 1957, **40**, 683–702.

Kupfer, C. The distribution of cell size in the lateral geniculate nucleus of man following transneuronal cell atrophy. *Journal of Neuropathology and Experimental Neurology,* 1965, **24**, 653–661.

Kupfer, C., & Palmer, P. Lateral geniculate nucleus: Histological and cytochemical changes following afferent denervation and visual deprivation. *Experimental Neurology,* 1964, **9**, 400–409.

Larsell, O. The effect of experimental excision of one eye on the development of the optic lobe and opticus layer in larvae of the treefrog (*Hyla regilla*). *Journal of Comparative Neurology*, 1929, **48**, 331–353.

Le Gros Clark, W. E. A morphological study of the lateral geniculate body. *British Journal of Ophthamology*, 1932, **16**, 264–284.

Le Gros Clark, W. E. The anatomy of cortical vision. *Transactions of the Ophthalmologic Society of the United Kingdom,* 1943, **62**, 229–245.

Le Gros Clark, W. E. Inquiries into the anatomical basis of olfactory discrimination. *Proceedings of the Royal Society of London, Series B*, 1957, **146**, 299–319.

Le Vay, S. On the neurons and synapses of the lateral geniculate nucleus of the monkey, and the effects of eye enucleation. *Zeitschrift für Zellforschung und Mikroskopische Anatomie*, 1971, **113**, 396–419.

Levick, W. R. & Williams, W. O. Maintained activity of lateral geniculate neurons in darkness. *Journal of Physiology* (London), 1964, **170**, 582–597.

Levi-Montalcini, R. The development of the acousticovestibular centers in the chick embryo in the absence of the afferent root fibers and of descending fiber tracts. *Journal of Comparative Neurology,* 1949, **91**, 209–242.

Lindner, I., & Umrath, K. Veränderungen der Sehsphäre I und II in ihrem monokularen und binokularen Teil nach Extirpation eines Auges beim Kaninchen. *Deutsche Zeitschrift für Nervenheilkunde,* 1955, **172**, 495–525.

Liu, C. N., Bailey, H. L., & Windle, W. F. An attempt to produce structural changes in nerve cells by intense functional excitation induced electrically. *Journal of Comparative Neurology*, 1950, **92**, 168–181.

Loeser, J. Some properties of deafferented spinal neurons. *Proceedings of the Annual Clinical Spinal Cord Injury Conference,* 1967, **16**, 9–11.

Loewy, A. D. The effects of dorsal root lesions on Clarke neurons in cats of different ages. *Journal of Comparative Neurology*, 1972, **145**, 141–163.

MacNeill, M., & Zubek, J. P. Effects of prolonged deprivation (dark-rearing) on the weight of the sensory cortex of the rat. *Canadian Journal of Psychology,* 1967, **21**, 177–183.

Maletta, G. J., & Timiras, P. S. Acetylcholinesterase activity in optic structures after complete light deprivation from birth. *Experimental Neurology*, 1967, **19**, 513–518.

Mann, G. Histological changes induced in sympathetic, motor, and sensory nerve cells by functional activity. *Journal of Anatomy and Physiology*, 1894–1895, **29**, 100–108.

Maraini, G., Carta, F., Franguelli, R., & Santori, M. Effect of monocular light-deprivation on leucine uptake in the retina and the optic centers of the newborn rat. *Experimental Eye Research,* 1967, **6,** 299–302.

Matthews, M. R. Further observations on transneuronal degeneration in the lateral geniculate nucleus of the macaque monkey. *Journal of Anatomy,* 1964, **98,** 225–263.

Matthews, M. R., Cowan, W. M., & Powell, T. P. S. Transneuronal cell degeneration in the lateral geniculate nucleus of the macaque monkey. *Journal of Anatomy*, 1960, **94**, 145–169.

Matthews, M. R., & Powell, T. P. S. Some observations on transneuronal cell degeneration in the olfactory bulb of the rabbit. *Journal of Anatomy,* 1962, **96**, 89–102.

McMahan, U. J. Fine structure of synapses in the dorsal nucleus of the lateral geniculate body of normal and blinded rats. *Zeitschrift für Zellforschung und Mikroskopische Anatomie*, 1967, **76**, 116–146.

Mendelson, J. H., & Ervin, F. R. Influences of afferent neurons on efferent neurons. In R. G. Grenell (Ed.), *Neural physiopathology*. New York: Harper, 1963. Pp. 178–210.

Mikeladze, A. L. Characterization of the postsynaptic structures of the brain. *Folia Morphologica*, 1969, **17**, 420–431.

Møllgaard, K., Diamond, M. C., Bennett, E. L., Rosenzweig, M. R., & Lindner, B. Quantitative synaptic change with differential experience in rat brain. *International Journal of Neuroscience,* 1971, **2,** 113–128.

Mouren-Mathieu, A. M., & Colonnier, M. The molecular layer of the adult cat cerebellar cortex after lesion of the parallel fibers: An optic and electron microscope study. *Brain Research*, 1969, **16**, 307–323.

Penman, J., & Smith, M. C. Degeneration of the primary and secondary sensory neurons after trigeminal injection. *Journal of Neurology, Neurosurgery and Psychiatry*, 1950, **13**, 36–46.

Pinching, A. J. Persistance of post-synaptic membrane thickenings after degeneration of olfactory nerves. *Brain Research*, 1969, **16**, 277–281.

Pinching, A. J., & Powell, T. P. S. Ultrastructural features of transneuronal cell degeneration in the olfactory system. *Journal of Cell Science,* 1971, **8**, 253–287.

Powell, T. P. S. Transneuronal cell degeneration in the olfactory bulb shown by the Golgi method. *Nature*, 1967, **215**, 425–426.

Powell, T. P. S., & Erulkar, S. D. Transneuronal cell degeneration in the auditory relay nuclei of the cat. *Journal of Anatomy,* 1962, **96**, 249–268.

Rasch, E., Riesen, A. H., & Chow, K. L. Altered structure and composition of the retinal cells in dark-reared cat. *Journal of Histochemistry and Cytochemistry,* 1959, **7**, 321–322.

Rasch, E., Swift, H., Riesen, A. H., & Chow, K. L. Altered structure and composition of retinal cells in dark-reared mammals. *Experimental Cell Research*, 1961, **25**, 348–363.

Recordon, E., & Griffitsh, G. M. A case of primary bilateral anophthalmia (clinical and histological report). *British Journal of Ophthalmology*, 1938, **22**, 353–360.

Riesen, A. H. Brain and behavior: Session I. Symposium, 1959. Effects of stimulus deprivation on the development and atrophy of the visual sensory system. *American Journal of Orthopsychiatry,* 1960, **30**, 23–36.

Riesen, A. H. Stimulation as a requirement for growth and function in behavioral development. In D. W. Fiske & S. R. Maddi (Eds.), *Functions of varied experience.* Homewood, Illinois: Dorsey Press, 1961. Pp. 57–80.

Riesen, A. H. Effects of visual deprivation on perceptual function and the neural substrate. In J. de Ajuriaguerra (Ed.), *Symposium Bel Air II, Geneva,* 1964. *Désafférentation expérimentale et clinique.* Geneva, Switzerland: Georg, 1965. Pp. 47–66. (a)

Riesen, A. H. Effects of early deprivation of photic stimulation. In S. F. Osler & R. E. Cooke (Eds.), *The biosocial basis of mental retardation.* Baltimore: Johns Hopkins University Press, 1965. Pp. 61–85. (b)

Riesen, A. H. Sensory deprivation. In E. Stellar and J. Stellar (Eds.), *Progress in physiological psychology.* New York: Academic Press, 1966. Pp. 117–147.

Rodieck, R. W., & Smith, P. S. Slow dark discharge rhythms of cat retinal ganglion cells. *Journal of Neurophysiology*, 1966, **29**, 942–953.

Röhlich, P., & Török, L. J. The effect of light and darkness on the fine structure of the retinal clubs of *Dendrocoelum lacteum. Quarterly Journal of Microscopial Science*, 1962, **4**, 543–548.

Rosenzweig, M. R. Environmental complexity, cerebral change, and behavior. *American Psychologist*, 1966, **21**, 321–332.

Rosenzweig, M. R., Bennett, E. L., Diamond, M. C., Wiu, S. Y., Slagle, R. W., & Saffran, E. Influences of environmental complexity and visual stimulation on development of occipital cortex in rat. *Brain Research*, 1969, **14**, 427–445.

Ruiz-Marcos, A., & Valverde, F. Dynamic architecture of the visual cortex. *Brain Research*, 1970, **19**, 25–39.

Schapiro, S., & Vukovich, K. R. Early experience effects upon cortical dendrites: A proposed model for development. *Science*, 1970, **167**, 292–294.

Scheibel, M. E., & Scheibel, A. B. The inferior olive: A Golgi study. *Journal of Comparative Neurology*, 1955, **102**, 77–131.

Scheibel, M. E., & Scheibel, A. B. On the nature of dendritic spines—report of a workshop. *Communications in Behavioral Biology*, 1968, **1**, 231–265.

Schimke, R. T. Effects of prolonged light deprivation on the development of retinal enzymes in the rabbit. *Journal of Biological Chemistry*, 1959, **234**, 700–703.

Schüpbach, P. Beiträge zur Anatomie und Physiologie der Ganglienzellen in Zentralnervensystem der Taube. *Zeitschrift für Biologie*, 1905, **47**, 437–474.

Shabadash, A. L. The histochemistry of the nucleoproteins of the neurones in relation to their functional activity. In A. V. Palladin (Ed.), *Problems of the biochemistry of the nervous system.* New York: Macmillan, 1964. Pp. 196–204.

Sherman, S. M., Hoffman, K. P., & Stone, J. Loss of a specific cell type from dorsal lateral geniculate nucleus in visually deprived cats. *Journal of Neurophysiology,* 1972, **35**, 532–541.

Sherman, S. M., & Sanderson, K. J. Binocular interaction on cells of the dorsal lateral geniculate nucleus of visually deprived cats. *Brain Research*, 1972, **37**, 126–131.

Siou, G. Changements morphologiques des neurones collicularies consécutifs a l'énucleation oculaire chez le lapin nouveau né. *Archives d'Anatomie Microscopique*, 1963, **2**, 53–73.

Sotelo, C. Permanence of postsynaptic specializations in the frog sympathetic ganglion cells after denervation. *Experimental Brain Research*, 1968, **6**, 294–305.

Sternschein, E. Das ganglion cervicale supremum nach prae- und postganglionäer durchschneidung. *Arbeiten aus dem Neurologischem Institut an der Wiener, Universitaet Leip* 39, *Wien,* 1921, **23**, 155–176.

Szentágothai, J. The use of degeneration methods in the investigation of short neuronal connections. *Progress in Brain Research*, 1965, **14**, 1–32.

Terry, R. J., & Gordon, J., Jr. The effects of unilateral and bilateral enucleation on the optic lobe development and pigmentation of the skin in *Rana catesbiana* larvae. *Journal of Experimental Zoology,* 1960, **143**, 245–258.

Terry, R. J. Roland, A. L., & Race, J., Jr. Effect of eye enucleation and eyelid closure upon the brain and associated visual structures in the mouse. I. A report on degeneration changes. *Journal of Experimental Zoology*, 1962, **150**, 165–183.

Thompson, W. R., & Schaefer, T. J. Early environmental stimulation. In D. W. Fiske & S. R. Maddi (Eds.), *Functions of varied experience.* Homewood, Illinois: Dorsey, 1961. Pp. 81–105.

Torvik, A. Transneuronal changes in the inferior olive and pontine nuclei in kittens. *Journal of Neuropathology and Experimental Neurology*, 1956, **15**, 119–145.

Tower, S. S., Howe, H., & Bodian, D. Fibrillation in skeletal muscle in relation to denervation and to inactivation without denervation. *Journal of Neurophysiology,* 1941, **4**, 398–401.

Tsang, Y. C. Visual centers in blinded rats. *Journal of Comparative Neurology,* 1937, **66**, 211–261.

Umrath, K. van, Histologische Veränderungen im Gehirn von Tieren nach Ausschaltung von Augen durch Vernahen der Lider oder durch Extirpation. *Zeitschrift für Biologie*, 1965, **115**, 99–118.

Valverde, F. Apical dendritic spines of the visual cortex and light deprivation in the mouse. *Experimental Brain Research,* 1967, **3**, 337–352.

Valverde, F. Structural changes in the area striata of the mouse after enucleation. *Experimental Brain Research*, 1968, **5**, 274–292.

Valverde, F. Rate and extent of recovery from dark rearing in the visual cortex of the mouse. *Brain Research*, 1971, **33**, 1–11.

Valverde, F., & Estéban, M. E. Peristriate cortex of mouse: location and effects of enucleation on the number of dendritic spines. *Brain Research*, 1968, **9**, 145–148.

Van der Loos, H., & Woolsey, T. A. Somatosensory cortex: Structural alterations following early injury to sense organs. *Science*, 1973, **179**, 395–397.

Volkmar, F. R., & Greenough, W. T. Rearing complexity affects branching of dendrites in the visual cortex of the rat. *Science*, 1972, **176**, 1445–1447.

Walberg, F. Role of normal dendrites in removal of degenerating terminal boutons. *Experimental Neurology*, 1963, **8**, 112–124.

Walberg, F. The fine structure of the cuneate nucleus in normal cats and following interruption of afferent fibres. An electron microscopical study with particular reference to findings made in Glees and Nauta sections. *Experimental Brain Research*, 1966, **2**, 107–128.

Weiskrantz, L. Sensory deprivation and the cat's optic nervous system. *Nature*, 1958, **181**, 1047–1050.

West, R. W., & Greenough, W. R. Effect of environmental complexity on cortical synapses of rats: Preliminary results. *Behavior Biology*, 1972, **7**, 1–6.

Westman, J. The lateral cervical nucleus in the cat III. An electron microscopical study after transection of spinal afferents. *Experimental Brain Research*, 1969, **7**, 32–50.

Westrum, L. E. Electron microscopy of degeneration in the prepyriform cortex. *Journal of Anatomy*, 1966, **100**, 683–685.

White, L. E., Jr., & Westrum, L. E. Dendritic spine changes in prepyriform cortex following olfactory bulb lesions—rat, Golgi method. *Anatomical Record,* 1964, **148**, 410–411.

Wiesel, T. N., & Hubel, D. H. Effects of visual deprivation on morphology and physiology of cells in the cat's lateral geniculate body. *Journal of Neurophysiology*, 1963, **26**, 978–993.

Wiesel, T. N., & Hubel, D. H. Comparison of the effects of unilateral and bilateral eye closure on cortical unit responses in kittens. *Journal of Neurophysiology*, 1965, **28**, 1029–1040. (a)

Wiesel, T. N., & Hubel, D. H. Extent of recovery from the effects of visual deprivation in kittens. *Journal of Neurophysiology,* 1965, **28,** 1060–1072. (b).

Wilson, P. D., & Riesen, A. H. Visual development in rhesus monkeys neonatally deprived of patterned light. *Journal of Comparative Physiological Psychology,* 1966, **61**, 87–95.

Young, I. J., & Rowley, W. F. Structural and histochemical change in ventral-horn cells resulting from sensory deprivation. *Recent Advances in Biological Psychiatry*, 1968, **10**, 53–73.

CHAPTER III

Neurochemical Correlates of Sensory Deprivation

J. P. Walker, Judith Boas Walker

Andrus Gerontology Center
University of Southern California, Los Angeles

R. L. Kelley, A. H. Riesen

Department of Psychology
University of California, Riverside

I. Introduction

Although there is less known about the biochemical characteristics of the various sensory systems than about their electrophysiological, morphological, or behavioral characteristics, new techniques, and an increasing interest in neurochemical mechanisms are rapidly increasing our knowledge. The study of the biochemistry of sensation is becoming an important field of research. The effect of afferent input on brain metabolism has recently received wide attention; for instance, see reviews of the neurochemical correlates of learning and experience by Agranoff (1971), Horn, Rose, and Bateson (1973), and Hydén and Lange (1971), and a review of changes in brain biochemistry during various functional states by Talwar and Singh (1971). The biochemical effects of sensory deprivation, however, have not received such widespread notice, probably because the effects are subtle, only partially studied, and less controversial. Biochemical and morphological effects of unilateral deprivation in the chick visual system have been reviewed by Bondy and Margolis (1971), and will not be reexamined here.

Sensory deprivation, as used herein, will mean the prolonged reduction of stimulation. This treatment is often begun neonatally, as the biochemical effects of deprivation in the young are often different or more severe than in older animals, implying the need for afferent input during the development of the organism. Because the overwhelming majority of papers have dealt with the effects of visual deprivation, most of this review will concentrate on the importance of afferent input to visual function. This research emphasis is due in part to the relative ease with which visual deprivation can be manipulated, and in part to the anatomy of the visual system. Input arrives via a single pathway, the optic tract, and the amount of input can be better controlled than in other sensory systems. It is thus possible to compare the effects of different types of deprivation, from the more subtle, such as pattern and wave length, through intermediate, such as eyelid suture, to the most severe, that is, enucleation.

The study of the biochemical correlates of deprivation rests on several premises. Some investigators are interested in the biochemical correlates of "learning to see" (Rose, 1967; DeBold, 1967); while others are interested in labile changes as a function of light without consideration of the history of the animal (Talwar, Chopra, Goel, D' Monte, 1966). Others (for example, Kupfer & Downer, 1967) have concentrated upon the differential effects of different types of deprivation and some (Gyllensten, Malmfors, & Norrlin, 1965) have been more concerned with the effects of different durations of deprivation upon a given morphocytochemical measure. Phylogenetic differences in the response to deprivation have also been noted (Rasch Swift, Riesen, & Chow, 1961; Riesen, 1966). Other questions being asked focus on specific effects of deprivation, that is, does deprivation delay cytochemical differentiation—the orderly maturation of biochemical systems—or does it cause atrophy in already existing systems? The multiplicity of approaches to the problem and the wide spectrum but relatively small volume of publication have made it necessary to separate these questions.

In discussing the biochemistry of deprivation we have adopted a biochemical categorization, retaining the sensory systems and the animal species distinctions. There is good reason to believe that similar visual functions can be subserved by different biochemical mechanisms in different species. For example, the rabbit retina may depend more heavily on glycolysis than the cat retina (Lowry, 1964), in which case the effects of deprivation on retinal enzymes may be different in the two species. A second factor arguing for a species-specific approach is that species-specific characteristics, such as functional anatomy and maturity at birth, may explain differences in the effectiveness of deprivation. Within the subsections we have treated the data in the order: mouse, rat, rabbit, cat, and primate.

II. Glycolysis and the Phosphogluconate Pathway

A. Production of Energy in the Brain

The rates of respiration of brain tissues *in vitro,* as determined by measuring oxygen consumption, are known to increase as much as 100% when electrical stimulation is applied as a means for inducing higher levels of activity (reviewed in McIlwain & Bachelard, 1971, pp. 68–72). In the process of glucose utilization, the glycolytic pathway alone involves the production of ten intermediate substances, each stage requiring a different enzyme. The overall result is conversion of 20% of consumed glucose to lactic acid. The remaining 80% of glucose is oxidized to CO_2.

The first stage enzyme, hexokinase, is thought to be the limiting factor in the pathway from glucose to lactate in the brain, *in vivo.* The brain is dependent upon glucose both for energy and for structural carbon in a great variety of complex molecules; this glucose must be constantly supplied by the bloodstream as relatively small amounts are stored in brain tissue. Blood volume in the brain is sensitive to metabolic demands, both acutely and over the longer term.

Few of the relevant stages of glycolysis have been examined in relation to sensory deprivation. A need for studies of this process is emphasized by the observation of Cohen and Noell (1960) that the retinas of neonatal rats show a sudden increase in glycolytic activity when their eyes open. The same correlation was reported for rabbits. In the following sections we will discuss under each biochemical topic the visual system prior to any of the other sensory systems and take up the pathway by level, in ascending order, from retina to cortex, for example.

B. Retina

Liberman (1962) raised S-3 Tryon rats in the dark from birth to sacrifice at age 17 weeks to determine the effect on the glycolytic activity of the rat retina. Using the Barker and Summerson technique to determine lactic acid production, he found no differences between the dark-reared and normally reared groups. From this finding Liberman (1962) deduces " . . . that the glycolytic process, necessary for normal visual function, is not influenced by lowered retinal excitation [p. 372]." Evaluating the entire glycolytic process by lactate production does not permit the detection of relative contributions from separate biochemical pathways. The importance of distinguishing between the contribution of the two major pathways to lactate is underlined by the finding by Graymore and Towson (1965) that the phosphogluconate path has relatively greater importance in the retina of the immature rat than in the adult.

Schimke (1958) kept albino rabbits in the dark from birth for 26, 60, or 120 days, at which point they were sacrificed and their whole retinas examined to determine the activity of various enzymes. There was a significant difference in the activity of lactate dehydrogenase in both the 60- and 120-day-old animals. Dark-reared animals failed to show the increase with age found in light-reared controls. Adults kept in darkness for 120 days showed no effects. Glucose 6-phosphate dehydrogenase was found to be higher in the dark-reared animals at 26 and 60 days.

C. Optic Tract and Nuclei of the Visual System

Iida and Schiebler (1968) examined the development of different parts of the visual system of the rat to determine whether complete darkness influences the postnatal chemodifferentiation of the optic system. During fetal life, the superior colliculus becomes laminated and the lateral geniculate nucleus develops into two regions. From the tenth postnatal day onward, there was an increase in the activity of lactate dehydrogenase as well as of other enzymes described below. By the end of the first month of life, the visual system was histochemically that of an adult rat. Myelination began around day 13 and was completed by day 30. This process was accompanied by enzyme activity increases in optic tract glial cells. No effect of dark-rearing on the activity of lactate dehydrogenase by using the histochemical techniques of this study was found with light deprivation up to 24 days after birth. Neither did these authors find effects of dark-rearing on the activity of glucose 6-phosphate dehydrogenase in optic chiasm, optic tract, superior colliculus, or lateral geniculate nucleus.

Kupfer (1963) noted a decrease in the activity of 6-phosphogluconate dehydrogenase in the laminae of lateral geniculate nucleus receiving fibers from the eye of kittens monocularly enucleated at 10 weeks and sacrified two months later. He also found a reduction in lactate dehydrogenase activity.

Kupfer and Palmer (1964) confirmed the observation above in kittens enucleated at 5 weeks and sacrificed 5 days to 2 months later, but found no change in 6-phosphogluconate dehydrogenase in kittens whose eyelids were sutured at 5 weeks and sacrificed 3–4 weeks later. There was no noticeable decrease in enzyme activity, in spite of the fact that the cells of the appropriate LGN laminae showed a 30% to 40% decrease in mean area, a decrease similar to that of the enucleates. The eyelid-sutured kittens, however, showed normal staining properties for 5-week-old kittens, suggesting that the 3–4-week period following suture produced a failure to grow rather than degeneration. This arrest was also seen in two kittens with unilateral lid closure prior to eye opening, within 10 days of lid closure.

Kupfer and Downer (1967) have looked at some of the metabolic correlates of transynaptic degeneration in the monkey using optic nerve transection. Carbon-14–glucose uptake in the LGN was measured from 1 to 23 days after nerve transection. During the first 2 days, glucose oxidation increased, but subsequently decreased to levels below control values.

Increased metabolic activity in the LGN shortly after deafferentation has also been reported in the cat (Deffenu, Bertaccini, & Pepeu, 1967) and in the rabbit (Vander Eecken & Fautrez, 1965; de Vos & Fautrez, 1967). Metabolic and morphological consequences of enucleation occur most rapidly in the LGN of the monkey, followed by the cat, and then by the rabbit. The mechanism underlying the metabolic disturbances is not known. The orderly progression of changes, and the reports of degeneration occurring preferentially on one side after binocular enucleation represent phenomena yet to be explained. An initial phase of glial cell proliferation is probably involved.

III. The Tricarboxylic Acid Cycle

A. Retina

Schimke (1958) found a reduced rate of development of malate dehydrogenase activity in retinas of albino rabbits dark reared from birth and studied at 26, 60, and 120 days of age. Water homogenates of whole brain showed no effect of dark rearing in these same animals.

B. Superior Colliculus and Lateral Geniculate

Iida and Schiebler (1968) found no difference in the activity of succinate dehydrogenase of the optic tract, colliculus, or LGN of their dark-reared rats at up to 24 days of deprivation.

Kupfer (1963) reported decreases of succinic dehydrogenase activity in the LGN laminae receiving fibers from the cat enucleated at 10 weeks of age and sacrificed after 2 months.

Kupfer and Palmer (1964) showed, by cytochemical investigation, a decrease in succinate dehyrdogenase activity of LGN cells of kittens beginning 5 days after unilateral enucleation at 5 weeks, with further decrease to 2 months postoperatively. Unilaterally lid-sutured kittens showed no noticeable decrease when sutured at 5 weeks and examined 3–4 weeks later. This was the finding even in cells that had ceased normal growth and therefore were smaller in diameter than control cells.

IV. Pyridine Nucleotide Oxidation-Reduction

Nicotine adenine dinucleotide (NAD) and nicotine adenine dinucleotide phosphate (NADP) play important roles in glycolysis, respiration, and biosynthetic activities. Kupfer and Downer (1967) found that after optic nerve transection in the adult monkey (*Macaca mulatta*) NAD: lipoamide oxidoreductase activity increased during the first 2 days, and subsequently decreased. These changes paralleled changes in levels of RNA.

Iida and Schiebler (1968) found no differences in the concentration of NADH and NADPH in the optic chiasm, optic tract, superior colliculus, and lateral geniculate of dark-reared rats when compared with light-reared rats.

Kupfer (1963) found that the LGN laminae receiving fibers from the deafferented side of kittens enucleated at 10 weeks and killed 2 months later showed a decrease in NADH and NADPH oxidoreductase activities.

In the same study, Kupfer found no change in the activity of alpha-glycerophosphate dehydrogenase (α-GPD). This failure is subject to a number of interpretations. Since this enzyme can be important in the synthesis of phospholipids, and since phospholipids are important constituents of myelin, it may be the case that myelination of transneuronal fibers is not affected by enucleation. It should also be noted that myelination of cat brain fibers is essentially complete prior to the age at which these animals were killed. The story may be even more complex than this, however. This enzyme catalyzes the reversible reaction: L-glycerol 3-phosphate $\rightleftharpoons$ dihydroxyacetone phosphate, but is known to work with two different electron acceptors, NAD and cytochrome c. The latter reaction takes place in the mitochondria (the general activity of which is affected by enucleation), whereas the former reaction is cytoplasmic. It is entirely possible, then, that the activity of this enzyme is decreased in mitochondria of LGN cells following enucleation while being increased in the cytoplasm.

Kupfer and Palmer (1964) replicated these findings in kittens monocularly enucleated at 5 weeks and sacrificed 2 days to 2 months later, but there was no noticeable effect on enzyme activity in kittens monocularly eyelid-sutured at 5 weeks and sacrificed 3 to 4 weeks later.

Gay and Silberberg (1964) studied histochemical correlates of transynaptic degeneration in the lateral geniculate after enucleation of one eye in the cynomolgus monkey. The animals were sacrificed 3, 4, 11, or 30 days after surgery. A decrease in the activity of NADH oxidoreductase and NADPH oxidoreductase was found at all survival times. These laminar effects were slight at 3 days but strong by the eleventh day. The enzymic decreases preceded noticeable changes in the amount of Nissl substance and can be considered leading indicators of transynaptic degeneration.

V. Nucleic Acids: Synthesis and Turnover

A. Retina

The most cogent argument for the necessity of functional activity in stimulating cytochemical differentiation of nerve cells was made by Brattgård (1952), using X-ray microradiography to study the postnatal maturation of several cytoplasmic constituents in the individual retinal ganglion cells of rabbits. He found that normally the pentose nucleoprotein (PNP) fraction per unit volume, and, presumably, cytoplasmic RNA, increased from 11 days after birth to a stabilized value at 10 weeks.

In studying the effects of deprivation, he used the following groups: rabbits reared to 10 weeks under a diurnal light cycle, dark-reared rabbits reared to 10 weeks of age, and 13-week-old rabbits reared from birth in darkness for 10 weeks but then exposed to 3 weeks of diurnal stimulation. Microchemical analysis revealed that in the deprived ganglion cells the PNP fraction was undetectable at 10 weeks. After 3 weeks of stimulation, the PNP fraction had increased but did not reach average control levels. The mean value attained, however, is not fully descriptive. The ganglion cells after three weeks of recovery showed far greater variability than those of control animals. Some cells yielded a PNP of the magnitude found in normally stimulated cells, while others showed little or no recovery, and perhaps were no longer responsive to normal synaptic input.

Rasch *et al.* (1961) studied retinal cytological and cytochemical changes resulting from visual deprivation in a number of mammals: rats, cats, and chimpanzees. The experiment with rats included the following conditions: (1) rats reared in total darkness from birth to sacrifice at 65 days of age; (2) rats reared in normal diurnal lighting from birth to sacrifice at 130 days; and (3) rats reared in total darkness from birth to 90 days followed by 60 days of diurnal lighting, at which time they were sacrificed. Although no marked histological differences between the retinas of dark-reared and control animals were found, photometric estimates of azure B binding in individual cells revealed an RNA concentration seven to ten times lower in the retinas of rats never exposed to light. Those returned to diurnal lighting after 90 days in the dark were intermediate in RNA concentration.

Rasch *et al.* (1961) reared cats under the following conditions: (1) normal diurnal variations of light and darkness; (2) total darkness; and (3) total darkness except for 1 hour of light stimulation per day. The rearing period lasted 3.5, 6, 19, 36, or 40 months.

Cytological observation after staining with azure B bromide revealed changes in cell structure in the dark-reared cats. These included differences in the staining intensity and distribution of the Nissl bodies of the ganglion cells, a reduced nucleolar volume, and alterations in the cytoplasmic nucleoproteins. Lower total RNA concentrations were reported in the ganglion, amacrine, and bipolar cells, and in the inner segments of cells of the receptor layer.

Rasch *et al.* (1961) also found depressed RNA levels in the surviving cells of darkreared chimpanzee retinas. Winsberg and Riesen (1966) found diminished basophilia in both the bipolar and ganglion cell layers of the macaque monkey after prolonged light deprivation. A large part of basophilic properties presumably reflects RNA content.

The above-outlined changes in chemical composition were associated with reduced thickness of the inner plexiform layer.

B. Lateral Geniculate Nucleus

Cook, Walker, and Barr (1951) found that the effects of monocular enucleation on the morphology of the LGN in the adult rabbit and cat are very similar, but that the effects take longer to develop in the rabbit. The gradual diminution in Nissl substance and the decrease in the volume of the nucleus and nucleolus in cells receiving input from the deafferented side suggest a depression of nucleic acid and nucleoprotein metabolism. These findings are at variance with the work of Vander Eecken and Fautrez (1965) who found an increase in the DNA stained by the Feulgen reaction in the LGN and cortex of rabbits which were monocularly enucleated as adults. The increases, paradoxically, occurred on both sides. We are reminded that monocular deprivation may change the structure and function of cells both ipsilateral and contralateral to the deprived side (Fifková, 1972; Yinon & Auerbach, 1973).

The distribution of DNA stained by the Feulgen reaction is not homogeneous and only the chromatin associated with the nucleolus is stained. It is impossible to say whether the finidings represent an increase in nuclear DNA, a redistribution of nuclear DNA, or a modification of stainability of the DNA. The first possibility would seem unlikely by current opinion (Garcia, 1970).

Gay and Silberberg (1964) studied the LGN of the monkey 3, 4, 11, or 30 days after monocular enucleation. Decreases in Nissl substance were noted at 11 days, increasing in degree thereafter.

Kupfer and Downer (1967) studied RNA levels of the LGN after optic nerve transection in the monkey. RNA increased in the denervated layers of the LGN as compared with contralateral LGN during the first and second postoperative days. At 3 days the RNA decreased from its peak, reaching a steady value below initial levels by 23 days. Examination of neurons undergoing transneuronal atrophy 1–28 days following denervation demonstrated a marked decrease in both the staining and the size of Nissl granules. Since Nissl granules have been identified with the rough endoplasmic reticulum, including ribosomal RNA, one would expect a decrease in the level of RNA. The decrease was confirmed by a modified Hess and Thalheimer assay.

C. Cortex

More subtle changes in RNA have been reported by several authors to result from variation of early visual experience. One such report is that of De Bold *et al.* (1967) who found no effects of darkness and other lighting conditions on the total amount of cortical RNA, but who did find evidence suggesting an influence on the species of RNA produced in the visual cortex. One high molecular weight fraction yielded the highest density values, and another the lowest values in rats reared to about 3 months in darkness and then another month in light. The comparisons are with rats reared for similar periods under the other permutations of continuous light and continuous darkness. A diurnally reared group was not exceptional. The effect was absent in the frontal cortex. The authors suggested that the changes may have reflected permanent alterations of function in response to light. The hypothesis provided by this exploratory study is in need of further substantiation.

Appel, Davis, and Scott (1967) found that 15 min of light after 3 days of darkness in otherwise normally reared 30-day-old rats produced increased numbers of polysomes, and, thus, ribosomal RNA, in both visual and remaining cortex. Over a longer period of stimulation, Dewar and Reading (1970) observed clear differences in the labelling of visual and motor cortex RNA in adult rats of two strains, one blind, when both were exposed to a flashing light. The blind rats were normal in motor cortex. As compared with a continuous light source, a flashing light hastened the progressive labelling of heavier RNAs in the seeing animals. This finding implies that an optimal stimulus will increase the turnover of larger RNAs which normally have a slower turnover rate than do smaller species.

Using split-brain chicks with one eye covered during exposure to a rotating flashing light Bateson, Rose, and Horn (1973) found maximum incorporation of uracil into macromolecules in the forebrain roof on the side receiving input from the stimulated eye. These effects were concentrated in the first four hours of exposure on the first day, and the longer the exposure on day 1 the less the incorporation rate on the second day. Since other brain regions did not show the effect these authors regard their results as indicating that the anterior part of the forebrain roof is the locus of the imprinting process.

VI. Protein Synthesis and Turnover

A. Retina

1. Total Proteins

Brattgård (1952) studied the protein content of the ganglion cells of dark-reared rabbits as well as their nucleic acid content. The protein fraction in such animals 10-weeks-old was one-half of the control values. After 3 weeks of light stimulation, protein as well as other cytoplasmic components increased, but not to the levels of normal controls. As with the pentose nucleoprotein fraction, the variability was greater than in cells from control retinas.

Rasch *et al.* (1961) noted alterations in the cellular RNA levels of cats which were accompanied by a decrease in the protein content of the cytoplasm and nucleoli of ganglion cells. Since the volume of these organelles was reduced, as well as their stainability by the Millon reaction and fast green, total protein differences may have been more marked than could be judged visually. No observations on the protein contents of cells of the rat retinas were reported.

Rasch *et al.* (1961) interpreted their findings as an indication that peripheral stimulation may lead to an altered capacity for nucleoprotein synthesis. Koenig (1958) demonstrated a rapid incorporation of labeled precursors into RNA and protein in mature neurons of mammals. He suggested that protein metabolism of the cell body may serve in the maintenance of axonal proteins through axoplasmic flow. By mechanisms presently unknown, lack of peripheral stimulation may lead to incomplete differentiation of the cell. Proteins, as putative regulators of transcription of nuclear DNA and as the products of translation of messenger RNA, are likely to be involved both early and late in the chain of consequences resulting from sensory input.

Rasch *et al.* (1961) found depressed protein levels in chimpanzee ganglion cells after dark-rearing and in one animal (Faik) placed in darkness from 8 months of age to 24 months.

Although many of the biochemical studies of visual deprivation have employed the techniques of ocular enucleation or of dark-rearing, relatively few have used monocular lid suture, which has been popular in both electrophysiological and structural studies. An exception is that of Maraini, Carta, Franguelli, and Santori (1967). These investigators measured the incorporation of the essential amino acid, leucine, into the retinal proteins of Wistar rats with one eyelid sutured shut from 14 days of age until sacrifice 4–7 months later. Tritiated leucine was administered intravenously

1.5 hr before sacrifice, and incorporation was subsequently assessed by autoradiography. The grain counts for various layers of the deprived retina did not differ from those of the normal eye, nor did the various layers of left visual cortex differ from those of the right. The eye of the rat may be less affected by visual deprivation than in other species, but techniques more sensitive and better controlled than autoradiography are needed to prove the point.

Fluctuations of dry weights of retinal ganglion cells in mice reared to 2 months of age showed strong effects of rearing in darkness (Sankova & Aref'eva, 1973). The ganglion cells of the unstimulated eyes were lower in mass than those of light reared controls, and when stimulated the prompt rise in protein of normal ganglion cells did not occur. A slow rise followed by a much delayed fall as stimulation by flashing light was continued characterized the response of deprived ganglion cells. The direction of these effects are what would be expected from the results of Brattgård (1952) and Rasch *et al.* (1961). The exact time course of the fluctuating changes is a new finding.

Raising the question of whether all protein fractions show enhancement of incorporation of precursors into retina following first exposure to light, Richardson and Rose (1973a) measured incorporation of lysine into 41 fractions and found significant differences emerging after 1 hr in 13 of these fractions. The authors propose that these differential effects may be associated with synaptic modifications related to retinal function.

2. *Protein-Bound Sulfhydryl Groups*

Measures of the amount of sulfhydryl (—SH) bound to protein are of interest since this chemical group has been implicated in various functions. These include the maintenance of chemical structure by disulfide (—SS—) linkages, the biological activity of a molecule by the presence of reactive sulfhydryl groups, and the adjustment of the oxidation-reduction balance of the cell by the oxidation of sulfhydryl to disulfide (Bahr, 1966). Of the common amino acids, only cysteine contains the free sulfhydryl group.

Hellström and Zetterström (1956) and Svanidze (1965) measured the level of protein-bound sulfhydryl in the retina of the dark-reared cat. Hellström and Zetterström, using Bennett's mercury orange method, found no difference during the first few days of life between light- and dark-reared animals. After a week, there was a decrease in the stainability of the dark-reared retina, relative to controls. The difference increased with greater periods of dark-rearing.

Svanidze (1965), using the sensitive dihydroxy–dinaphthyl–disulfide method, studied protein-bound sulfhydryl groups in the retina of cats 54–55 days old whose eyelids had been sutured at 9–10 days. Retinas studied 24 hr after opening of the eyes showed a marked increase of sulfhydryl groups in all layers. The sulfhydryl content of the unopened eye was largely restricted to the external segments of the photoreceptor layer.

Winsberg and Riesen (1966) found a reduction of protein-bound sulfhydryl groups in the bipolar and ganglion cell layers of the retina of the dark-reared macaque monkey.

Experiments on the squid axon indicate that protein synthesis and the existence of sulfhydryl groups are important in the kinetics of conduction (Agin, 1966). Further research may establish whether and in what way the subnormal levels of proteins, and of cysteine-containing proteins in particular, may be responsible for such phenomena as the fatigability and low amplitude of the electroretinogram (ERG) in light-deprived cats (Baxter & Riesen, 1961; Cornwell & Sharpless, 1968). The coincident recovery of the chemical and the electrophysiological events add strength to the association, as does the observation that the guinea pig shows both a mature ERG (Van Hof & Usami, 1968) and high level of protein-bound sulfhydryl groups (Svanidze, 1965).

3. *Axonal Transport in the Optic Nerve*

Karlsson and Sjöstrand (1971) studied the effects of dark-rearing on the composition of and axonal transport of proteins of the retinal ganglion cells of 2.5 month-old rabbits. The animals received injections of tritiated leucine intraocularly, and the radioactivity of LGN proteins so labelled was determined at various time intervals after the injection. Comparisons of the migration rate and subcellular distribution of the transported proteins in light and dark-reared animals showed no differences. The authors concluded that "both rapid and slow axonal transport are at least qualitatively independent of an adequate stimulation of the retinal ganglion cells."

Noting that although spontaneous activity in the optic nerve can continue undiminished in darkness, Grafstein, Murray, and Ingolia (1972) studied axonal transport in a strain of mice (C57BL/6J le rd) whose visual receptors degenerate at about 10 days of age. Determining the time of appearance in the superior colliculus of protein labelled by intraocular injection of tritiated proline or tritiated leucine, the authors discovered a 35% reduction in the rate of slow axonal transport, but no effect on fast transport. As these investigators point out, the possibility that protein flow is linked to the transient electrical activity of cells remains open, and has not been separated from the changes in ganglion cell size and protein synthesis that were observed in the adult mice. It is not yet known whether spontaneous activity in optic neurons in darkness is as vigorous in the neonate as in the adult. Such a determination may be of special importance in species such as the chimpanzee whose ganglion cells can disappear in prolonged darkness.

B. Superior Colliculus

Maletta and Timiras (1968) measured the protein content of various brain areas of male Long–Evans hooded rats at 21 days of age. The experimental treatments included total dark-rearing, eyelid suture prior to eye opening, or normal diurnal rearing. The totally deprived rats showed a significantly smaller amount of protein in the superior colliculi. The mothers of the experimental litters, which had shared the same environments as their pups, were not distinguishable.

C. Lateral Geniculate Nucleus

Maraini *et al.* (1967) used autoradiography to study protein synthesis in the rat LGN after monocular suture from 14 days of age to sacrifice, 4–7 months later. Grain counts in the LGN cells receiving reduced input from the deprived eye showed a "small but constant" decrease in the incorporation of tritiated leucine. Retinas were not statistically different. The 20% decrease in geniculate protein synthesis was correlated with a similar decrease in cellular surface. Hubel and Wiesel (1963) observed a similar reduction of size in the cat. The authors observed that their findings support the idea that monocular deprivation has its most dramatic effects in the LGN and suggested that the relationship between protein synthesis and cellular size is a direct one. No direct confirmation of the involvement of proteins was sought, nor, as common to autoradiographic studies, were corrections for precursor pools possible.

Kupfer and Downer (1967) studied the incorporation of tritiated leucine into protein of the monkey LGN after optic nerve transection. Incorporation values rose the first 2 days, and subsequently declined as did RNA levels.

It is not clear to what extent deprivation effects in the LGN may depend on afferent impulses, or on trophic substances which could be liberated at the synapse. Degeneration or failure to differentiate would be characterized intracellularly in either case by changes in protein synthesis.

D. Visual Cortex

Biochemical changes have been described for the visual cortex of the deprived rat. Svanidze (1965) reported that some cortical pyramidal cells of Layer IV of lid-sutured cats showed an increase in the content of protein-bound sulfhydryl groups after a day's normal light experience.

Rose (1967) exposed rats to various periods of light after dark-rearing them to 50 days of age. The incorporation of tritiated lysine into protein, corrected for the precursor pool soluble in trichloracetic acid (TCA), was measured in visual and frontal cortex. Both cortical areas, but not liver, showed significant effects with 3 hr of light stimulation, as compared with those of littermates left in darkness. Rose's measure of relative incorporation, the ratio of incorporation of the light-exposed group to that of the group remaining in darkness, increased for the visual cortex, but decreased in the motor cortex. After 24 hr of light, however, the light–dark incorporation ratio fell to a minimum in both cortical areas, and, thereafter, with up to 99 hr of light exposure, tended upward toward unity. Unfortunately there was no light-reared but dark-adapted control group with which to compare this apparently transient effect of first stimulation. The interpretation of Rose's biphasic curve remains uncertain, and its correlation with changes in the fine structure of the cortex unperformed.

In a subsequent study (Rose, Sinha, & Broomhead, 1973) the elevated incorporation into proteins of the visual cortex was found to be occurring only in the neuronal fraction and the depressed incorporation after prolonged exposure was not found under somewhat different behavioral conditions. With gel electrophoresis using double-labeling technique (Richardson & Rose, 1973b) these investigators showed that two fractions of the soluble proteins and seven fractions of insoluble proteins were involved in the differential lysine incorporation.

Maraini *et al.* (1967) found that 4–7 months of eyelid suture from birth produced no change in the incorporation of tritiated leucine into cortical cells, although geniculate changes had been observed.

Measures of cell density in neurons of the visual cortex (Gomirato & Baggio, 1962) as a function of 3 hr of darkness or of dazzling light failed to show significant effects, a contrast to highly significant effects on retinal ganglion cells. This study used adult rabbits. In monkeys, Singh and Talwar (1969) have reported increased protein incorporation during exposure to flickering light.

VII. Phosphatases

A. Retina

Iida and Schiebler (1968) found no effect of dark-rearing on the normal increase in the activity of acid and alkaline phosphatases in the rat retina. Such an increase is evident on the tenth postnatal day and subsequently. Alkaline phosphatase is present in high concentrations in the fetal brain and decreases or shows little change during brain development (Seiler, 1969).

Schimke (1968), who reared albino rabbits in the dark from birth for 26, 60, or 120 days, found decreases at all ages in the activity of retinal acid phosphatase in comparison with light-reared controls. No significant changes were noted in alkaline phosphatase activity.

B. Lateral Geniculate Nucleus

Gay and Silberberg (1964) found a drop in the acid phosphatase activity of the LGN of enucleated monkeys sacrificed 3, 11, or 30 days after surgery. At the earliest age, only ipsilateral laminae were affected.

VIII. Neurotransmitters and Related Enzymes

A. Retina

One functional characteristic of any neuron is the utilization and probably the manufacture of transmitter substances. It is not unreasonable to suppose that a reduction of functional input to a neuronal system might lead to a decrease in the synthesis of such substances. Liberman (1962) has investigated the effect of light deprivation on presumed substrates of neural transmission in the rat retina. He measured the activity of retinal acetylcholinesterase (AChE) of S-3 Tryon rats reared in darkness from birth to 17 weeks of age. Total cholinesterase activity of deprived animals was diminished 19%. As the activity of nonspecific cholinesterase was much smaller and similar in deprived and control rats, it was concluded that the effect was due to changes in AChE activity.

On the assumption that AChE activity is related to acetylcholine (ACh) utilization, and that the ACh is functioning as synaptic transmission, Liberman suggested that there may be cholinergic synapses in the retina which are more active in light than in dark. The status of ACh as a retinal transmitter, however, remains uncertain. Nichols and Koelle (1968) found that rat retinal AChE is limited to the amacrine cells of the inner plexiform layer. They suggested that since these cells may play an inhibitory role, the high levels of AChE may indicate that ACh is a precursor in the release of a second and inhibitory transmitter. Koelle (1967) noted that many noncholinergic neurons contain relatively high levels of AChE. As with other substances, a proper interpretation of the effects of light deprivation must await a more definitive discussion of their function.

The decline of retinal cholinesterase activity, whatever its significance, has been observed by others. Chang, Lee, and Li (1941) found that after a few days, monocular blindfolding resulted in less ChE activity in the dog. Glow and Rose (1964) confirmed Liberman's findings in adult rats placed in the dark. Glow and Rose (1966) reported that rats wearing opaque occluders show a drop in retinal ChE activity in only 14 days. After such treatment, 7 days in a normally lighted environment were sufficient to produce recovery. Whether there are developmental consequences of altered acetylcholine metabolism is uncertain.

B. Superior Colliculus and Lateral Geniculate Nucleus

Hess (1960), assuming that the postnatal increase in AChE is related to the development of visual function, investigated the effects of monocular enucleation at birth on the normal postnatal increase of AChE activity in the contralateral superior colliculus.

In the mouse, AChE activity was detected as early as 6 days of age. Even at this age, a difference in the staining of the two colliculi was evident after enucleation. Although the AChE staining intensity rose with time, the affected colliculus never reached the levels of the other side, through 222 days of age. Such differences did not arise in enucleated adults examined 60 days postoperatively. After 222 days, the colliculi of the mouse binocularly enucleated at birth and stained for AChE are difficult to distinguish from those of the normal adult, suggesting another example of normalization.

The area of the colliculus showing the AChE changes lies dorsally and includes the stratum zonale and the stratum griseum superficiale. The stratum opticum, containing optic nerve fibers, degenerates and shows gliosis after enucleation, but never stains for AChE. The stratum griseum superficiale shows an increase in cell number after enucleation, which Hess attributes to gliosis.

Rabbits similarly treated and examined at 18–243 days showed similar and striking differences in the colliculi. In guinea pigs enucleated at a fetal age of 42 days and examined 9 days later, AChE differences between the two colliculi were evident. However, one guinea pig enucleated at birth and examined at 66 days showed no differences between the colliculi, like the adult mouse.

Hess speculated that in the immature animal—neonatal mouse or fetal guinea pog—the synaptic input to the colliculi derive overwhelmingly from the optic nerve. Enucleation would effectively terminate stimulation. In the adult mouse and rabbit or in the relatively mature neonatal guinea pig there would exist a sufficient number of synapses of cortical or other origin to maintain the functional integrity of the colliculi despite enucleation.

To underscore our ignorance of the precise significance of variations of acetylcholine levels and of related enzymes, we may note several paradoxes. In the rabbit retina, cholinergic synapses have been found only at the somas of amacrine cells (Nichols & Koelle, 1968). Despite Hess' (1960) observations, optic fiber terminations are generally not considered cholinergic (Hebb, Silver, Swan, & Walsh, 1953). Himwich, Davis, and Agrowal (1967) consider the development of evoked potentials to light in the superior colliculus to be correlated as much with GABA levels as with AChE activity (Himwich & Aprison, 1955; Siou, 1958). Although ACh is released in the visual cortex in response to light flashes (Collier & Mitchell, 1967), it was found that the magnitude of the response depended largely on the state of arousal of the intact animal. Selective interruption of collicular efferents suggested that ACh release is due to nonspecific midbrain reticular system stimulation of large areas of the cortex and to nonprimary afferent stimulation of the visual cortex by thalamic nuclei.

Maletta and Timiras (1967) studied AChE and nonspecific ChE activity of the brain after dark-rearing male Long–Evans hooded rats to 21 days. The AChE activity of tissue taken from the LGN and the superior colliculus of the experimental animals was roughly half that of light-reared controls. The mothers of the experimental animals, which had also spent 21 days in the dark with their young, failed to show this change when compared with the mothers of rats reared in diurnal lighting. Nonspecific ChE levels were unaffected in any group.

The same animals failed to show changes in other brain areas, including visual cortex. The authors concluded that the changes in AChE levels are related to the developmental stage of the animal and to only some visual centers. The LGN and superior colliculus are far more dependent upon a single input system, the optic tract, whereas the visual cortex has other innervation as well.

In a subsequent study, Maletta and Timiras (1968) measured the cholineacetyltransferase (ChAc) activity of various brain areas of rats similarly reared. An additional group was subjected to eyelid suture prior to eye opening. ChAc activity was determined in *in vitro* slices by utilizing radioactively labeled sodium acetate, a precursor of ACh. While the eyelid-sutured and normal groups were comparable, the dark-reared animals were found to have significantly lower levels of ChAc activity in the LGN and superior colliculus. No significant differences between light- and dark-housed mother rats were present. While all groups had similar body and brain weights, the groups totally deprived of light, mothers and pups alike, had adrenal weights significantly greater than those of the control or lid-sutured groups.

Since marked changes in the cell structure of neither LGN nor superior colliculus were found histologically, the decrease in ChAc was interpreted to be ". . . due to reduced neural function, rather than to general morphological or metabolic degeneration of the CNS areas considered [p. 793]." The authors also felt that the strong similarity of the results using AChE activity and ChAc activity provide some assurance of the validity of their data as a measure of ACh content, which in turn appears to be correlated with functional demands made upon the visual system.

Iida and Schiebler (1968) found no histochemical effect of dark-rearing upon the activity of AChE, nonspecific esterase, or monoamine oxidase (MAO). They dark-reared their rats to 7–14 days.

Karlsson (1967) reported a gradual postnatal increase in the number of synaptic profiles in the LGN of the rat which contain vesicles. It would be a worthwhile confirmation of the results of Maletta and Timiras should the rate of growth of the number of vesicles parallel that of enzymic activity.

Wawrzyniak (1969) examined the effect of monocular section of the optic nerve on the AChE activity of the LGN and superior colliculus of the rabbit over periods from 3 days to 7 months postoperatively. His study is distinctive in correlating the biochemical analyses with cytochemical observations of synaptic changes during the degeneration period.

In the superior colliculus the AChE activity of the contralateral side dropped immediately and remained below unoperated control levels thereafter. Ipsilaterally, AChE activity fell but gradually rose to a level above that of controls.

In the LGN, AChE activity on the contralateral side showed little change initially, then dropped to a level below controls. The ipsilateral side responded with an immediate and sustained increase in enzymic activity. Such quantitative observations again demonstrate that both sides of the brain are changed after monocular deprivation. The biochemical changes were small and indicate nondegenerating sources of AChE.

The histochemical observations are instructive. Type 1 synapses, small and distributed at regular intervals along nerve fibers, demonstrated increased AChE activity during degeneration before then disappearing. Type 4, the glomerular synapses, showed more intense staining and a blurring of structure before degenerating. Type 2 synapses, irregularly distributed, shrank during degeneration, losing the strongly stained border of the normal state. Type 3 or axosomatic synapses showed no change. The fifth type, claw-like, was too rarely seen to characterize.

Wawrzyniak interpreted the findings to support the idea that the noncholinergic fibers of the optic tract form cholinergic synapses in the LGN. His study can also be cited as a caution against the immediate extrapolation of results with whole tissue homogenates to cellular or subcellular components. Such a warning is no doubt unnecessary, but the problem posed has not yet been technically solved, even with modern techniques of producing fractions enriched in neurons or glia or synaptosomes.

C. Visual Cortex

Maletta and Timiras (1967, 1968) found no reduction in either ChAc activity or AChE activity in the visual cortex of the 21-day-old mouse reared in the dark, although changes in lower optic centers were found, as already indicated.

D. Drug and Deafferentation Studies

One of the effects of sensory deprivation that might reasonably be expected is a change in the concentration of the suspected chemical transmitters subserving a given sensory system. This hypothesized correlation of neurohumoral concentration and functional activity has been examined in the LGN, superior colliculus, and occipital cortex of enucleated cats by Deffenu *et al.* (1967) for both ACh and serotonin. Barbiturate anesthetics could not be used because of their depressive effects on cholinergic neurons, and, therefore, transections were made. ACh determinations were made in four groups of animals: controls that received a midpontine pretrigeminal section only; an experimental group which received the same transection as well as enucleation; a second experimental group which was enucleated, transected, and given an IV injection of DOPA, which causes cortical desynchronization; and a fourth group which received a *cerveau isolé* section only. All determinations of ACh concentration in the LGN were made 3 hr following the various operations.

ACh content, measured in micrograms per gram, was found to be considerably higher in the LGN of those cats receiving both enucleation and the pretrigeminal section than in the LGN of the pretrigenimal-only preparations. No significant differences were found in the superior colliculus between these two groups and, while they did show a difference in occipital cortex similar in direction to that found in the LGN, the difference was smaller, irregular, and possibly attributable to the fact that cortical dissection was delayed until LGN and superior colliculus had been dissected. Since the deafferented group showed a long lasting EEG synchronization, a second deafferented group was given IV injections of DOPA (to produce long-lasting activation) 30 min before the ACh concentrations were measured, to test the hypothesis that the difference between the visually intact and the enucleated groups were correlated with the synchronization effect. This correlation did seem to exist, as the DOPA administered group showed ACh levels essentially the same as those found in the visually intact animals. The hypothesis received further support from the finding that visually intact *cerveau isolé* cats showed steady EEG synchronization with ACh levels as high as those found in the enucleated cats. From these data, supported by electrophysiological, morphological, and pharmacological data of other experimenters, the authors suggest that much of the ACh found in the LGN may well be associated with afferents from the reticular formation; and, that, because ACh levels in the DOPA enucleated cats were the same as those in the visually intact cats, there is little likelihood that the optic nerve is a cholinergic system.

Th 5-HT concentration determinations were carried out in a control group of midpontine-pretrigeminal preparations and in a similarly sectioned group which had been enucleated as well. Measures taken 3 hr after the operations showed no significant differences in serotonin levels between the two groups. The authors suggest that it is unlikely that serotonin plays a direct role in visual impulse transmission through the LGN. This conclusion, however, seems unwarranted in view of the fact that several experiments have demonstrated, by microelectrophoresis, an inhibitory role for 5-HT on the firing of LGN neurons to optic nerve impulses (Curtis & Davis, 1962; Phillis, Tebecis, & York, 1967a).

This study has interesting implications for sensory deprivation. If ACh is a modulator/transmitter serving fibers from the reticular formation to the LGN, the increase in ACh levels following deafferentation suggests that sensory deprivation of this type influences not only the direct visual pathway, but those neurons which have modulating effects on the classical sensory pathway as well. ACh, applied to LGN microelectrophoretically, has been shown to cause the firing of approximately 50% of the neurons in nonbarbiturate anesthetized cats (Phillis, Tebecis, & York, 1967b) and to depress a small percentage of the neurons. In the decerebrate cat a much greater proportion of LGN units fired to ACh application (Satinsky, 1967).

IX. Histological, Cytological, and Circulatory Changes

A. Retina

Several studies above can be interpreted to indicate that short term light deprivation delays biochemical maturation while prolonged deprivation produces no further deficit. Similar conclusions can be drawn from morphological studies. Gyllensten and Malmfors (1963) found that mice placed in the dark at birth for 20–30 days had fewer thick optic fibers and fewer myelinated fibers than controls, although the overall thickness of the optic nerve was unaffected. A more prolonged stay in the dark did not prevent eventual normal myelination (Gyllensten *et al.,* 1966b).

Rasch *et al.* (1961) reported histological and cytochemical changes (see p. 99) resulting from visual deprivation in the rat, cat, and chimpanzee. No marked histological differences were found among the retinas of dark-reared rats, normal controls, and rats reared to 90 days in darkness followed by 60 days of diurnal lighting.

In cats dark-reared 3.5–40 months, on the other hand, they observed cytoplasmic hypotrophy of the bipolar and ganglion cell layers accompanied by a comparative reduction in the thickness of the inner plexiform layer. The mean nucleolar volume of ganglion cells was significantly reduced, as was the mean cytoplasmic cross-sectional area.

Rasch *et al.* (1961) noted that the chimpanzee, which loses over 90% of the cells in the ganglion cell layer with dark-rearing, has fewer receptor cells per ganglion cell than the rat or cat, which show no cell loss. If photoreceptor stimulation exerts a trophic effect on ganglion cells, the chimpanzee retina might be expected to suffer from fewer opportunities for summation of the residual spontaneous activity of its dark-adapted rods and cones.

Svanidze (1965) sewed shut the eyelids of 9- to 10-day-old kittens. Some parts of the retinas of animals were incompletely differentiated 45 days later, as manifested by the incomplete division of the outer and inner nuclear layers, the arrangement of the ganglion cells, and continued mitotic migration of the central cells. These results do not agree with those of Hellström and Zetterström (1956) who found that the division into outer and inner nuclear layers was complete by the seventh to twelfth day. The inner and outer segments could be distinguished by the twelfth to seventeenth day. There was no difference between light- and dark-reared animals with respect to such histological criteria of maturity.

The reasons for these conflicting findings are unclear. However, in some cases precise measurement is necessary in order to detect subtle differences. The criteria for maturity employed by some authors is not clear. Donovan's (1966) description of retinal development indicates that maturity, even after morphological differentiation, may be judged by different criteria.

Donovan showed that the morphological differentiation of the cat retina is incomplete at birth. Development proceeds from the center to the periphery. At birth, the ganglion cell layer is present but, although both large and small cells are seen, they do not have the adult distribution of Nissl substance, and the cells are smaller than their adult counterparts. Ganglion cells appear to be fully developed at 2½ weeks. The inner nuclear layer is difficult to distinguish at birth and consists largely of immature neuroblasts. The external plexiform layer, which divides the neuroblastic layer into outer and inner nuclear layers, is present at birth in the area centralis, but does not appear at the periphery until 7 days. The nuclei of the inner nuclear layer mature in the central region at about 2 weeks and in the periphery at about 4 weeks. The nuclei of the receptor cells, that is, in the outer nuclear layer, are slower to develop but seem mature in all areas by 5 weeks of age. The outer segments of receptors cannot be distinguished as a clearly defined layer until 8–10 days postnatally. The outer segments of the area centralis reach their adult length between 30 and 35 days of age, while similar growth in the periphery is incomplete until 9 weeks of age.

Criteria of maturity may thus include the distribution of Nissl substance, cellular size, lamination, and the comparison of such attributes in the central and peripheral portions of the retina. As Donovan cautions, however, developmental morphology may appear to follow an altered time course with other techniques of examination, for example, electron microscopy which has detected the separation of the inner and outer segments as early as the first postnatal day.

A reduced blood flow in neural centers that receive lowered levels of sensory stimulation has characterized the observations of all visual stations from retina to cortex. Such loss, clearly a consequence of the sensory deprivation, may in turn contribute to neurochemical and morphological changes, as suggested by several workers (for example, Bondy & Morelos, 1971). The reduced vascularity of chimpanzee retinal tissue was seen to precede loss of ganglion cells following prolonged dark-rearing (Riesen, 1950; Chow, Riesen, & Newell, 1957).

B. Higher Centers: Optic Nerve and Tract, Superior Colliculus, Lateral Geniculate, and Visual Cortex

Gyllensten and Malmfors (1963) found that the myelination of the optic nerve is retarded in mice reared in darkness. After 20–30 days of dark-rearing the number of fibers myelinated is reduced 12–13% by comparison with normal controls. The coarse fibers are the most affected, so that at 30 days, the number of fibers at least 1 μm in diameter that are myelinated is reduced 60%. These authors also noted that dark-rearing retarded the growth and the change of shape of ganglion cell nuclei which occur postnatally.

Atrophic changes have been demonstrated in the superior colliculus after neonatal enucleation. Terry, Roland, and Race (1962) reported degeneration of the optic tract and reduction in the volume of the *stratum griseum* of the colliculus as the result of enucleation at 4–6 days of age. The prevention of opening of the eyelids had no comparable effect. DeLong and Sidman (1962) found that monocular enucleation of the mouse at birth resulted in the loss of 40% of the neurons of the superior colliculus 7 days later. Glial cells of the colliculus, in contrast to neurons, proliferate postnatally, but they failed to do so in enucleated animals when examined 3 days later. The number of cells in the undersized adult colliculus of enucleated mice was near normal, implying both an eventual replacement of the cells which degenerated or which failed to appear on schedule and a smaller size of the replacing cells.

Cook *et al.* (1951) found that monocular enucleation has effects on the morphology of the rabbit LGN similar to those in the cat, but that the effects take longer to develop in the rabbit. The volumes of nuclei and nucleoli of affected cells were seen to decrease, as did the amount of Nissl substance, suggesting a net depression of synthesis of nucleic acids and nucleoproteins.

Gyllensten *et al.* (1965) examined the effects of dark-rearing on the nuclear diameters of cells and on the volume of internuclear material in the mouse brain. The results and their time course are summarized in the preceding chapter by Globus.

The greatest reduction was found in the LGN, about 20%, while a 9.5% reduction was found in the colliculus. The effect in both nuclei showed no tendency to diminish after more prolonged rearing.

In the visual cortex, the effect was much more pronounced in the granular layer (Layer IV) and those more superficial. This finding is in agreement with the fact that the outer layers of the mouse cortex develop later (Angevine & Sidman, 1961), and with the principle that they should therefore be more susceptible to modification by the postnatal environment. The cortical differences in nuclear size were most pronounced at about 1 month of deprivation, rapidly declining thereafter. The cortical differences in internuclear material were most pronounced after 2 months of deprivation, and were minimal after 4 months of deprivation. The "normalization" seen in the cortex does not seem to be entirely a shifting of the time axis of the growth curve in that adult rats placed into darkness from 4 months of age to 7 months of age show a decline in the volume of internuclear material, but not of nuclear size.

Comparison of the effects of enucleation immediately after birth with those of dark-rearing (Gyllensten, Malmfors, & Norrlin-Grettve, 1967) revealed that enucleation produced similar changes in the visual system; however, the hypotrophy was more severe with enucleation, and normalization of cortical tissue did not occur. Such findings suggest that enucleation reduces the trophic value of the optic nerve on higher structures below some threshold, but the mechanism, both biochemical and anatomical, has not been elucidated. Complicating factors include input to the visual cortex from nonvisual sources, and output from the cortex to LGN and colliculus.

Cerebral blood circulation responds within 1 hr to monocular lid suturing in both newly hatched and older birds (Bondy & Davis, 1972). On the side opposite the sutured eye, to which there is full crossing over in birds, there is reduced blood flow in the optic lobe (tectal) and in the cerebral hemisphere. The differences between the two sides of the brain are reversed within 1 hr after removal of the lid suture. This recovery actually overshoots following 16 days of monocular deprivation, and "resulted in a significantly *greater* blood flow to the previously deprived cerebral hemispheres, relative to corresponding visual regions [Bondy & Davis, 1972, p. 607]." With continuous monocular occlusion, the reduced blood flow persisted for the duration of the experimental treatment of 15 days in optic lobe measurements, but not in the cerebral hemispheres. The authors suggested that impaired neural development during crucial periods of growth may result from such decreased blood flow.

In view of the rapid time course of the changes in blood circulation, and recalling the Brattgård (1952) finding of an equally rapid fall in the PNP fraction during dark adaptation, the suggested relation between these faster responses to reduced sensory input and the longer term changes in structure and function must be seriously considered, and merits further investigation. Gyllensten (1959) studied the vascular changes in the visual cortex of mice reared to 20 or 30 days in darkness, arriving at the conclusion that they were secondary to retarded development of the nervous structures. By his measuring techniques, relative vascularity was not an early change, appearing between 20 and 30 days after the initiation of dark-rearing.

X. Nonvisual Modalities

Deafferentation results in similar effects regardless of sensory modality. The nuclei of the auditory and olfactory systems require stimulation for normal cellular morphology and biochemical activity. Destruction of the cochlea in the cat led to cell shrinkage and to reduced Nissl substance in the medial trapezoid and ventral cochlear nuclei 30–60 days after the lesion, and a similar pattern of changes after 60 days in the superior olive (Powell & Erulkar, 1962). Utley (1966) showed that lesions of the brachium of the medial geniculate nucleus resulted in a decrease of ChE and glial proliferation within 6 weeks. Short-term effects of sound stimulation were studied by Yakovlev, Titova, Bronshtein, and Vinnikof (1961). After 15–30 min of stimulation, hair cells of the organ of Corti contained increases in —SH, SS, and COOH groups, and in total protein. Continued stimulation of from 1 to 6 hr brought about decreases in these values.

Transection of the olfactory peduncle resulted in a diminution of Nissl substances in the prepyriform cortex (Allison, 1965). Experimental sectioning of the olfactory bulb in rats resulted in a reduction of higher order branching of dendrites after 91 days, with no cell loss noted with survival times up to 1 year (Jones & Thomas, 1962).

Torvik (1956) reported that in kittens unilateral lesions of the spinal cord, brain stem, or cortex resulted in cell loss in appropriate unilateral nuclei of the pons, superior olive, lateral reticular nucleus, and external cuneate nucleus. Also, in the samatosensory system Penman and Smith (1950) found degeneration in the secondary neurons of the trigeminal pathway after biochemical lesions in man.

Multimodal stimulation was involved in the finding of Ferchmin, Eterovic, and Caputto (1970) that 4 days of exposure to a more complex environment resulted in an increase in total RNA of the cerebrum of albino rats. This increase was paralleled by brain weight increases as reported also for blinded rats (Krech, Rosenzweig, & Bennett, 1963).

Transneuronal degeneration of great clinical significance has been the subject of extensive investigation (Windle, 1968; Faro & Windle, 1969). In human cerebral palsy and in experimental studies of asphyxiated infant monkeys (*Macaca mulatta*) certain of the degenerative changes are delayed for 10 months or more. When the asphyxia produces lesions in afferent relay centers, the delayed brain damage is seen most clearly in areas of the cortex to which thalamic centers normally project. Other areas in delayed transneuronal degeneration included additional thalamic nuclei and the brain stem reticular formation (Faro & Windle, 1969). A fascinating aspect of this series of studies lies in the degree of behavioral improvement sometimes observed even while brain areas were deteriorating. Neurochemical correlates of these important observations are still to be investigated.

XI. Discussion of Issues

The metabolic correlates of dark adaption and of more prolonged visual deprivation seem to be similar in kind, if not in degree. As neural activity is increased or decreased, a complex system responds involving blood flow, biochemical events, and electrical changes. It is perhaps meaningless to say that one component precedes another once the change in sensory input has initiated a shift in the rates and directions of interacting demand and supply processes. Since, over the longer term of sensory deprivation, some of these processes reach a point of no return, the search for differences in early and late changes in morphology, neurochemistry, and electrophysiology, as well as consequent behavioral alterations, is necessary to an understanding of how sensory nervous systems function.

More work is required in which the support mechanisms are investigated in relation to sensory deprivation. Blood supply and glial cells have been implicated, but thus far have received only occasional attention. Brazovskaya (1967) reported an increase in the perineural and pericapillary glia, and in the density of the capillary network in the LGN and in layer IV of the visual cortex as a result of light stimulation. Closer attention to the effects of precisely specified stimulating conditions is needed. In the Singh and Talwar (1967, 1969) experiments, intermediate levels of light intensity increased protein synthesis, while extreme levels depressed the uptake of tritiated lysine. Flicker rates of 7/sec were more effective than lower frequencies. This corresponds well with the findings of Jung (1964) that the summed responses of light-sensitive neurons in the occipital cortex are maximal at frequencies of 7–12/sec.

Dark adaptation and dark-rearing have not always been distinguished since appropriate control groups have been missing in previous studies. Brattgård did supply the needed information in his work on retinal ganglion cells, and found that dark-rearing resulted in a more severe depression of nucleoproteins than dark adaptation, and that recovery was slower and highly variable from cell to cell. Future workers would do well to include a dark adapted control group when studying effects of visual deprivation.

The study of brain-specific proteins in relation to sensory activation has received encouraging support by the finding (Singh & Talwar, 1969) that the S-100 type of protein is among the group of low molecular weight proteins synthesized rapidly in the visual cortex in response to flickering lights. Further identification of such proteins and their role in cell and membrane functions will be of great interest to students of behavior.

The effects of changes in one sense mode upon the development of another (Krech *et al.*, 1963; Gyllensten, Malmfors, & Norrlin, 1966a) should be looked into further from the neurochemical standpoint.

Two studies in amphibian species have run counter to the vertebrate studies of visual deprivation. The discrepancy remains to be resolved. Winsberg (1966, 1968) found an initial fall in RNA levels during dark adaptation, followed by an increase, in her studies of the inner segments of the eyes of *Xenopus*. After a more prolonged stay in the dark all retinal layers of salamander eyes showed an increase in alkaline phosphatase activity (Tewari & Tyagi, 1968). This finding was interpreted to reflect increased nucleic acid synthesis.

Neurochemical effects of sensory deprivation should be studied in the context of ongoing biochemical processes common to neural systems. Such studies are capable of yielding a wealth of information regarding the importance of afferent input in supporting cell growth and in maintaining a fully functioning sensory system.

Acknowledgment

This study was supported by Grant No. EY-00573 from the National Institutes of Health, USPHS.

References

Agin, D. Macromolecules and electrical activity of nerve cells. In J. Gaito (Ed.), *Macromolecules and behavior.* New York: Appleton, 1966. Pp. 13–19.

Agranofi, B. W. Memory. In A. Lajtha (Ed.), *Handbook of neurochemistry,* Vol. 6. New York: Plenum, 1971. Pp. 203–220.

Allison, A. C. The second olfactory areas in the human brain. *Journal of Anatomy,* 1954, **88**, 381–488.

Angevine, J. B., & Sidman, R. L. Autoradiographic study of cell migration during histogenesis of the cerebral cortex in the mouse. *Nature*, 1961, **192**, 766–768.

Appel, S. H., Davis, W., & Scott, S. Brain polysomes: Response to environmental stimulation. *Science*, 1967, **157**, 836–838.

Bahr, G. F. Introduction to the cytochemisty of sulfhydryl and disulfide groups. In G. L. Wied (Ed.), *Introduction to quantitative cytochemistry.* New York: Academic Press, 1966. Pp. 469–488.

Bateson, P. P. G., Rose, S. P. R., & Horn, G. Imprinting: Lasting effects on uracil incorporation into chick brain. *Science,* 1973, **181**, 576–578.

Baxter, B. L., & Riesen, A. H. Electroretinogram of the visually deprived rat. *Science,* 1961, **134,** 1626–1627.

Bondy, S. C., & Davis, F. N. Reversible responses of the cerebral circulation to visual deprivation. *Brain Research*, 1972, **43**, 606–609.

Bondy, S. C., & Margolis, F. L. *Sensory deprivation and brain development: The avian system as a model.* Jena: Fischer, 1971.

Bondy, S. C., & Morelos, B. S. Stimulus deprivation and cerebral blood flow. *Experimental Neurology,* 1971, **31**, 200–206.

Brattgård, S. O. The importance of adequate stimulation for the chemical composition of retinal ganglion cells during early postnatal development. *Acta Radiologica Supplementum*, 1952, **96,** 1–80.

Brazovskaya, F. A. Quantitative changes in the structure of the visual analyzer due to functional deafferentation. *Zhurnal Vyssheĭ Nervoĭ Deiatel'nosti*, 1967, **17**, 548–552.

Chang, H. C., Lee, L. Y., & Li, T. H. Studies on tissue acetylcholine IX. Diminution of acetylcholine of the retina during functional disuse. *Chinese Journal of Physiology*, 1941, **6**, 373–378.

Chow, K. L., Riesen, A. H., & Newell, F. W. Degeneration of retinal ganglion cells in infant chimpanzees reared in darkness. *Journal of Comparative Neurology,* 1957, **107**, 27–40.

Cohen, L. H., & Noell, W. K. Glucose catabolism of rabbit retina before and after development of visual function. *Journal of Neurochemistry,* 1960, **5**, 253–276.

Collier, B., & Mitchell, J. F. The central release of actetylcholine during consciousness and after brain lesions. *Journal of Physiology (London)*, 1967, **188**, 83–98.

Cook, W. H., Walker, J. H., & Barr, M. L. A cytological study of transneuronal atrophy in the cat and rabbit. *Journal of Comparative Neurology,* 1951, **94**, 267–291.

Cornwell, A. C., & Sharpless, S. K. Electrophysiological retinal changes and visual deprivation. *Vision Research*, 1968, **8**, 389–401.

Curtis, D. R., & Davis, R. Pharmacological studies upon neurons of the lateral geniculate nucleus of the cat. *British Journal of Pharmacology*, 1962, **18**, 217–246.

De Bold, R. C., Firshein, W., Carrier, S. C., III, & Leaf, R. C. Changes in RNA in the occipital cortex of rats as a function of light and dark during rearing. *Psychonomic Science*, 1967, **7**, 379–380.

Deffenu, G., Bertaccini, G., & Pepeu, G. Acetylcholine and 5-hydroxytryptamine levels of the lateral geniculate bodies and superior colliculus of cats after visual deafferentation. *Experimental Neurology,* 1967, **17**, 203–209.

DeLong, G. R., & Sidman, R. L. Effects of eye removal at birth on histogenesis of the mouse superior colliculus: an autoradiographic analysis with tritiated thymidine. *Journal of Comparative Neurology,* 1962, **118**, 205–223

de Vos, M., & Fautrez, J. Modification de la teneur en acid désoxyribonucleique des noyanes des atrocytes du lapin après énucléation de l'oeil. *Compte Rendu Academie de Science* (Paris), 1967, **161**, 198–200.

Dewar, A. J., & Reading, H. W. Nervous activity and RNA metabolism in the visual cortex of rat brain. *Nature*, 1970, **225**, 869–870.

Donovan, A. The postnatal development of the cat retina. *Experimental Eye Research*, 1966, **5**, 249–253.

Faro, M. D., & Windle, W. F. Transneuronal degeneration of brains of monkeys asphyxiated at birth. *Experimental Neurology*, 1969, **24**, 38–53.

Ferchmin, P. A., Eterovic, V. A., & Caputto, R. Studies of brain weight and RNA content after short periods of exposure to environmental complexity. *Brain Research*, 1970, **20**, 49–57.

Fifková, E. Effect of visual deprivation and light on synapses of the inner plexiform layer. *Experimental Neurology*, 1972, **35**, 458–469.

Garcia, A. M. Stoichiometry of dye binding versus degree of chromatin coiling. In G. L. Wied & G. F. Bahr (Eds.), *Introduction to quantitative cytochemistry,* Vol. II. New York: Academic Press, 1970. Pp. 153–170.

Gay, A. J., & Silberberg, D. H. Histochemical correlates of transynaptic degeneration. *Archives of Neurology,* 1964, **10**, 85–90.

Glow, P. H., & Rose, S. Effects of light and dark on the acetylcholinesterase activity of the retina. *Nature*, 1964, **202**, 422–423.

Glow, P. H., & Rose, S. Activity of cholinesterase in the retina with different levels of physiological stimulation. *Australian Journal of Experimental Biology and Medical Science*, 1966, **44**, 65–72.

Gomirato, G., & Baggio, G. Metabolic relations between the neurons of the optic pathway in various functional conditions. *Journal of Neuropathology and Experimental Neurology*, 1962, **21**, 634–644.

Grafstein, B., Murray, M., & Ingoglia, R. L. Protein synthesis and axonal transport in retinal ganglion cells of mice lacking visual receptors. *Brain Research,* 1972, **44**, 37–48.

Graymore, C., & Towson, M. Oxidized and reduced pryidine nucleotides and oxidation of the carbon-1 and carbon-6 in the developing retina. *Nature*, 1965, **206**, 1361–1362.

Gyllensten, L. Postnatal development of the visual cortex in darkness (mice). *Acta Morphologica Neerlando-Scandinavica*, 1959, **2**, 331–345.

Gyllensten, L., & Malmfors, T. Myelinization of the optic nerve and its dependence on visual function—a quantitative investigation in mice. *Journal of Embryology and Experimental Morphology*, 1963, **11**, 225–266.

Gyllensten, L., Malmfors, T., & Norrlin, M-L. Effect of visual deprivation on the optic centers of growing and adult mice. *Journal of Comparative Neurology,* 1965, **125**, 149–160.

Gyllensten, L., Malmfors, T., & Norrlin, M-L. Growth alteration in the aduitory cortex of visually deprived mice. *Journal of Comparative Neurology,* 1966, **126**, 463–469. (a)

Gyllensten, L., Malmfors, T., & Norrlin-Grettve, M-L. Developmental and functional alterations in the fiber composition of the optic nerve in visually deprived mice. *Journal of Comparative Neurology,* 1966, **128**, 413–418. (b)

Gyllensten, L., Malmfors, T., & Norrlin-Grettve, M-L. Visual and nonvisual factors in the centripetal stimulation and postnatal growth of the visual centers in mice. *Journal of Comparative Neurology*, 1967, **131**, 549-557.

Hebb, C. O., Silver, A., Swan, A. B., & Walsh, E. G. A histochemical study of cholinesterases of the rabbit retina and the optic nerve. *Quarterly Journal of Experimental Physiology,* 1953, **38**, 185–191.

Hellström, B., & Zetterström, B. The effect of light on the manifestation of the electroretinogram and on histochemically demonstrable SH-groups in the retina. *Experimental Cell Research*, 1956, **10**, 248–251.

Hess, A. The effects of eye removal on the development of cholinesterase in the superior colliculus. *Journal of Experimental Zoology*, 1960, **144**, 11–19.

Himwich, W. A., & Aprison, M. H. The effect of age on cholinesterase activity of rabbit brain. In H. Waelsch (Ed.), *Biochemistry of the developing nervous system*. New York: Academic Press, 1955. Pp. 301–307.

Himwich, W. A., Davis, J. M., & Agrawal, H. C. Biochemical substrates for the development of the matured evoked potential. *Recent Advances in Biological Psychiatry*, 1967, **9**, 271–277.

Horn, G., Rose, S. P. R., & Bateson, P. P. G. Experience and plasticity in the central nervous system. *Science*, 1973, **181**, 506–514.

Hubel, D. H., & Wiesel, T. N. Effects of visual deprivation on morphology and physiology of cells in the cat's lateral geniculate body. *Journal of Neurophysiology*, 1963, **26**, 978–992.

Hydén, H., & Lange, P. W. Do specific biochemical correlates to learning exist in brain cells? In A. Lajtha (Ed.), *Handbook of neurochemistry*, Vol. 6. New York: Plenum, 1971. Pp. 221–240.

Iida, T., & Scheibler, T. H. Über die Chemodifferenzierung der Sehbahn der Ratte. *Histochemie,* 1968, **12**, 265–284.

Jones, W. H., & Thomas, D. B. Changes in the dendritic organization of neurons in the cerebral cortex following deafferentation. *Journal of Anatomy*, 1962, **92**, 375–381.

Jung, R. Neuronal integration in the visual cortex and its significance for visual information. In W. A. Rosenblith (Ed.), *Sensory communications.* Cambridge, Massachusetts: MIT Press, 1964.

Karlsson, U. Observations on the postnatal development of neuronal structures in the lateral geniculate nucleus of the rat by electron microscopy. *Journal of Ultrastructure Research*, 1967, **17**, 158–175.

Karlsson, J. O., & Sjöstrand, J. Effect of deprivation of light on axonal transport in retinal ganglion cells of the rabbit. *Brain Research,* 1971, **29**, 315–332.

Koelle, G. B. Synaptic functions of acetylcholine and acetylcholinesterase. In D. H. Efron (Ed.), *Psychopharmacology: A review of progress,* 1957–1967. Washington, D. C.: U. S. Gov't Printing Office, USPHS publication #1836. PP. 77–79.

Koenig, H. An autoradiographic study of nucleic acid and protein turnover in mammalian neuroaxis. *Journal of Biophysical and Biochemical Cytology,* 1958, **4**, 785–792.

Krech, D., Rosenzweig, M. R., & Bennett, E. L. Effects of complex environment and blindness on rat brain. *Journal of Neurology,* 1963, **8**, 403–412.

Kupfer, C. Changes of dehydrogenase activity during transneuronal atrophy. *Nature,* 1963, **200**(4901), 80–81.

Kupfer, C., & Downer, J. L. deC. Ribonucleic acid and metabolic activity of lateral geniculate nucleus in monkey following afferent denervation. *Journal of Neurochemistry*, 1967, **14**, 257–263.

Kupfer, C., & Palmer, P. Lateral geniculate nucleus: Histological and cytochemical changes following afferent denervation and visual deprivation. *Experimental Neurology*, 1964, **9**, 400–409.

Liberman, R. Retinal cholinesterase and glycolysis in rats raised in darkness. *Science,* 1962, **135**, 372–373.

Lowry, O. H. Biochemical studies on layered structures. In M. M. Cohen & R. S. Snyder (Eds.), *Morphological and biochemical correlates of neural activity.* New York: Harper, 1964.

Maletta, G. J., & Timiras, P. S. Acetylcholinesterase activity in optic structures after complete light deprivation from birth. *Experimental Neurology*, 1967, **19**, 513–518.

Maletta, G. J., & Timiras, P. S. Choline acetyltransferase activity and total protein content in selected optic areas of the rat after complete light-deprivation during CNS development. *Journal of Neurochemistry*, 1968,**15**, 787–793.

Maraini, G., Carta F., Franguelli, R., & Santori, M. Effect of monocular light-deprivation on leucine uptake in the retina and the optic centers of the newborn rat. *Experimental Eye Research*, 1967, **6**, 299–302.

McIlwain, H., & Bachelard, H. S. *Biochemistry and the central nervous system.* (4th ed.) Baltimore: Williams & Wilkins, 1971.

Nichols, W. N., & Koelle, G. W. Comparison of the localization of acetylcholinesterase and nonspecific cholinesterase activities in mammalian and avian retina. *Journal of Comparative Neurology,* 1968, **133**, 1–16.

Penman, J., & Smith, M. C. Degeneration of primary and secondary neurons after trigeminal injection. *Journal of Neurology, Neurosurgery, and Psychiatry,* 1950, **13**, 36–46.

Phillis, J. W., Tebecis, A. K., & York, D. H. The inhibitory action of monoamines on lateral geniculate neurons. *Journal of Physiology,* 1967, **190**, 563–581. (a)

Phillis, J. W., Tebecis, A. K., & York, D. H. A study of cholinoceptive cells in the lateral geniculate nucleus. *Journal of Physiology*, 1967, **192**, 695–713. (b)

Powell, T. P. S., & Erulkar, S. D. Transneuronal cell degeneration in the auditory relay nuclei of the cat. *Journal of Anatomy,* 1962, **96**, 249–268.

Rasch, E., Swift, H., Riesen, A. H., & Chow, K. L. Altered structure and composition of retinal cells in dark-reared mammals. *Experimental Cell Research,* 1961, **25**, 348–363.

Richardson, K., & Rose, S. P. R. Differential incorporation of lysine into retinal protein fractions following first exposure to light. *Journal of Neurochemistry,* 1973, **21**, 521–530. (a)

Richardson, K., & Rose, S. P. R. Differential incorporation of [^{3}H] lysine into visual cortex protein fractions during first exposure to light. *Journal of Neurochemistry,* 1973, **21**, 531–537. (b)

Riesen, A. H. Arrested vision. *Scientific American,* 1950, **183**, 16–19.

Riesen, A. H. Sensory deprivation. In E. Stellar & J. M. Sprague (Eds.), *Progress in physiological psychology*. New York: Academic Press, 1966. Pp. 117–148.

Rose, S. P. R. Changes in the visual cortex on first exposure of rats to light. *Nature,* 967, **215**, 253–255.

Rose, S. P. R., Sinha, A. K., & Broomhead, S. Precursor incorporation into cortical protein during first exposure of rats to light; cellular localization of effects. *Journal of Neurochemistry*, 1973, **21**, 539–546.

Sankova, E. I., & Aref'eva, A. M. Effect of light deprivation on formation of the metabolic reaction of the retinal ganglion cells. *Bulletin of Experimental Biology and Medicine*, 1973, **74**, 1454–1456.

Satinsky, D. Pharmacological responsiveness of lateral geniculate nucleus neurons. *International Journal of Neuropharmacology*, 1967, **6**, 387–397.

Schimke, R. T. Effects of prolonged light deprivation on the development of retinal enzymes in the rabbit. *Journal of Biological Chemistry*, 1958, **234**, 700–703.

Seiler, N. Enzymes. In A. Lajtha (Ed.), *Handbook of neurochemistry,* Vol. 1. New York: Plenum, 1969.

Singh, V. B., & Talwar, G. P. Effect of the flicker frequency of light and other factors on the synthesis of proteins in the occipital cortex of monkey. *Journal of Neurochemistry*, 1967, **14**, 675–680.

Singh, V. B. & Talwar, G. P. Identification of a protein fraction in the occipital cortex of the monkey rapidly labelled during exposure of the animal to rhythmically flickering light. *Journal of Neurochemistry*, 1969, **16**, 951–959.

Siou, G. Distribution normal et variation expérimental de l'activité cholinestérasique au niveau des tubercules quadrijumeaux antérieurs chez la Souris. *Compte Rendu Academic de Science,* 1958, **246**, 315–317.

Svanidze, E. K. [Morphocytochemical features of the cells of the retina and visual cortex during the period when an animal regains vision.] *Trudy Instituta Fiziologii Akademiya Nauk Gruzinskoi SSR*, 1965, **14**, 199–211.

Talwar, G. P., Chopra, S. P., Goel, B. K., & D'Monte, B. Correlation of the functional activity of the brain with metabolic parameters. III. Protein metabolism of the occipital cortex in relation to light stimulus. *Journal of Neurochemistry*, 1966, **13**, 109–116.

Talwar, G. P., & Singh, U. B. Excitation. In A. Lajtha (Ed.), *Handbook of Neurochemistry*, Vol. 6. New York: Plenum, 1971. Pp. 29–62.

Terry, R. J., Roland, A. L., & Race, J. Effect of eye enucleation and eyelid closure upon the brain and associated visual structures in the mouse. *Journal of Experimental Zoology*, 1962, **150**, 165–183.

Tewari, H. B., & Tyagi, H. R. On the Alkaline phosphatase activity amongst the constituents of the eye of *Calotes versicolor* in light and dark environments. *Experimental Eye Research*, 1968, **7**, 200–204.

Torvik, A. Transneuronal changes in the inferior olive and pontine nuclei in kittens. *Journal of Neuropathology and Experimental Neurology*, 1956, **8**, 119–145.

Utley, J. D. Acetylcholinesterase and pseudocholinesterase in neural and non-neural tissue in the medical geniculate body of the cat. *Biochemical Pharmacology*, 1966, **15**, 1–6.

Vander Eeken, H., & Fautrez, J. Cellular modifications in the rabbit's visual system after unilateral ocular enucleation. *Nature,* 1965, **206**(4982), 423–424.

Van Hof, M. W., & Usami, E. The ERG in the normal and dark-reared guinea pig. *Acta Societatis Opthalmologicae Japonicae,* 1968, **72**, 283–286.

Wawrzyniak, M. Acetylcholinesterase activity in certain areas of the rabbit brain following the unilateral excision of the optic nerve. *Folia Histochemica et Cytochemica*, 1969, **7**, 213–232.

Winsberg, G. R. Effects of light and dark on RNA and protein synthesis in *Xenopus* retinal cells. *Journal of Cell Biology*, 1966, **31**, 4125.

Winsberg, G. R. RNA synthesis in the retina of *Xenopus* during early dark adaptation. *Experimental Cell Research*, 1968, **52**, 555–564.

Winsberg, G. R., & Riesen, A. H. Cytochemical changes in the nucleoproteins of macaques reared in differing visual environments. *Journal of Histochemistry and Cytochemistry*, 1966, **14**, 798–799.

Yakovlev, V. A., Titova, L. K., Bronshtein, A. A., & Vinnikov, Ya. A. Localization and cytochemical properties of the proteins of the hair cells of the organ of Corti in a state of relative rest and during exposure to sound. *Doklady Akademii Nauk SSSR, Biological Sciences Section*, 1961, **136**, 73–77. (Translation)

Yinon, U., & Auerbach, E. Deprivation of pattern vision studied by visual evoked potentials in the rat cortex. *Experimental Neurology*, 1973, **38**, 231–251.

CHAPTER IV

Disuse Supersensitivity

Seth K. Sharpless

Department of Psychology
University of Colorado

I. Disuse Supersensitivity: The Phenomenon

Elliott's 1905 paper, which laid the foundations for the modern theory of neurohumoral transmission, demonstrated that epinephrine mimics the action of sympathetic nerve impulses. In that same paper, it was shown that effector organs become far more sensitive to epinephrine when denervated. Over and over, in the ensuing years, similar phenomena were observed until, in 1939, Cannon felt justified in pronouncing his "Law of Denervation": When in a series of efferent neurons a unit is destroyed, an increased irritability to chemical agents develops in the isolated structure or structures, the effects being maximal in the part directly denervated. This phenomenon, "denervation supersensitivity," has since been invoked to account for a variety of changes occurring in central nervous structures deprived by various means of normal patterns of nervous influence (Cannon & Rosenblueth, 1949; Heron, 1961; Stavraky, 1961; Jaffe & Sharpless, 1968; Sharpless 1964, 1969). It has been suggested that some form of denervation supersensitivity may play a role in the etiology of epilepsy, thalamic causalgia, bizarre effects of sensory deprivation, withdrawal symptoms following chronic intoxication by depressant drugs, restitution of function after injury to the nervous system, and other like phenomena.

A. Spread of the Chemosensitive Surface of Denervated Skeletal Muscle Fibers

Perhaps the best-known phenomenon associated with denervation supersensitivity in effector organs is an increase in the chemosensitive area of denervated striated muscle fibers. Except for the sole-plate region and the muscle tendon junction, adult mammalian fast muscle fibers are insensitive to acetylcholine (ACh). Iontophoretic application of ACh elicits a depolarizing response only within a few hundred microns of the sole plate. Within a few days after denervation, ACh-sensitive spots develop in the extrajunctional region, and eventually the entire fiber seems to become sensitized to ACh (Thesleff, 1960; Albuquerque & McIsaac, 1970). According to Axelsson and Thesleff (1959), the end plate region itself does not increase in sensitivity, and most investigators agree with this. However, it will be appreciated that a precise quantitative measure of end-plate sensitivity by the iontophoretic technique is difficult. Possible changes in remaining intact neuromuscular junctions following partial denervation have been investigated by Frank and Inoue (1966) in frog sartorius. This muscle is unique in that each fiber is dually innervated, receiving an axon from each of two distinct nerve bundles. If one nerve bundle is transected, the ACh sensitivity spreads somewhat more slowly and less completely than in completely denervated mammalian muscle. However, in this preparation, the innervated end plate also seems to become sensitized. Thus, Frank and Inoue were able to show an increase in the amplitude of miniature end-plate potentials at the innervated end plate of the partially denervated frog sartorius fibers over and above that which could be accounted for on the basis of a change in membrane resistance. Transmission at the remaining intact junction would thus be expected to become more efficient following partial denervation.

Not all striated muscle fibers exhibit the limited chemosensitive area found in adult, mammalian fast fibers. Mammalian slow muscle (such as rat soleus) is normally sensitive along its entire length, although the sensitivity is greater at the end plate. Fetal muscle fibers are also sensitive along their entire length, the ACh-sensitive area shrinking to the end plate region only after a functional myoneural connection is established. This has suggested that denervation results in dedifferentiation and reversion to a more primitive state (Diamond & Miledi, 1962).

B. Spread of the Chemosensitive Surface of Denervated Neurons

There would appear to be little point in dwelling on the changes that occur in denervated striated muscle fibers, from the viewpoint of this monograph, unless similar changes occur in neurons. Until recently, there has been no direct evidence that neurons undergo similar changes. Indeed, most of the evidence suggesting something akin to denervation supersensitivity in neurons has been indirect, although taken as a whole, persuasive. The earlier work has been reviewed by Stavraky (1961). It is exceedingly difficult to map the chemosensitive surface of a nerve cell by the local application of ACh or other transmitters. Indeed, this has only recently been done in an exquisite series of experiments by Kuffler and his associates (McMahan & Kuffler, 1971; Dennis, Harris, & Kuffler, 1971; Harris, Kuffler, & Dennis, 1971; Kuffler, Dennis, & Harris, 1971). These investigators used neurons, parasympathetic ganglion cells, in the interatrial septum of the frog's heart. This preparation can be placed on a microscope stage, and the neurons can be visualized and maintained in good condition for long periods of time. The neurons have the additional advantage of being sparsely invested with synaptic knobs, which cover only about 3% of the surface. This is important, because it is necessary to compare the responses of synaptic and extrasynaptic regions of ACh applied through a micropipette. In the normally innervated neurons, sensitivity is confined to subsynaptic zones; however, after denervation, the entire surface appears to become sensitized to ACh. This represents the first well-controlled demonstration of a phenomenon in neurons closely resembling the expansion of the chemosensitive surface of denervated muscle fibers. Whether it occurs in other classes of neurons, and if so, whether the phenomenon may be expected to have functional significance in the changes wrought in the central nervous system by injury or disuse, are matters to be considered below. In the meantime, the existence of the phenomenon in neurons justifies considering the denervated muscle fiber as a potential model of the deafferented neuron.

II. Disuse versus Denervation as Causative Factors in the Development of Supersensitivity in Effector Organs

It is convenient to distinguish between two kinds of problems: first, the conditions giving rise to supersensitivity (for example, disuse versus denervation), and second, the chemical and morphological changes underlying the development of supersensitivity (for example, *de novo* synthesis of receptors versus other changes that may result in increased sensitivity). Opinion on the first problem has vacillated during the last decade and now seems to be converging toward the view that disuse per se is a causative factor in the development of supersensitivity.

A. Disuse Supersensitivity in Skeletal Muscle

Since at least one class of neurons exhibits a form of supersensitivity similar to that occurring in skeletal muscle, and since the myoneural junction has often been taken as a model of central synapses in the past, with some success, it may be worthwhile considering factors causing supersensitivity in skeletal muscle in more detail.

During the 1960s, the prevalent view ascribed the spread of the chemosensitive region of skeletal muscle to the withdrawal of some "trophic" factor normally liberated from the nerve ending. An alternative hypothesis, that the degenerating nerve ending released some compound which transformed the muscle, was excluded by the observation of Katz and Miledi (1964) that transection of the muscle and excision of the end plate region, thus removing influences emanating from the degenerating nerve terminal, does not prevent the remainder of the muscle from becoming supersensitive. That a trophic factor released from the intact nerve is responsible for restricting the sensitive region to the sole plate and immediate surrounds was supported by the fact that the chemosensitive area of fetal muscle shrinks to the sole plate region when the myoneural contact is formed (Diamond & Miledi, 1962).

If some neurogenic trophic factor were responsible for the restricted sensitivity of adult mammalian muscle, a logical candidate might be the transmitter itself. This was suggested by Thesleff (1960b), who found that botulinum toxin, which prevents the release of ACh, results in a spread of ACh sensitivity quite as dramatic as that following denervation. However, it has always been conceded that botulinum toxin may prevent the release of other substances than ACh. When a severed motor nerve is allowed to regenerate, the chemosensitive zone of the skeletal muscle fiber begins to shrink before the frequency of miniature end plate potentials increase significantly (Miledi, 1960). Furthermore, isolated frog muscle maintained in an organ bath develops supersensitivity even if the bathing medium contains ACh (Miledi, 1960). From data of this sort, it was argued that the "trophic" factor was unlikely to be ACh. Korr and associates (1967) have shown that labeled amino acids applied to the hypoglossal nucleus are incorporated into materials which are transported down the axon, the radioactivity eventually appearing in tongue muscles.

If some trophic factor other than ACh is released from the intact nerve ending, it is still necessary to specify the features of skeletal muscle structure and function that are controlled by this factor, for it may be that certain features, for example, invagination of the sarcolemma in the end plate region, accumulation of sole-plate acetylcholinesterase, etc., are controlled by a trophic factor, whereas other features, including the relative insensitivity to acetylcholine of regions remote from the end plate, are not. The evidence relating to trophic influence of nerve on muscle has been set forth in detail in Guth's landmark review of 1968.

We shall see below that disuse per se may be responsible for some forms of supersensitivity in smooth muscle and glands. In the 1960s, however, it appeared that skeletal muscle might be different in this respect. Johns and Thesleff (1961) found that decentralization of motoneurons by section of the cord and dorsal roots yields only a slight spread of ACh sensitivity compared with that produced by denervation. Sokoll and associates (1968) attempted to block muscle activity by periodic injection of a long-acting local anesthetic in the vicinity of the muscle. This treatment paralyzed the muscle and produced the usual spread of ACh sensitivity accompanied by profound atrophic changes. However, periodic application of the drug to the sciatic nerve at the site where it leaves the pelvis also resulted in paralysis but failed to produce either atrophy or spread of sensitivity. In 1970, Robert and Oester described a new technique for producing long-term conduction block without apparent damage to the muscle nerve, employing for this purpose a silicone rubber cuff containing a local anesthetic. This treatment also, in their hands, failed to produce supersensitivity in skeletal muscle. However, Jones and Vrbová (1970) reported that exercise of muscle in an organ bath reduces supersensitivity, and they pointed out that the development of supersensitivity seems to be curtailed when denervated muscle becomes active through fibrillation. The problem was again taken up by Lømo and Rosenthal (1972). Using both the silicone cuff technique of Robert and Oester (1970) and local injection of diphtheria toxin (which produces a local demyelinization and conduction block), they found that muscular inactivity led to supersensitivity equivalent to that observed in denervated muscle. That the distal part of the nerve remained intact and functional was shown by the appearance of normal spontaneous miniature end plate potentials, and also by stimulation of the nerve block. The supersensitivity could be reversed, or prevented from developing, by stimulating the nerve distal to the conduction block through permanently indwelling electrodes. Moreover, Lømo and Rosenthal (1972) found that the supersensitivity of denervated muscle could be prevented, or reversed, by direct stimulation of the muscle fibers. The sensitivity of the directly stimulated denervated muscles was 100–1000 times less than that of unstimulated denervated muscles, although still somewhat higher than normal. The sensitivity of the original end plate region remained high. The work of Lømo and Rosenthal, particularly the stimulation procedures, strongly support the view that the spread of chemosensitivity in skeletal muscle is largely due to disuse.

Muscle in tissue culture would appear to provide a good preparation for investigating the effects of use and disuse upon ACh sensitivity. Cohen and Fischbach (1973) found that muscle fibers developing from myoblasts in culture can be made less sensitive to iontophoretically applied ACh by intermittent electrical stimulation; furthermore, the stimulated fibers bind less α-bungarotoxin than inactive fibers. Thus, the accumulated evidence would appear to entitle us to speak of "disuse supersensitivity" of skeletal muscle as well as of smooth muscle and glands. The failure of previous attempts to produce supersensitivity by procedures designed to render the muscle inactive may have been due to the persistence of some motor impulse activity in the "blocked" or decentralized nerves.

B. Disuse Supersensitivity in Smooth Muscle and Glands

Although the skeletal myoneural junction is more often taken as a model of central synapses than autonomic neuroeffector junctions, this seems to be due to historic accident rather than a considered argument. In fact, skeletal myoneural junctions are highly differentiated structures, quite different from most central synapses. In mammals, most skeletal muscle fibers receive but a single nerve ending, whereas most neurons, and most autonomic effector cells, are multiply innervated. Central cholinoceptive neurons, with a few exceptions (such as the Renshaw cell), appear to resemble autonomic effector organs more than skeletal muscle fibers with respect to their sensitivity to parasympathamimetic or parasympatholytic drugs. It can never be assumed, without proof, that principles governing transmission in a peripheral junction will be operative in central synapses, but to the degree that it is useful to argue from this kind of analogy, the autonomic neuroeffector junction would appear to be at least as representative of some central synapses as the myoneural junction.

It is therefore interesting that disuse per se produces a form of supersensitivity in autonomic effector organs. Thus, smooth muscles and glands, whether they normally receive adrenergic or cholinergic input, or both, show a gradual increment in irritability following any measure that blocks the flow of motor impulses to the effector cell. This form of supersensitivity has been called "disuse" (Sharpless, 1969) and "unspecific" (Fleming, 1968) supersensitivity. The evidence relating to disuse supersensitivity is extensive and has been reviewed several times (Emmelin, 1961; Sharpless, 1964, 1969; Trendelenburg, 1963). Here, it will be necessary only to summarize the salient features of disuse supersensitivity in autonomic effector organs, most of which have been known from the early 1960s:

1. It is produced by any agent that blocks the flow of nerve impulses to the effector organ, including ganglionic blockade or destruction of pre-

ganglionic fibers, compounds which prevent the liberation of neurohumor from the nerve ending (for example, bretylium, reserpine, xylocholine, botulinum toxin), and blocking agents that occupy postjunctional receptors on the effector organ (atropine, etc.)

2. Disuse supersensitivity is slow to develop, requiring several weeks to approach an asymptote.

3. Disuse supersensitivity is nonspecific, in the sense that the disused cell becomes more reactive to many agents other than the transmitter. The smooth muscle of the nictitating membrane of the cat, for example, which is normally innervated only by adrenergic fibers, becomes sensitized after prolonged disuse to adrenomimetic agents, cholinomimetic agents, 5-hydroxytryptamine, potassium, and even to direct mechanical stimulation in the presence of blocking agents which would prelude indirect humoral excitation (Rothballer & Sharpless, 1961; Schaeppi, 1963; Trendelenburg, 1963). A lack of specificity has been observed in other autonomic effector organs subjected to disuse by pharmacological blockade, including salivary glands (Emmelin, 1961), guinea pig ileum (Fleming, 1968), and aortic strips (Taylor & Green, 1971). However, it should not be supposed that the sensitization is equal for all agents that normally excite the cell. Thus, after reserpine blockade of adrenergic activity, aortic strips become sensitized to ACh, norepinephrine and potassium, but not to histamine, 5-hydroxytryptamine or angiotensin (Hudgins & Harris, 1970). It has been suggested that it is the interaction between the agent and various pools of calcium in the disused cell that determines the degree of sensitization (Hudgins & Harris, 1970; Carrier & Jurevics, 1973).

4. Denervation may have effects in addition to those produced by disuse per se. For example, in the case of adrenergic neuroeffector junctions, denervation results in a rapid increase in sensitivity to norepinephrine and closely related amines, at about the time the nerve terminal degenerates, and a more slowly developing nonspecific supersensitivity, presumably due to disuse. This rapidly developing, specific supersensitivity has been attributed to the fact that adrenergic nerve terminals actively take up and sequester norepinephrine (Hertting, Axelrod, & Whitby, 1961). The intact nerve ending thus competes with postjunctional receptors for norepinephrine which diffuses into the junctional region; when the nerve ending degenerates, the concentration at the site of action would rise to a higher level and give the appearance of supersensitivity. The difference between the two forms of supersensitivity has been subjected to extensive analyses by Trendelenburg and his associates (Trendelenburg, 1963). It should be noted parenthetically that certain drugs blocking transmission across adrenergic junctions (for example, bretylium, phenoxybenzamine) affect the catecholamine uptake mechanism as well, and thus may mimic the effects of denervation as well as produce disuse.

5. Disuse supersensitivity is reversible, sensitivity reverting to normal when input is restored. The development of disuse supersensitivity in denervated or decentralized glands has been prevented by exercising the glands with daily injections of pilocarpine (Emmelin, 1961; Reas & Trendelenburg, 1967).

6. Disuse supersensitivity is apparently produced by withdrawal of excitatory influences only. Thus, pharmacological blockade of inhibitory adrenergic input to guinea pig ileum does not produce supersensitivity (Fleming, 1968; Green, Fleming, & Schmidt, 1968). In the early literature summarized by Cannon and Rosenblueth (1949), it was shown that smooth muscle inhibited by epinephrine became more sensitive to these inhibitory influences after denervation. A similar effect was not observed after decentralization (for example, Modern & Thienes, 1936; Youman, Karstens, & Aumann, 1942). This discrepancy can now be accounted for, since denervation would destroy the catecholamine uptake mechanism in the nerve ending, and thus give the appearance of supersensitivity. Decentralization of inhibitory nerves, on the other hand, would not decrease the activity of the smooth muscle, which is the necessary condition for the development of disuse supersensitivity.

III. Disuse Supersensitivity: Mechanisms

A. Proliferation of Receptors

Authors who invoke denervation supersensitivity as an explanatory concept for changes occurring in the central nervous system often seem to be thinking of a proliferation of receptors of the type that is believed to occur in skeletal muscle. However, it should be emphasized that receptor proliferation is not the only phenomenon associated with denervation or disuse supersensitivity in effector organs, and, indeed, receptor proliferation may not account adequately for supersensitivity, even in skeletal muscle.

Several steps intervene between the binding of an agonist (ACh) to its receptor and the physiological consequences of this binding (for example, activation of an ionophore or of contractile elements). Receptologists distinguish between the affinity of the receptor for various ligands and its intrinsic activity (Ariëns, 1954) or efficacy (Stephenson, 1956). Receptor proliferation implies a change in the affinity of the membrane for the appropriate ligands. However, it is also possible that the entire membrane is sparsely covered with ACh binding sites, not necessarily identical with those at the end plate; but these receptors are normally lacking in intrinsic activity, and they achieve the capacity to open ionophores or otherwise affect the response of the cell as a consequence of prolonged disuse.

Most of the work in this area has been concerned with the intrinsic activity rather than the affinity of the newly manifested receptive sites. Thus, in their original work, Axelsson and Thesleff (1959) argued that the newly formed receptors were identical to those in the vicinity of the end plate because the ionophores activated by ACh at the two sites appeared similar. This was shown by the fact that the reversal or "equilibrium" potentials during the action of ACh was the same whether it was applied to the end plate region of an innervated muscle or along the surface of the denervated fiber. The work of Axelsson and Thesleff (1959) was carried out on cat tenuissimus. More recently, Feltz and Mallart (1970), studying frog muscle, obtained a different result. In this preparation, even normally innervated fibers appear to show two kinds of ionic permeability. At the end plate itself, the reversal potential during the response to locally applied ACh is about −15 mV, whereas the reversal potential in the region immediately surrounding the end plate (the "extrajunctional" receptors) is about −44 mV. After denervation, the entire fiber becomes sensitive as usual, and the newly effective receptive sites show an equilibrium potential of about −41 mV, similar to that of the extrajunctional receptors of the innervated muscle. Interestingly, even in the innervated muscle, the extrajunctional sites appeared to be labile, becoming conspicuous during hibernation and tending to disappear during the summer.

Pharmacological attempts to identify the newly formed receptive sites have also yielded ambiguous results. Axelsson and Thesleff (1959) observed that the effects of ACh on denervated muscle membrane could be blocked by curare, which might be expected if the new receptive sites are similar to those of the end plate region. However, curare may have quite different effects on denervated muscle, in some instances, causing a depolarizing response (Bowman & Raper, 1964). This is somewhat reminiscent of the effects of methonium compounds in denervated neurons of the sympathetic ganglia. Normally, such compounds block the effects of ACh on the ganglionic neurons, without activating the neurons themselves. However, after denervation, neurons in perfused sympathetic ganglia may be excited by methonium compounds (Perry & Reinert, 1954; Perry & Reinert, 1955). One way of characterizing nicotinic receptors is to measure the relative blocking action of curare and atropine (since the latter, in high concentrations, exerts a curare like blocking effect). Nicotinic receptors appear to differ with respect to their susceptibility to these two blocking agents. Beránek and Vyskočil (1967) found that the ratio of potencies of the two agents differed in denervated and innervated rat diaphragm. They believed that the difference could not be attributed to an action of the drugs on presynaptic endings (in the innervated diaphragm), that it indicated rather a difference in receptors.

Ultimately, the receptor as a chemical entity must be identified by its affinity for various ligands and by its presence in the correct concentrations at the appropriate sites. Waser and Hadorn (1960) attempted to identify ACh receptors in muscle by radioautographic study of binding sites ^{14}C-curare. They found some increased binding after denervation, but only in the end plate region. The expected expansion of binding sites to the entire surface of the fiber did not occur. It is not certain, however, that curare binds to the same receptors as ACh; it may block the action of ACh through allosteric reactions, as pointed out by Miledi and Potter (1971). These investigators employed α-bungarotoxin labeled with radioactive iodine to label nicotinic receptive sites in normal and denervated muscle. α-Bungarotoxin appears to be bound irreversibly by nicotinic sites. Ten to fifteen percent of the radioactivity was bound to end-plate free regions of normal rat diaphragm. After denervation, the amount of α-bungarotoxin bound by the end-plate free region increased about 200 times, but the concentration did not appear to approach that of the end-plate region. Thus, it appears that receptors closely resembling those of the end-plate region with respect to affinity for this toxin are either unmasked or generated *de novo* in the end-plate free part of denervated muscle. However, from a quantitative point of view, it is difficult to account for the very high ACh sensitivity of denervated muscle in terms of the observed increase in toxin-receptive sites alone.

B. Changes in Coupling

The occupation of receptors is but the first step in a complex series of reactions that eventuate in the contraction of the muscle fiber. Preoccupation with this initiating step may have caused us to neglect other changes possibly contributing to supersensitivity. These have been reviewed often (for example, Gutmann, & Hník, 1963; Guth, 1968). In some cases, such changes can be dissociated from the expansion of the chemosensitive surface, either not developing contemporaneously, or being produced by conditions which do not give rise to supersensitivity.

In the older literature, it was reported that denervated muscle becomes sensitized to caffeine, potassium, and epinephrine, as well as nicotinic agents (Cannon & Rosenblueth, 1949). The responses were probably contractures (that is, contractions not associated with conducted impulses). Recently, contracture responses to caffeine and other agents have been studied more carefully *in vitro*. Gutmann and Hanzlíková (1966) observed that the addition of either caffeine or acetylcholine to the bathing solution produces contractures in "slow" mammalian muscle and in denervated "fast" muscle. These agents also produced contractures in innervated "fast" muscle during early stages of development. Thus, skeletal muscle fibers which are sensitive to ACh throughout their length appear also to be hypersensitive to the contracture-producing effects of ACh and caffeine. This might be expected when ACh is added to the organ bath, since it would depolarize the entire muscle and thus produce contraction without the necessity of setting up a propagated action potential. However, hypersensitivity to the contracture-producing effects of caffeine is observed even if the muscle membrane is initially depolarized by the addition of potassium salts to the bathing medium (Gutmann & Sandow, 1965; Gutmann & Hanzlíková, 1966). Caffeine causes release and inhibits uptake of calcium by the isolated sarcoplasmic reticulum (Herz & Weber, 1965). Caffeine increases the influx and efflux of calcium in depolarized muscle fibers (Bianchi, 1961). Isaacson and Sandow (1967) found that chronically denervated muscle showed a much greater increase in radiocalcium flux in response to caffeine than innervated muscle. Howell and associates (1966) reported that chronically denervated muscle is able to sequester more calcium than normal muscle, an effect attributed to the sarcoplasmic reticulum. More recently, Thorpe and Seeman (1971) have inferred from somewhat indirect evidence that it is the sarcolemma itself (rather than the sarcoplasmic reticulum) which binds more calcium after denervation. These authors suggested that "release of a greater number of calcium ions by the plasma membrane of denervated skeletal muscle might account for its greater contractile response to ACh and caffeine."

Certain forms of supersensitivity in smooth muscle may be associated with a change in excitation–contraction coupling, possibly involving an alteration in calcium binding or mobilization. Supersensitivity following decentralization of smooth muscle is relatively nonspecific, the effector organ becoming sensitized to any agent that is normally capable of exciting it. Nonspecific supersensitivity cannot be attributed to the proliferation of a specific (cholinotropic or adrenotropic) receptor. Hudgins and Fleming (1966) have suggested that the supersensitivity of aortic strips after reserpinization (which reduces adrenergic input to the affected cell) depends on a change beyond the receptor level. An analysis of dissociation constants and efficacy for various agonists and antagonists indicated that a change in efficacy rather than affinity for receptors is responsible for nonspecific supersensitivity in smooth muscle (Green & Fleming, 1967; Taylor & Green, 1971).

Hudgins and Harris (1970) and Carrier and Jurevics (1973) have investigated calcium mobility in aortic strips from animals treated with reserpine. They found a change in ^{45}Ca mobility and also a tendency for the treated (supersensitive) aortae to bind ^{45}Ca more tightly, presumably at intracellular sites. Carrier and Jurevics (1973) found that the reserpinized aortae were supersensitive to calcium in a depolarizing medium. The supersensitivity of the aortic strips to ACh and potassium depended upon extracellular concentrations of calcium; that to norepinephrine and isoproterenol was exhibited even in calcium-free media. It was suggested that the supersensitivity to ACh and potassium depended upon facilitated entry of extracellular calcium, whereas that to norepinephrine and isoproterenol depended upon an increase in the availability of intracellular calcium to the contractile elements. An increased sensitivity to barium ions, believed to act at a site where calcium is involved in excitation–contraction coupling, was observed by Taylor and Green (1971).

All of this points to structures responsible for binding or mobilization of calcium as probable sites of changes induced by denervation or disuse, changes which may contribute to the apparent supersensitivity of the affected cell to excitatory chemical agents. As yet, the data are merely suggestive, but it seems probable that mechanisms involved in excitation–contraction coupling will be the focus of research on denervation and disuse supersensitivity in muscle during the next few years.

It would thus appear that two mechanisms may be involved in denervation supersensitivity. In mammalian skeletal muscle fibers and in one class of neurons (the parasympathetic ganglion cell of the frog), new nicotinic receptors develop or are unmasked in the nonjunctional regions of the denervated cell. In skeletal muscle, this effect is evidently produced by disuse per se. Hitherto, only nicotinic receptors have been shown to spread in this fashion. In both skeletal and smooth muscle, denervation appears to affect excitation–contraction coupling, probably owing to a change in the binding or distribution of calcium. In smooth muscle, the latter change is produced by disuse per se and results in a nonspecific increase in the contraction-producing effects of all agents that normally excite the cell. In skeletal muscle, the change is manifested in an increased sensitivity to the contracture-producing effects of caffeine.

IV. Effects of Disuse and Denervation on Neurons

Study of disused or denervated effector organs has focused attention on two processes, receptor proliferation and increased excitation-contraction coupling, the latter owing probably to changes in the mobility of calcium. Do such changes occur in neurons? If so, how would they be manifested?

The latter question is especially interesting in connection with possible changes in calcium kinetics in disused neurons. In view of the ubiquitous role of this ion in neuronal excitation and transmission, it would be gratuitous to present a detailed hypothesis as to how such a change would affect neuronal function. However, this line of thought does focus attention on mechanisms coupling excitation to the executive apparatus of the cell—the contractile or secretory apparatus. In muscle, a change in excitation–contraction coupling brought about by prolonged disuse may give the appearance of increased sensitivity, less excitation being required to produce a contractile response. In nerve, the chemoreceptive zone is separated from the neurosecretory apparatus by a conductile axon. Here, calcium mediates between the arrival of a nerve impulse at the nerve terminal and secretion of the transmitter, a process which seems similar in several respects to excitation–contraction coupling in muscle. Thus, even supposing that denervation or disuse engage similar chemical mechanisms in all excitable cells, this might be manifested in different ways in muscle and neuron, in the one causing an apparent increase in sensitivity, and in the other, an increase in quantity of transmitter released per nerve impulse. We refer to the latter as disuse potentiation, to distinguish it from changes in the chemoreceptivity of the cell. There is evidence that some neurons exhibit disuse potentiation, although there is as yet no evidence linking disuse potentiation in neurons with a change in calcium binding or mobilization.

A. Sensitization

The spread of chemosensitivity characteristic of disused muscle fibers has been observed in only one class of neurons, the parasympathetic ganglion cells in frog's heart studied by Kuffler and associates (1971). The technical difficulties associated with measuring the extrajunctional sensitivity of neurons to excitatory agents are so formidable that it is unlikely that this technique will soon be extended to other classes of neurons, particularly in the vertebrate central nervous system. One might expect that an expansion of the chemosensitive surface of a neuron would be manifested by an increased sensitivity to excitatory agents applied in bulk form, either by topical application, diffusion from a near micropipette, or diffusion from the blood stream. As will be shown below, neither neurons of the mammalian sympathetic ganglia nor neurons of cerebral cortex exhibit this kind of supersensitivity when surgically isolated from input. Investigators have therefore concluded that these neurons do no conform to Cannon's law.

However, the idea that bulk application of excitatory agents will reveal an increase in chemosensitivity of the type observed in skeletal muscle fibers involves certain assumptions. First, it must be assumed that the agonist is acting only, or principally, on the affected element. If it acts on both pre- and postsynaptic sites, as ACh and certain sympathomimetic amines are believed to do in some structures, then the effects of denervation become unpredictable, since the gain in active postsynaptic receptors may be counterbalanced by the loss of indirect sites of action on presynaptic terminals. Diffusion barriers encountered by the agonist may be altered in such a way as to reduce the concentration achieved at postsynaptic sites of action. Uptake by neighboring elements, including glia, may also confound the effects. For these reasons, in the absence of the kinds of control achieved by Kuffler and his associates (1971) in parasympathetic ganglion cells, it is difficult to obtain conclusive evidence pro or con the spread of chemosensitive surface in denervated neurons.

B. Neurons of Autonomic Ganglia

In the earlier literature reviewed by Cannon and Rosenblueth (1949), it had been claimed that denervated neurons of the mammalian sympathetic ganglia become sensitized to ACh following denervation. The evidence was indirect, since the investigators used the response of an effector organ (usually the nictitating membrane of the cat) as an index of the activity of ganglion cells. Since the disused nictitating membrane becomes sensitized to norepinephrine liberated from the sympathetic nerve terminals (Langer, Draskoczy, & Trendelenburg, 1967), a larger response elicited by ganglionic stimulation might be due either to an increased sensitivity of the ganglion cells themselves or to an increased sensitivity of the effector organ to norepinephrine released from the nerve terminals.

Another approach involves expressing the response of an effector organ to chemical stimulation of the ganglion in terms of the amount of electrical stimulation of postganglionic stimulation required to mimic the effects of ganglionic stimulation. Using this technique, Vickerson and Varma (1969) found that denervated ganglion cells appeared to become less sensitive to nicotinic stimulation and somewhat more sensitive to muscarinic stimulation. Green (1969), using a similar technique, found a reduction in sensitivity to both nicotinic and muscarinic stimulants after denervation.

Experiments in which the electrical activity of the postganglionic nerve has been measured have also revealed only subsensitivity of denervated ganglion cells to ACh (Volle & Koelle, 1961). Brown (1966) measured demarcation potentials of ganglion cells exposed to cholinergic agents *in vitro,* and found a reduction in sensitivity following chronic denervation.

Thus, the bulk of the recent evidence on neurons of mammalian sympathetic ganglia implies that these elements do not conform to Cannon's law and that they are dissimilar in this respect to the parasympathetic ganglion cells of the frog's heart studied by Kuffler and his associates. However, the caveat mentioned above may be relevant: a loss of presynaptic sites of action of ACh in the denervated ganglion might mask an increase in sensitivity of the postsynaptic elements.

The discrepancy between the early and later literature cannot be dismissed on the grounds of faulty technique alone. Both Chein (1960) and Murray and Thompson (1957) confirmed the earlier findings of Cannon and Rosenblueth (1949), quantitating the response of the nictitating membrane to ganglionic stimulation in terms of the amount of intravenous norepinephrine required to mimic that response. Their results showed that more norepinephrine was required to mimic the effects of ganglionic stimulation by ACh after chronic denervation of the ganglion cells.

One possible explanation of this discrepancy has apparently been overlooked. It may be that the disused postganglionic fibers release more norepinephrine per nerve impulse, and thus exhibit disuse potentiation. If this were the case, more norepinephrine would be required to mimic the response to ganglionic stimulation after a period of disuse, even if the ganglion cells themselves did not increase in sensitivity. Brown and his associates (1965, 1967) presented evidence that the capacity of adrenergic fibers of the splenic nerve to release transmitter increased following a period of disuse. These investigators used phenoxybenzamine to block uptake by adrenotropic receptors, permitting the liberated norepinephrine to diffuse into the venous effluent from the spleen. Under these conditions, the quantity of norepinephrine released during stimulation of the splenic nerve increased following section of preganglionic fibers or pharmacological blockade of the ganglion. The store of norepinephrine in the disused nerve terminals also increased (Brown *et al.*, 1967). The increased store could not be depleted by a few nerve impulses, provided the catecholamine uptake mechanism in the nerve ending was allowed to function. Apparently, the disused nerve ending was able to cycle more norepinephrine through the system made up of terminal storage sites and tissue receptors. The adrenergic nerve endings in the smooth muscle of the cat's nictitating membrance do not store more neurohumor when disused (Kirpekar, Cervoni, & Furchgott, 1962; Smith, Trendelenburg, Langer, & Tsai, 1966). It is nevertheless conceivable that the fraction of total transmitter released per nerve impulse increases as a consequence of disuse.

C. Spinal Neurons

A number of investigators have observed increases in the response of spinal motoneurons to various forms of stimulation after partial denervation (early work reviewed by Stavraky, 1961). In these studies, it has generally been impossible to determine either the site of the change or the condition responsible for it—that is, disuse versus some other effect of injury. One of the first attempts to study the effects of disuse per se was that of Eccles and McIntyre (1953), who sectioned the dorsal roots distal to the ganglion cells, leaving the intraspinal projections of the latter presumably intact. This resulted in a decrease in transmission efficacy in monosynaptic spinal pathways, leading to Eccles' (1953) view that disuse weakens and use strengthens excitatory synapses. However, it was acknowledged that the changes may have been due to degenerative changes and shrinking of dorsal root fibers whose peripheral processes had been severed.

One might expect that section of a muscle tendon would relieve the tension on stretch receptors and thereby reduce impulse traffic in the Ia fibers supplying the muscle spindle. This method of achieving disuse in the afferent limb of the monosynaptic arc was utilized by Beránek and Hník (1959) and Kozak and Westerman (1961). By several weeks after tenotomy, monosynaptic compound action potentials recorded either from ventral roots or the dorsal spinocerebellar tract during stimulation of Group I fibers from the tenotomized muscle had increased greatly in size. Assuming that tenotomy is, indeed, an effective way of silencing the Ia fibers, these results would imply that the disused synapses increased in strength. However, Kozak and Westerman (1961) suggested that the Ia afferent fibers might actually be subjected to greater use after tenotomy, owing to some compensatory increase in gamma efferent activity. This was ruled out by Spencer and April (1970), who showed that the monosynaptic discharges increased after tenotomy, even if the ventral roots had been cut at the time of tenotomy, preventing any activation of annulospiral endings by gamma efferent activity. Recently, Yellin and Eldred (1970) measured the discharge of spindle units in tenotomized ankle extensors and found a reduction at most positions of ankle extension. They concluded that the use of tenotomy to chronically reduce sensory inflow from spindles was justified. The evidence thus strongly implies that disuse of the afferent limb of the monosynaptic spinal reflex tends to strengthen that reflex.

Robbins and Nelson (1970) sought to determine whether the enhancement of transmission efficacy was due to a presynaptic (potentiation) or a postsynaptic (sensitization) change. Motoneurons projecting to the tenotomized muscle did not appear to be more sensitive, as judged by their response to tetanizing stimuli delivered to afferent fibers from intact muscles. Goldfarb and Muller (1971) found that single stimuli to the muscle nerve from tenotomized muscle were capable of evoking heteronymous monosynaptic discharges, which almost never occur in normal circumstances. Thus, the increased efficacy of transmission in monosynaptic spinal pathways subjected to a period of reduced usage is evidently due to a presynaptic change—a form of disuse potentiation.

Robbins and Fischbach (1971) attempted to determine whether disused motoneurons are capable of releasing more transmitter per nerve potential at the neuromuscular junction. Disuse was achieved by immobilizing knee and ankle joints with pins, which results in a profound decrease in motoneuron activity as judged by the electromyogram of ankle extensors (Fischbach & Robbins, 1969). The disused motor nerve fibers released more transmitter per nerve impulse at low frequencies of stimulation. The evidence indicated that the fraction of the available store released by a single impulse increased, and also that this store was replenished more rapidly. However, at high frequencies of stimulation, the disused terminals released less transmitter than controls. This form of disuse potentiation, measurable at low frequencies of stimulation, might account for the finding of Goldfarb and Sharpless (1971) that antidromic activation of motoneurons produces more recurrent inhibition after a period of disuse, possibly releasing more ACh from the recurrent collateral fibers ending on Renshaw cells.

D. Isolated Cerebral Cortex

Isolated cerebral cortex, undercut with its superficial blood supply intact, gradually becomes more susceptible to agents eliciting epileptiform activity (Echlin & McDonald, 1954; Grafstein & Sastry, 1957; Sharpless & Halpern, 1962). According to Spehlmann and associates (1970), destruction of the optic tract or lateral geniculate nucleus produces similar changes in occipital cortex. Fentress and Doty (1971) observed a dramatic increase in the excitability of striate cortex following enucleation. Desmedt and Franken (1963), recording evoked potentials, observed increased excitability in auditory cortex following destruction of the medial geniculate. Spiegel and Szekely (1955), also using evoked potentials, obtained evidence of increased excitability in posterior sigmoid cortex of cat following destruction of the specific sensory nucleus of the thalamus. There are literally hundreds of other examples of apparent increases in excitability of central nervous structures, at all levels of the nervous system, following surgical or pharmacological procedures that would be expected to deprive the affected structures of some source of input. It would be unrewarding to enumerate central nervous changes that are thus superficially analogous to changes induced in peripheral structures of denervation or disuse. The difficulty is that in every case, the affected elements are embedded in a complex matrix of cells, and it is the response of the system that is measured and appears to increase in excitability. Such a change in the system might result from the occurrence of phenomena quite different from those observed in isolated or disused peripheral structures, including, for example, changes in connectivity due to collateral growth or rearrangement of synaptic terminals, selective degeneration of inhibitory elements, changes in the capacity of certain neurons to sustain repetitive activity, and the like.

An interesting feature of chronically isolated cortex is the fact that the increased susceptibility to seizures can be prevented from developing, and possibly reversed, by exercise of the disused neural elements. Rutledge and co-workers (1967) found that daily stimulation at subconvulsive levels (20 applications of a 2-sec pulse train) through implanted electrodes prevented the development of increased susceptibility to epileptiform afterdischarges. This was confirmed by Vazquez and associates (1969), who reported that twice-weekly stimulation sessions (parameters unspecified) prevented the effects of isolation. Sharpless and Halpern (1962) had earlier noted that the capacity of the isolated region to sustain long epileptiform afterdischarges declined to almost normal following experimental sessions in which afterdischarges were repeatedly elicited by stimulation through implanted electrodes; several days might then be required for the reemergence of the effects of isolation. It is not yet known whether subconvulsive stimulation of the type used by Rutledge and associates (1967) will reverse the effect.

It may appear curious that the effects of isolation can be prevented by subconvulsive stimulating pulses applied to a small part of the isolated slab of cortex. However, a moderately intense subconvulsive pulse initiates a response which slowly spreads to all areas of the slab. This is the "burst" response of Burns (1958), during which there is a surface positive shift accompanied by intense unit firing. In the intervals between bursts, the slab tends to be electrically silent, showing very little unit activity. The bursts often recur spontaneously following a single stimulus, so that the amount of "exercise" to which the slab is subjected may be greater than would be supposed from the small amount of stimulation required. In any case, the work of Rutledge and associates (1967) tends to bring the increased seizure susceptibility of isolated cortex into the realm of disuse phenomena with which we are concerned.

Echlin and McDonald (1954) first observed that isolated cortex becomes more susceptible to epileptiform activity induced by topical application of ACh, and they suggested that the effect might be another manifestation of denervation supersensitivity in the central nervous system. Chu and associates (1971a, b) found that subcellular "membrane" fractions from chronically isolated cortex have an increased capacity to bind [^{14}C]-D-tubocurarine. Long-term electrical stimulation of the isolated area appreciably reduced the increase in binding sites. Measurement of radiocurarine binding in subcellular fractions from cerebral cortex is not a wholly convincing technique for demonstrating an increase in physiological ACh receptors. It will be recalled that denervated skeletal muscle shows some dispersal of binding sites for radiocurarine, but that these sites do not spread as the ACh sensitivity does. Titriated atropine binding did not increase in the subcellular fractions from isolated cortex, although the effects of ACh on cortical neurons is often blocked by atropine (Krnjević & Phillis, 1963).

A number of investigators have found a marked decrease in the cholinesterase content of isolated cortex (Duncan, Rutledge, & Domino, 1968;

Green, Halpern, & Van Niel, 1970; Hebb, Krnjević, & Silver, 1963; Rosenberg & Echlin, 1968). Rosenberg and Echlin found that the fall in cholinesterase occurs *pari passu* with the increased susceptibility to seizures. Chu and associates (1971) reported that long-term stimulation prevented the fall in acetylcholinesterase and protein in the cholinesterase-rich membrane fraction from isolated cortex. The increased acetylcholine sensitivity might thus be ascribed to a loss of inactivating enzyme. Support for this was provided by Reiffenstein and Triggle (1972), who observed that isolated cortex did not become more sensitive to cholinomimetic agents that were not broken down by cholinesterase.

Although the fall in cholinesterase may account for the lower concentration of ACh required to initiate seizure activity in isolated slabs, it is unlikely that increased cholinergic activity plays an important role in the prolongation of epileptiform discharges, particularly those induced by electrical stimulation. There is very little acetylcholine remaining in chronically isolated slabs, and acetylcholinetransferase, the enzyme required to produce ACh, falls to low levels after isolation (Hebb *et al.*, 1963). Furthermore, atropine does not curtail epileptiform discharges in chronic slabs, even those discharges initiated by cholinomimetic agents (Reiffenstein *et al.*, 1972).

A more direct test for ACh sensitization of neurons in isolated cortex was undertaken by Krnjević and associates (1970b), using microiontophoretic techniques. These investigators found a reduction in the number of neurons yielding spike discharges in response to ACh. In small slabs of cortex, particularly, ACh-sensitive cells were almost absent, and the few remaining did not appear hypersensitive. L-Glutamate sensitivity was also reduced.

Thus, it would appear that the increased susceptibility of disused cortex to epileptiform activity is probably not due to denervation or disuse sensitization. There are numerous morphological changes in chronically isolated cortex. Purpura and Housepian (1961) replicated Cajal's observation of extensive collateral growth from injured axons in undercut cortex of kittens. They suggested that the increased connectivity due to new recurrent collaterals might account for increased susceptibility to seizures. But attempts to measure collateral growth in mature, undercut cortex, although beset with technical problems, have yielded disappointing results (Rutledge, 1969; Rutledge, Duncan, & Beatty, 1969; Szentágothai, 1965). It is difficult to accept the idea that a gross morphological change accounts for the prolongation of seizures, since the latter can be prevented by daily electrical stimulation. Rutledge (1969) observed a reduction in dendritic spines in chronically isolated cortex, which he considered partly due to disuse, since the spines were better retained in slabs subjected to daily electrical stimulation. However, Rutledge and his associates consider that the effects of isolation are due to some form of supersensitivity following deafferentation, the amount of deafferentation possibly being affected by the degree of disuse (Chu *et al.*, 1971a, b).

Certainly the most conspicuous change in chronic slabs is in the ability to sustain intense, epileptiform activity for long periods. Normally, epileptiform afterdischarges are strictly limited, rarely exceeding 20 sec and averaging about 10 sec in acute slabs. In intact suprasylvian cortex also, epileptiform afterdischarges are short unless they spread into adjacent regions (in which case, they may last for minutes, possibly because of a shifting focus). However, after a few weeks, the average duration of epileptiform afterdischarges in chronic slabs increases five- to tenfold. Occasionally, an intense epileptiform discharge may go on for minutes in a small chronic slab, eventually giving way to sporadic epileptiform spiking which continues for hours (Sharpless & Halpern, 1962). It is as if a mechanism which normally terminates seizure activity becomes defective as a consequence of disuse.

A decrease in gamma-aminobutyric acid and a concomitant rise in glutamine has been observed in chronic slabs (Berl & McMurtry, 1967). There is no significant change in the sensitivity of neurons in isolated cortex to the inhibitory effects of gamma-aminobutyric acid, applied by microiontophoresis (Krnjević *et al.,* 1970a). Krnjević and associates also found that glutamate-induced firing could be inhibited by surface stimulation in chronic slabs, the inhibitory pause lasting somewhat longer than in acute slabs. Creutzfeldt *et al.* (1962) were able to obtain good inhibitory postsynaptic potentials by intracellular recording from chronic slabs, and suggested even that inhibition may be predominant after degeneration of corticopetal afferants (Creutzfeldt, Lax, & Watanabe, 1966). Thus, the evidence available does not favor the idea that there is a substantial loss of inhibitory circuits in chronic slabs.

There is one remarkable feature of epileptiform activity in chronic slabs that may provide an important clue. Unit responses, recorded from neurons by extracellular electrodes, actually diminish during the intense epileptiform activity recorded from the surface by macroelectrodes. Halpern, Ward, Black, and Lockhard (1969) were able to detect very little unit activity during full-blown epileptiform afterdischarges. Reiffenstein and Triggle (1972) found a reduction in the recordable number of unit discharges to about half during seizures elicited by cholinergic agents. Ferguson and Jasper (1971) also reported little unit firing during ACh-induced epileptiform activity. A reasonable explanation for the lack of unit discharges during a seizure was suggested by Reiffenstein and Triggle (1972). They noted that the spike generator in somatodendritic membrane may become inactivated while the axon continues to fire. Field potentials generated by axonal spikes would be more difficult to detect than those generated by somatic spikes. Electrophysiological studies of seizure activity in hippocampus and other structures often show an intense, "paroxysmal" depolarization of cells during early phases of the seizure (Spencer & Kandel, 1969). During this phase, the spike generator in the somatic–dendritic membrane is inactivated, but it is possible that the axon continues to fire, driven by current flowing into the depolarized soma. Synaptic bombardment through recurrent pathways would help to maintain the cellular depolarization and also produce the fluctuations in membrane potentials responsible for the large surface potentials associated with the seizure. This explanation helps to account for the otherwise paradoxical fact that chronic slabs exhibit at once an increased susceptibility to convulsoid activity induced by topical application of ACh and a decrease in the unit firing induced by microiontophoresis of ACh onto cortical cells.

This explanation focuses attention on the axonal spike generator and the nerve terminals as possible sites for the defect in the mechanism terminating seizure activity, for it would suggest that seizure activity is normally terminated either by inactivation of the axonal spike generator (perhaps by accommodation at the initial segment) or by a decline in the quantity of transmitter released per nerve impulse. Both events would remove the synaptic drive on the somatic–dendritic membrane and permit the cell to repolarize, thus terminating the seizure. The ability of chronic slabs to sustain seizure activity for long periods might then be attributed to some form of disuse potentiation, resulting from increased stores of transmitter or more rapid recovery of the transmitter release mechanism. Alternatively, there may be a derangement of the accommodation mechanism. In spinal motoneurons, accommodation is generally more rapid in the initial segment than in the somatic-dendritic membrane (Sasaki & Otani, 1961). But neurons differ greatly in the accommodative mechanisms (Bullock, 1965), and the accommodative process appears to be labile (Bradley & Somjen, 1961). The effects of use and disuse on neuronal accommodation have apparently not been studied.

V. Conclusions

1. It now seems probable that a large part, if not all, of the spread of ACh sensitivity that occurs in skeletal muscle is due to disuse.

2. Smooth muscle and glands also show a form of supersensitivity when disused for long periods, but this appears to involve a change in excitation–contraction coupling rather than a proliferation of specific receptors. There is indirect evidence that calcium binding and mobility may be altered by disuse.

3. Denervated skeletal muscle also exhibits an alteration in calcium binding and mobility, which probably accounts for an increased sensitivity to the contracture-producing effects of caffeine.

4. We have noted that if a similar change (in calcium binding and translocation) occurs in disused neurons, the effect might be manifested at the nerve ending, where calcium translocation mediates between the arrival of a nerve impulse and the liberation of transmitter. It is desirable to distinguish between disuse sensitization and disuse potentiation, the latter being manifested by an increase in the quantity of transmitter released per nerve impulse.

5. The only clear example of denervation sensitization in neurons is the demonstration of Kuffler and associates (1971) that parasympathetic ganglion cells in the interatrial septum of frog heart exhibit an expansion of ACh-sensitive membrane following denervation.

6. Recent evidence has failed to confirm early work purporting to demonstrate supersensitivity to ACh in denervated mammalian sympathetic ganglion cells. There is some evidence, mostly indirect, that denervated sympathetic ganglion cells exhibit a form of disuse potentiation, releasing more transmitter per nerve impulse.

7. Monosynaptic spinal pathways undergo an increase in transmission efficacy following a period of disuse, which can be attributed largely to presynaptic changes—that is, disuse potentiation.

8. Surgically isolated slabs of cortex, undercut so that the superficial circulation is left substantially unimpaired, gradually develop an increased susceptibility to epileptiform activity, the most conspicuous change being in the capacity to sustain an intense, epileptiform discharge for long periods. This change appears to be due to disuse of cortical neurons, since it can be prevented by daily subconvulsive stimulation.

9. Recent evidence, although not entirely conclusive, has tended to exclude supersensitivity, selective loss of inhibitory elements, or collateral growth as adequate explanations for the effects of isolation on cerebral cortex. Electrophysiological analyses of seizure activity in chronically isolated cortex points either to a derangement in accommodation or to some form of disuse potentiation as possible mechanisms for the effects of isolation.

10. Although there is ample evidence for compensatory reactions to prolonged disuse or denervation in the central nervous system, as in effector organs, the mechanisms responsible for these compensatory changes are still a matter for conjecture.

References

Albuquerque, E. X., & McIsaac, R. J. Fast and slow mammalian muscles after denervation. *Experimental Neurology,* 1970, **26,** 183–202.

Ariëns, E. J. Affinity and intrinsic activity in the theory of competitive inhibition. Part I. Problems and theory. *Archiv Internale Pharmacodynamie,* 1954, **99,** 32–49.

Axelsson, J., & Thesleff, S. A study of supersensitivity in denervated skeletal muscle. *Journal of Physiology* (*London*), 1959, **149**, 178–193.

Beránek, R., & Hník, P. Long-term effects of tenotomy on spinal monosynaptic response in the cat. *Science,* 1959, **130**, 981–982.

Beránek, R., & Vyskočil, F. The action of tubocurarine and atropine on the normal and denervated rat diaphragm. *J. Physiol.* **188**, 53–66.

Berl, S., & McMurty, J. C. Isolated cerebral changes in levels of glutamic acid, glutamine, aspartic acid and gamma-aminobutyric acid. *Archives of Biochemistry,* 1967, **118**, 645–648.

Bianchi, C. P. Calcium movements in muscle. *Circulation,* 1961, **24,** 518–522.

Bowman, W. C., & Raper, C. Spontaneous fibrillary activity of denervated muscle. *Nature,* 1964, **201**, 160.

Bradley, K., & Somjen, G. G. Accommodation in motoneurons of the rat and the cat. *Journal of Physiology,* 1961, **156**, 75–92.

Brown, D. A. Depolarization of normal and preganglionically denervated superior cervical ganglia by stimulant drugs. *British Journal of Pharmacology,* 1966, **26,** 511.

Brown, G. L. The release and fate of the transmitter liberated by adrenergic nerves. *Proceedings of the Royal Society, Series B,* 1965, **162**, 1.

Brown, G. L., Dearnaley, D. P., & Geffen, L. B. Noradrenaline storage and release in the decentralized spleen. *Proceedings of the Royal Society, Series B,* 1967, **168**, 48–56.

Bullock, T. Comparative neurology of excitability and conduction. In T. Bullock & G. Horridge (Eds.), *Structure and function in the nervous system of invertebrates.* Vol. I. San Francisco: Freeman and Co. 1965. Pp. 125–180.

Burns, B. D. *The mammalian cerebral cortex.* London: Edward Arnold, 1958.

Cannon, W. B., & Rosenblueth, A. *The supersensitivity of denervated structures.* New York: Macmillan, 1949.

Carrier, O., & Jurevics, H. A. The role of calcium in "nonspecific" supersensitivity of vascular muscle. *Journal of Pharmacology,* 1973, **184**, 81–94.

Chein, S. Supersensitivity of denervated superior cervical ganglion to acetylcholine. *American Journal of Physiology,* 1960, **198**, 949–954.

Chu, N.-S., Rutledge, L., & Sellinger, O. Z. The effect of cortical undercutting and long-term electrical stimulation on synaptic acetylcholinesterase. *Brain Research,* 1971, **29**, 323–330. (a)

Chu, N.-S., Rutledge, L., & Sellinger, O. Z. Tubocurarine binding in undercut cerebral cortex and the effect of long-term electrical stimulation. *Brain Research,* 1971, **29**, 331–337. (b)

Cohen, S. A., & Fischbach, G. D. Regulation of muscle acetylcholine sensitivity by muscle activity in cell culture. *Science,* 1973, **181**, 76–78.

Creutzfeldt, O. D., Lux, H. D., & Watanabe, S. Electrophysiology of cortical nerve cells. In D. P. Purpura & M. D. Yahr (Eds.), *The thalamus.* New York: Columbia University Press, 1966.

Creutzfeldt, O. D., & Struck, G. Neurophysiologie und Morphologie der cronisch isolierten Cortexinsel der Katze. *Archiv Psychiatrie Nervenkrankheit,* 1962, **203**, 708–731.

Dennis, M. J., Harris, A. J., & Kuffler, S. Synaptic transmission and its duplication by focally applied acetylcholine in parasympathetic neurons in the heart of the frog. *Proceedings of the Royal Society, London, Series B,* 1971, **177,** 509–539.

Desmedt, J., & Franken, L. Long-term physiological changes in auditory cortex following deafferentation. In E. Gutmann & P. Hník (Eds.), *The effect of use and disuse on neuromuscular functions.* Prague: Czechoslovakian Academy of Sciences, 1963. Pp. 264–276.

Diamond, J., & Miledi, R. A study of foetal and new-born rat muscle fibers. *Journal of Physiology (London),* 1962, **162,** 393–408.

Drachman, D. B., & Witzke, F. Trophic regulation of acetylcholine sensitivity of muscle: Effect of electrical stimulation. *Science,* 1972, 514–516.

Duncan, J. A., Rutledge, L. T., & Domino, E. F. Acetylcholinesterase activity in partially isolated cerebral cortex after prolonged intermittent stimulation. *Experimental Neurology,* 1968, **20,** 268–274.

Eccles, J. C. *The neurophysiological basis of mind.* Oxford: Clarendon Press, 1953.

Eccles, J. C., & McIntyre, A. K. The effects of disuse and of activity on mammalian spinal reflexes. *Journal of Physiology (London),* 1953, **121,** 492.

Echlin, F., & McDonald, J. The supersensitivity of chronically isolated and partially isolated cerebral cortex as a mechanism in focal cortical epilepsy. *Transactions of the American Neurological Association,* 1954, **79,** 75–79.

Emmelin, N. Supersensitivity following "pharmacological denervation." *Pharmacological Review,* 1961, **13,** 17–37.

Feltz, A., & Mallart, A. Differences in the action of acetylcholine on the denervated muscle fiber and on the normal end plate. *Brain Research,* 1970, **22,** 264–267.

Fentress, J., & Doty, R. Effects of tetanization and enucleation upon excitability of visual pathways in squirrel monkeys and cats. *Experimental Neurology,* 1971, **30,** 535–554.

Ferguson, J., & Jasper, H. Laminar D. C. studies of acetylcholine-activated epileptiform discharge in cerebral cortex. *Electroencephalography and Clinical Neurophysiology,* 1971, **30,** 305–320.

Fischbach, G. D., & Robbins, N. Changes in contractile properties of disused soleus muscles. *Journal of Physiology,* 1969, **201,** 305–320.

Fleming, W. W. Nonspecific supersensitivity of the guinea-pig ileum produced by chronic ganglion blockade. *Journal of Pharmacology,* 1968, **162,** 277–285.

Frank, G. B., & Inoue, F. Large miniature end plate potentials in partial denervated skeletal muscle. *Nature,* 1966, **212,** 596–598.

Goldfarb, J., & Muller, R. Occurrence of heteronymous monosynaptic reflexes following tenotomy. *Brain Research,* 1971, **28,** 553–555.

Goldfarb, J., & Sharpless, S. K. Effects of nicotine and recurrent inhibition on monosynaptic reflexes in acute and chronic spinal cats. Neuropharmacology, 1971, **10,** 413–423.

Grafstein, B., & Sastry, P. Some preliminary electrophysiological studies on chronic neuronally isolated cerebral cortex. *Electroencephalography and Clinical Neurophysiology,* 1957, **9,** 723–725.

Green, J. R., Halpern, L. M., & Van Niel, S. Alterations in the activity of selected enzymes in the chronic isolated cerebral cortex of the cat. *Brain,* 1970, **93,** 57–64.

Green, R. D., III. The effect of denervation on the sensitivity of the superior cervical ganglion of the pithed cat. *Journal of Pharmacology and Experimental Therapy,* 1969, **167,** 143–150.

Green, R. D., III & Fleming, W. W. Agonist–antagonist interactions in the normal and supersensitive nictitating membrane of the spinal cat. *Journal of Pharmacology,* 1967, **156,** 207–214.

Green, R. D., III, Fleming, W. W., & Schmidt, J. L. Sensitivity changes in the isolated ileum of the guinea pig after pretreatment with reserpine. *Journal of Pharmacology,* 1968, **162**, 270–276.

Guth, L. "Trophic" influences of nerve on muscle. *Physiological Review,* 1968, **48,** 645–687.

Gutmann, E., & Hanzlíková, V. Contracture responses of fast and slow mammalian muscles. *Physiologie Bohemoslovaca,* 1966, **15**, 404–414.

Gutmann, E., & Hník, P. (Eds.), *The effects of use and disuse upon neuromuscular function.* Prague: Czechoslovakian Academy of Sciences, 1963.

Gutmann, E., & Sandow, A. Caffeine-induced contracture and potentiation of contraction in normal and denervated rat muscle. *Life Sciences,* 1965, **4**, 1149–1156.

Halpern, L., Ward, A., Black, R., & Lockhard, J. The hyperexcitable neuron as a model for the laboratory analysis of anticonvulsant drugs. *Epilepsia,* 1969, **10,** 281–314.

Harris, A., Kuffler, S., & Dennis, M. Differential chemosensitivity of synaptic and extrasynaptic areas on the neuronal surface membrane in parasympathetic neurons of the frog, tested by micro application of acetylcholine. *Proceedings of the Royal Society of London Series, B,* 1971, **177**, 541–553.

Hebb, C., Krnjevic, K., & Silver, A. Effect of undercutting on the acetylcholinesterase and choline acetyltransferase activity in the cat's cerebral cortex. *Nature (London),* 1963, **198**, 692.

Heron, W. Cognitive and physiological effects of perpetual isolation. In Solomon, P., Kubzansky, P., Leiderman, P., Mendelson, J., Trumbullo, R., & Wexler, D. (Eds.), *Sensory deprivation.* Cambridge Massachusetts: Harvard University Press, 1961. Pp. 6–33.

Hertting, G., Axelrod, J., & Whitby, L. G. Effect of drugs on the uptake and metabolism of H^3-norepinephrine. *Journal of Pharmacology,* 1961, **134,** 146–153.

Herz, R., & Weber, A. Caffeine inhibition of Ca uptake by muscle reticulum. *Federation Proceedings,* 1965, **24**, 208.

Howell, J. N., Fairhurst, A. S., & Jenden, D. Alterations of the calcium accumulating ability of striated muscle following denervation. *Life Sciences,* 1966, **5**, 439–446.

Hudgins, P. M., & Fleming, W. W. A relatively nonspecific supersensitivity in aortic strips resulting from pretreatment with reserpine. *Journal of Pharmacology,* 1966, **153**, 70–80.

Hudgins, P. M., & Harris, T. M. Further studies on the effects of reserpine pretreatment on rabbit aorta: Calcium and histological changes. *Journal of Pharmacology,* 1970, **175**, 609–618.

Isaacson, A., & Sandow, A. Caffeine effects on radiocalcium movement in normal and denervated rat skeletal muscles. *Journal of Pharmacology,* 1967, **155**, 376–388.

Jaffe, J., & Sharpless, S. Pharmacological denervation supersensitivity in the central nervous system: A theory of physical dependence. In A. Wikler (Ed.), *The addictive states, Research Publication: Association for Research in Nervous and Mental Disease,* 1968, **46**, 226–243.

Johns, T. R., & Thesleff, S. Effects of motor inactivation on the chemical sensitivity of skeletal muscle. *Acta Physiologica Scandinavica,* 1961, **51,** 136–141.

Jones, R., & Vrbova, G. Effect of muscle activity on denervation hypersensitivity. *Journal of Physiology (London),* 1970, **210**, 144–145.

Katz, B., & Miledi, R. The development of acetylcholine sensitivity in nerve-free segments of skeletal muscle. *Journal of Physiology (London),* 1964, **170**, 389–396.

Kirpekar, S. M., Cervoni, P., & Furchgott, R. Catecholamine content of the cat nictitating membrane following procedures sensitizing it to norepinephrine. *Journal of Pharmacology,* 1962, **135**, 180–190.

Korr, I. M., Wilkinson, P. N., & Chornock, F. W. Axonal delivery of neuroplasmic components in muscle cells. *Science,* 1967, **155**, 342–345.

Kozak, W., & Westerman, R. Plastic changes of spinal monosynaptic responses from tenotomized muscles in cats. *Nature (London)*, 1961, **189**, 753–755.

Krnjević, K., & Phillis, J. Pharmacological properties of acetylcholine-sensitive cells in the cerebral cortex of cat. *Brain,* 1970, **93**, 57–64.

Krnjević, K., Reiffenstein, R., & Silver, A. Chemical sensitivity of neurons in long-isolated slabs of cat cerebral cortex. *Electroencephalography and Clinical Neurophysiology,* 1970, **29**, 269–282. (a)

Krnjević, K., Reiffenstein, R., & Silver, A. Inhibition and paroxysmal activity in long-isolated cortical slabs. *Electroencephalography and Clinical Neurophysiology,* 1970, **29**, 283–294. (b)

Kuffler, S., Dennis, M. J., & Harris, A. J. The development of chemosensitivity in extrasynaptic areas of the neuronal surface after denervation of parasympathetic ganglion cells in the heart of the frog. *Proceedings of the Royal Society of London, Series B,* 1971, **177**, 555–563.

Langer, S. Z., Draskoczy, P. R., & Trendelenburg, U. Time course of the development of supersensitivity to various amines in the nictitating membrane of the pithed cat after denervation of decentralization. *Journal of Pharmacology and experimental Therapy,* 1967, **157**, 255–273.

Lømo, T., & Rosenthal, J. Control of ACh sensitivity by muscle activity of the rat. *Journal of Physiology,* 1972, **221**, 493–513.

McMahan, U., & Kuffler, S. Visual identification of synaptic boutons on living ganglion cells and of varicosities in postsynaptic axons in the heart of the frog. *Proceedings of the Royal Society of London, Series B,* 1971, **177**, 485–508.

Miledi, R. The acetylcholine sensitivity of frog muscle fibers after complete or partial denervation. *Journal of Physiology,* 1960, **151**, 1–23.

Miledi, R., & Potter, L. T. Acetylcholine receptors in muscle fibers. *Nature (London)*, 1971, **233**, 599–603.

Modern, F., & Thienes, C. Vagal and sympathetic endings in the rabbit intestine. *Science,* 1936, **83**, 522.

Murray, J. G., & Thompson, J. W. The occurrence and function of collateral sprouting in the sympathetic nervous system of the cat. *Journal of Physiology (London)*, 1957, **135**, 133–162.

Perry, W. L. M., & Reinert, H. The effects of preganglionic denervation on the reactions of ganglion cells. *Journal of Physiology,* 1954, **126**, 101–115.

Perry, W. L. M., & Reinert, H. On the metabolism of normal and denervated ganglion cells. *Journal of Physiology,* **130,** 156–166.

Purpura, D. P., & Housepian, E. M. Morphological and physiological properties of chronically isolated immature neocortex. *Experimental Neurology,* 1961, **4**, 377–401.

Reas, H. W., & Trendelenburg, U. Changes in the sensitivity of the sweat glands after denervation. *Journal of Pharmacology and Experimental Therapy,* 1967, **156**, 126.

Reiffenstein, R., & Triggle, C. Sensitivity of denervated cerebral cortex to cholinomimetics. *Electroencephalography and Clinical Neurophysiology,* 1972, **33**, 215–220.

Robbins, N., & Fischbach, G. Effects of chronic disuse of rat soleus neuromuscular junctions on postsynaptic function. *Journal of Neurophysiology,* 1971, **34,** 570–578.

Robbins, N., & Nelson, P. G. Tenotomy and the spinal monosynaptic reflex. *Experimental Neurology,* 1970, **27,** 66–75.

Robert, E., & Oester, Y. T. Absence of supersensitivity to acetylcholine in innervated muscle subjected to a prolonged pharmacologic nerve block. *Journal of Pharmacology,* 1970, **174,** 133–140.

Rosenberg, P., & Echlin, F. Time-course of changes in cholinesterase activity of chronic partially isolated cortex. *Journal of Nervous and Mental Diseases,* 1968, **147,** 56–63.

Rothballer, A., & Sharpless, S. Effects of intracranial stimulation on denervated nictitating membrane of the cat. *American Journal of Physiology,* 1961, **200,** 901–908.

Rutledge, L. T. Effect of stimulation on isolated cortex. In H. Jasper, A. Ward, & A. Pope (Eds.), *Basic mechanisms of the epilepsies.* Boston, Massachusetts: Little, Brown, 1969. Pp. 349–355.

Rutledge, L., Duncan, J., & Beatty, N. A study of pyramidal cell axon collaterals in intact and partially isolated adult cerebral cortex. *Brain Research,* 1969, **16,** 15–22.

Rutledge, L., Ranck, J., & Duncan, J. Prevention of supersensitivity in partially isolated cerebral cortex. *Electroencephalography and Clinical Neurophysiology,* 1967, **23,** 256–262.

Sasaki, K., & Otani, T. Accommodation in spinal motoneurons of the cat. *Japanese Journal of Physiology,* 1961, **11,** 443–456.

Schaeppi, U. Comparison of serotonin with directly and indirectly acting compounds in their effect on the nictitating membrane of spinal cats. *Journal of Pharmacology and Experimental Therapy,* 1963, **139,** 330–336.

Sharpless, S. Reorganization of function in the nervous system — use and disuse. *Annual Review of Physiology,* 1964, **26,** 357–388.

Sharpless, S. Isolated and deafferented neurons: Disuse supersensitivity. In H. Jasper, A. Ward, & A. Pope (Eds.), *Basic mechanisms of the epilepsies.* Boston, Massachusetts: Little, Brown, 1969, Pp. 329–348.

Sharpless, S., & Halpern, L. The electrical excitability of chronically isolated cortex studied by means of permanently implanted electrodes. *Electroencephalography and Clinical Neurophysiology,* 1962, **14,** 224–255.

Smith, C. B., Trendelenburg, U., Langer, S., & Tsai, T. H. The relation of retention of norepinephrine-H^3 to the norepinephrine content of the nicititating membrane of the spinal cat during development of denervation supersensitivity. *Journal of Pharmacology,* 1966, **151,** 87–94.

Sokoll, M. D., Sonesson, B., & Thesleff, S. Denervation changes produced in an innervated skeletal muscle by long-continued treatment with a local anesthetic *European Journal of Pharmacology,* 1968, **4,** 179–187.

Spehlmann, R., Cheng, M., & Daniels, J. Excitability of partially isolated cortex. I. Macroelectrode studies. *Archives of Neurology,* 1970, **22,** 504–509.

Spencer, W. A., & April, R. Plastic properties of monosynaptic pathways in mammals. In G. Horn and R. Hinde (Eds.), *Short-term changes in neural activity and behavior,* London: Cambridge University Press, 1970. Pp. 433–474.

Spencer, W. A., & Kandel, E. R. Synaptic inhibition in seizures. In H. Jasper, A. A. Ward, & A. Pope (Eds.), *Basic mechanisms of the epilepsies.* Boston, Massachusetts: Little Brown, 1969. Pp. 575–603.

Spiegel, E. A., & Szekely, E. G. Supersensitivity of sensory cortex following partial deafferentation. *Electroencephalography and Clinical Neurophysiology,* 1955, **7,** 375–381.

Stavraky, G. W. *Supersensitivity following lesions of the nervous system.* Toronto: University of Toronto Press, 1961.

Stephenson, R. P. A modification of receptor theory. *British Journal of Pharmacology,* 1956, **11**, 379–393.

Szentágothai, J. The use of degenerative methods in the investigation of short neuronal connections. *Progress in Brain Research,* 1965, **14**, 1–32.

Taylor, J., & Green, R. D. Analysis of reserpine-induced supersensitivity in aortic strips of rabbits. *Journal of Pharmacology,* 1971, **177**, 127–135.

Thesleff, S. Effects of motor innervation on the chemical sensitivity of skeletal muscle. *Physiological Review,* 1960, **40**, 734–752. (a)

Thesleff, S. Supersensitivity of skeletal muscle produced by botulinum toxin. *Journal of Physiology* (*London*), 1960, **151**, 598–607. (b)

Thorpe, W., & Seeman, P. Effect of denervating skeletal muscle on calcium binding by isolated sarcolemma. *Experimental Neurology,* 1961, **30**, 277–290.

Trendelenburg, U. Supersensitivity and subsensitivity to sympathomimetic amines. *Pharmacological Review,* 1963, **15**, 225–275.

Vazquez, A. J., Krip, G., & Pinsky, C. Evidence for a muscarinic inhibitory mechanism in the cerebral cortex. *Experimental Neurology,* 1969, **23**, 318–331.

Vickerson, F. H. L., & Varma, D. R. Effects of denervation on the sensitivity of the superior cervical ganglion of the cat to acetylcholine and McN•A-343. *Canadian Journal of Physiological Pharmacology,* 1969, **47**, 255–259.

Volle, R. L., & Koelle, G. B. The physiological role of acetylcholinesterase (AChE) in sympathetic ganglia. *Journal of Pharmacology and experimental Therapy,* 1961, **133**, 223.

Waser, P. G., & Hadorn, J. Relations of cholinergic receptors to acetycholinesterase of end-plates in denervated muscle. *Bibliotheca Anatomy,* 1960, **2**, 155–160.

Yellin, H., & Eldred, E. Spindle activity of the tenotomized gastrocnemius muscle in the cat. *Experimental Neurology,* 1970, **29**, 513–533.

Youmans, W., Karstens, A., & Aumann, K. Effect of vagotomy and of sympathectomy on the sensitivity of intestinal smooth muscle to adrenalin. *American Journal of Physiology,* 1942, **137**, 87–93.

CHAPTER V

Electrophysiological Changes after Sensory Deprivation

Austin H. Riesen

Department of Psychology
University of California, Riverside

I. Problems of Neural Function after Deprivation

The functional physiology of a deprived sensory system is altered both peripherally and centrally, and not always in relation to correlated behavioral or anatomical effects. Serious investigations of electrophysiological changes following stimulus deprivation began scarcely more than a decade ago. They started with evidence for delayed maturation of retinal function following early dark-rearing, were then carried into measurable effects on gross evoked cortical potentials, and, more recently, entered the stage of threshold determinations and sophisticated measures of complex wave forms and single cell responses. Variations in the patterns and rates of presentation of test stimuli give evidence for long-term changes in neurophysiological functions.

Developmental studies began with little more than a strictly empirical question: What properties of the response will be altered? Now there are interesting theoretical questions concerning critical period, conditions for recovery, and whether the changes can be explained by such hypothetical concepts as competition for synaptic space or intersensory compensation. With just a few exceptions, the work has concentrated on visual systems.

II. Effects along the Visual Pathway

A. Changes in the Electroretinogram (ERG)

In newborn kittens reared in normal daylight surroundings the b-wave of the ERG first appears during the third week. Under conditions of dark-rearing this component of the response is delayed to the fourth week (Zetterström, 1955–1956). A series of light flashes accelerates the appearance of the b-wave in 21- to 24-day-old dark-reared kittens. (Hellström & Zetterström, 1956), and this effect is correlated in time with an increased sulfhydryl content of nuclear layers of the retina. In older cats, the b-wave is fatigued or is inhibited in its recovery following the elicitation of even a single ERG response when the eye has not had light stimulation for some days or longer (Baxter & Riesen, 1961; Cornwall & Sharpless, 1968). Again, a return to normal stimulation levels soon reverses the effects of withholding light.

Rearing cats in total darkness from birth to 12–18 months or suturing the lid of one eye up to 6 months of age reduced the amplitude of the b-wave about 40% below amplitudes measured in control animals (Ganz, Fitch, & Satterberg, 1968). In this study it was also reported that the longer periods of deprivation, beyond 12 months, resulted in a flicker ERG critical fusion frequency (CFF) that was below normal when small stimulus areas were used or when the intensity of light flash was relatively low. Parallel but delayed recovery functions for the b-wave responses were obtained from the cats with 12–18 months of dark-rearing (Fig. 1). No such effects appeared after monocular lid suturing. Closing the lid over one eye of rhesus monkeys (*Macaca mulatta*) failed to produce any reportable changes in the ERG in several animals kept under this condition up to 56 weeks of age (von Noorden, Dowling, & Ferguson, 1970). The difference in this outcome from that with the kittens in the Ganz *et al.* (1968) study is probably due to the large amounts of diffused light passing through the thin and unpigmented eyelids of the rhesus monkeys.

Effects of light deprivation on retinal responses in the rabbit eye contrast sharply with those for the cat or guinea pig. French investigators (Goswamy, Bonaventure, & Karli, 1967; Bonaventure, Goswamy, & Karli, 1971) discovered an opposite effect of darkrearing on b-wave amplitudes. With darkness from birth and beginning on about the twelfth day, the "total ERG amplitude" of rabbits becomes larger than in control animals. Reuter, Legein, van der Marc, and van Hof (1971) confirmed this early effect in 4-week-old light deprived rabbits, but then found that continuing light deprivation to 7 months resulted in a modest reduction of b-wave amplitudes over a series of intensities. Even at this age, however, response to the initial flash was larger in the dark-reared animals.

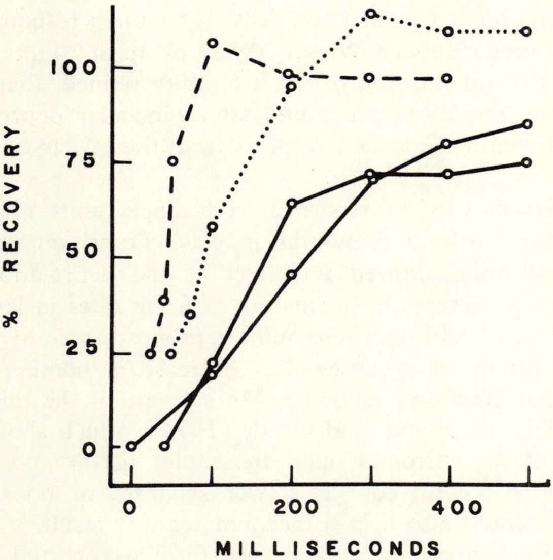

Fig. 1. Recovery functions for the b-wave of the ERG. Interstimulus intervals were varied. Magnitudes of the second b-wave were plotted as a percentage of the magnitude of the first b-wave of a pair. Broken lines are for two cats reared without visual deprivation. Solid lines are for two cats reared 15 and 18 months in darkness. (From Ganz *et al.*, 1968.)

The retinal changes as measured by the ERG have in all studies been found to normalize after a period of normal light stimulation. Whatever the metabolic processes are that underlie the effects, they do include both the sources of the late receptor potential and the standing potential across the eye (Hamasaki & Pollack, 1972), and apparently these metabolic alterations are dissimilar in rabbits and cats. Rhesus monkeys (unpublished data of Ramsey, see Riesen, 1965) respond like the cat, judging from changes in visually mature animals that have been put in darkness for two weeks or have had one eye covered with the other receiving normal light. All indications are that the changes are strictly retinal. They can be developed independently in each eye by monocular deprivation, and cutting the optic nerve has no immediate effects on the responses that are obtained. Depressed ERG amplitudes have been confirmed with human patients after eye patching (Hamasaki & Flynn, 1973).

B. Unit Responses in the Lateral Geniculate Nucleus

Morphological effects of visual deprivation in the lateral geniculate nucleus (LGN) are well established (see Chapter II). Only recently have electrophysiological changes been uncovered. The normal center–surround field organization holds true of LGN cells that remain responsive following either a few months (Hubel & Wiesel, 1963) or up to 20 months (Chow & Stewart, 1972) of lid suturing from birth. With refined quantitative measures, significant alterations are found after binocular deprivation, which are in turn different in important respects from the effects of suturing only one eyelid.

Eysel and Gaedt (1971) recorded from single units after monocular deprivation from birth to 6 months in cats. Transition probabilities in maintained unit firing showed no effect of the deprivation. Off-center neurons showed a decrease in fluctuation of firing rates in layers receiving input from the deprived eye. These authors propose three hypotheses: (1) heightened sensitivity of synapses, (2) decrease in number of synapses, and (3) reduced inhibitory influences. In support of the third hypothesis are the data of Eysel, Flynn, and Gaedt (1971), which show a reduction in the effects of the surround upon the center in the receptive field of neurons fed by the deprived eye. Fewer synapses or poor transmission across synapses could also help to account for this result.

Hamasaki, Rackensperger, and Vesper (1972) reported that 50% of cells from which they recorded, in layers fed by a deprived eye (monocular deprivation to 6 months of age), were abnormal in center-surround receptive field characteristics. For these cells the latency of peak firing rates was about twice the normal time, and the maximum rates were below normal.

Significant questions must be related to selective effects on specific types of cells. Two important studies from the Australian laboratory of P. O. Bishop and his group are the opening attack on this set of issues. Again working with cats, some reared with BD (binocular deprivation) and others with MD (monocular deprivation), Sherman and Sanderson (1972) found that BD produced a significant reduction in the degree of binocular interaction on cells of the LGN, and only a slight reduction resulted from MD. As we shall see, this result contrasts sharply with effects on cortical cells. Also reported in this study was a small reduction in the numbers of binocular units that could be found following lid suturing, whether monocular or binocluar.

Another fundamental distinction of cell types is that between X cells, which have slow axonal conduction rates and which sum center-surround receptive field effects linearly, and Y cells (fast conducting and nonlinear or transient). Comparing nondeprived, monocularly sutured, and BD cats, Sherman, Hoffman, and Stone (1972) obtained results that require going beyond the concept of binocular competition. In both groups of visually deprived cats there was a reduction in proportion of Y cells. With MD, this loss was confined to those laminae of the LGN that were receiving input from the deprived eye. Following BD, the loss was throughout the dorsal lateral geniculate nucleus and somewhat less severe than under MD. This last finding helps to explain some of the behavioral consequences of binocular form deprivation as well as being important for our understanding of changes in electrophysiological responses in the visual cortex. Measurable changes in cell growth have been reported only for geniculate cells of kittens where binocular competition across laminae occurs under MD (Guillery, 1972).

III. Changes in Cortical Responses

A. Visual Evoked Potentials (VEP)

The normal development of visual evoked potentials as recorded at the cortex has been fully described for rats, rabbits, and kittens (Marty, 1962; Callison & Spencer, 1968; Rose & Ellingson, 1970). Similar sequences of a shortening latency of the primary response and an increasing complexity of waveforms, accompanied by the development of individual characteristics of responses to visual patterns and to monochromatic light, are generally true of early mammalian visual development.

Wistar albino rats were reared in darkness or in light (schedule not specified) and studied at 12–45 days for maturation of the gross VEP and the ability of the cortex to follow higher frequencies of stimulation (Callison & Spencer, 1968). Differences in latencies were small and disappeared by 20 days. Cortical following of high-flash frequencies reached highest levels by 30 days in light-reared animals, and by 45 days in the dark-reared animals. "Normalization" in the electrophysiological responses by the visual cortex thus appears to parallel the morphological and biochemical effects of dark-rearing.

Dogs kept in darkness from birth to 5 weeks showed extreme variability of VEP latencies and wave form (Fox, 1971). Whereas latencies in some were longer in the dark-reared pups at 5 weeks of age, older animals kept in darkness for 5 weeks gave slightly shorter latencies than control animals. Biochemical changes were reported to occur only in the pups that were deprived from birth to 5 weeks, not in those deprived from 5 to 10 weeks, or as adults.

When rabbits are dark-reared (all light excluded), the longer latencies and the simplified wave forms in cortical VEPs are retained as long as the dark-rearing continues (Fourment & Scherrer, 1961; Scherrer & Fourment, 1964). Furthermore, a hypersensitivity to light stimulation appears in the nonspecific responses recorded from motor and somatosensory areas.

By contrast to the above, rearing with diffused light permits normal development of the gross visual evoked response. Dzidzishvili (1963) sutured the eyelids of newborn rabbits and obtained the normal developmental sequence. (When he removed the eyes at birth, he obtained what he described as a gradual silencing of the visual cortex.) The gross response to a light flash as measured over the primary visual cortex failed to show any effects of the early restriction of pattern vision or the changes that relate to monocular lid suturing.

Yinon and Auerbach (1973) sutured one eyelid of albino rats before the eyes opened and studied the VEP following this type of monocular pattern deprivation. In view of morphological differences described by Fifková (see Chapter II) some differences in the VEP from the right and left hemispheres were expected. The VEP to flash was indeed larger in the cortex contralateral to the nondeprived eye following stimulation of that eye than it was in the opposite (deprived) eye and cortex. However, even the nondeprived eye and cortex responded with lower amplitudes than did control rats that had both eyes open during rearing. This result and other data derived after eyelid suturing in albino rats require reexamination under rearing conditions that insure absence of retinal damage by light (Noell, Walker, Kang, & Berman, 1966; Fifková, 1972). Damage in the open eye when its mate has been deprived is found to be greater than in control animals receiving light binocularly.

Rearing cats under monocular deprivation by lid closure and thereby with some diffused light entering the eye does alter evoked response over motor cortex and over the suprasylvian area (Glass, 1971). The initial component of the response is present over the suprasylvian but later components are modified by the deprivation. The large positive response in the precruciate gyrus following stimulation of the normally stimulated eye is reduced by deprivation, an effect attributed by the investigator to alterations in the diffuse projection system. These are said to be a consequence of the differing behavioral demands associated with each monocular input.

Reversing the eye suture "effected a gradual acquisition of normal behavior" and development of the normal VER in the precruciate gyrus from the second eye (Glass, 1973). Deficits in late components of the marginal gyrus persisted even to 12 months. This result implies that the geniculocortical system is not involved in the behavioral recovery. These findings with the VER have been confirmed (Ganz & Haffner, 1973).

The effects of total exclusion of light from birth and for as long as 12 months in the rabbit or cat, as determined by cortical response to light flash, are reversed after 2 weeks of living in normally lighted environments (Scherrer & Fourment, 1964). Cortical response to flicker was used by

Baxter (1966) to show that in cats reared in darkness for 12 months the cortex is capable of "following" frequencies up to 50/sec. This compared favorably to results from normal controls. The enhancement of "on" and "off" responses to light in young monkeys tested at 16 months of age was reported by Lindsley *et al.* (1964). Visual deprivation consisted of 23 hr in darkness and 1 hr of diffused light daily. These monkeys showed behavioral "hunger" for visual stimulation (Chapter VII). They pressed levers at exceptionally high repetition rates in comparison with light-reared monkeys when the results of their effort was to turn on briefly unpatterned light. They did not press at unusually high rates to turn on sound or somatic stimulation (Wendt, Lindsley, Adey, & Fox, 1962).

B. Pattern Evoked Responses

Recent studies of vision in human infants are making use of flash exposures of visual patterns to obtain measures of the development of detail vision and the resolving power of the visual system. First found to be effective in evaluating the mature eye and brain (Spehlmann, 1965; Harter & White, 1968), the method provides a complex evoked response, the components of which are sensitive to checkerboard or other high contour patterns when presented to the eye of a human infant or the young of other mammals.

Kittens reared from birth to 6 months wearing diffusing percale hoods showed no evoked response to contour (or contour differences) when recordings were taken over the striate or the motor areas of the brain. Control-reared kittens given the same daily 3 hr of light exposures and playing actively with their experimental littermates without wearing hoods showed consistent differences in latencies of the second positive (P2) component to different amounts of contour (Siegel, Coleman, & Riesen, 1973) in recordings taken over the primary visual cortex. Responses evoked at the motor cortex consisted of a single positive wave peaking at 89 msec. Here the amplitude of the wave was significantly smaller in the kittens reared under the diffused light condition, but there was no effect of contour in either group.

Recordings were taken at a third location in this study. Over the suprasylvian gyrus, the normally exposed kittens showed amplitude differences in the P_2 component as a function of amount of contour. The pattern deprived group showed no such effect of contour. This wave form is more comparable to the contour responses that have been recorded in human subjects from scalp electrodes, inasmuch as amplitudes of P_2 and N_2 components are augmented by checkerboard or striped patterns of appropriate size (Harter & Suitt, 1970).

C. Cortical Single Cell Responses

Cells in the visual cortex that respond selectively to the orientation of a moving (light or dark) edge have shown a dramatic dependence upon early usage for the maintenance of and the further development of specificity of responsiveness. The work of David Hubel and Torsten Wiesel (Hubel & Wiesel, 1962, 1963, 1965, 1970b; Wiesel & Hubel, 1963a, b, 1965a, b) has generated most of the basic findings and inspired widespread interest and concentrated research efforts toward the unravelling of physiological substrates of the effects of monocular and binocular pattern deprivation as well as the consequences of strabismus.

The largest and most rapidly induced effects of monocular deprivation in kittens begin when they are in the fourth week after birth. The sensitive period continues through about 12 weeks of age, at which time several weeks of eye occlusion are required to produce the same deficits that require only a few days at the beginning of the sensitive period. The effect of unilateral eye closure is to reduce drastically the numbers of cells in the visual cortex that remain responsive to stimulation of the occluded eye (Wiesel & Hubel, 1963b, 1965a; Hubel & Wiesel, 1970b). Binocular eye closure results in losses of cells responsive to both eyes (binocular units) and moderate rather than severe losses of monocular units. Some cells also become less selective in their definition of the orientations of the moving edges (Wiesel & Hubel, 1965a, b).

Among binocularly sensitive units are those that are relatively insensitive to stimulation from either eye alone, requiring binocular stimulation and, furthermore, responding most strongly if the identically oriented edges that stimulate the two eyes have a small but precise degree of lateral disparity. These variations about points of exact correspondence are such as would be required for stereoscopic vision. Stereoscopic cells were first reported in the striate cortex of cats (Pettigrew, Nikara, & Bishop, 1968; Bishop, Henry, & Smith, 1971). In monkeys, similar units have been described only within peristriate regions (Hubel & Wiesel, 1970a).

The binocular cortical cells having a high degree of disparity specificity appear relatively late in development and they are highly dependent upon binocular visual experience. Barlow and Pettigrew (1971) studied 109 single cells in kittens at various stages of development. These units were responsive when activated through one eye or the other by stimuli moving along a particular axis, but with binocular stimuli at various disparities Barlow and Pettigrew state, "no sharply peaked responses were ever found in the cortex of kittens with no visual experience [p. 100]." When kittens have been lid-sutured before eye-opening for varying times up to the age of 6 weeks, units are found that show directional selectivity, but fewer than

10% show orientation selectively (Pettigrew, 1972). In these same visually inexperienced kittens "disparity-tuning curves cover a wide range of six degrees or more, even when the receptive field size is as small as two degrees [Pettigrew, 1972, p. 389]."

Synchronous inputs from the two eyes are required during early development if normal binocular function is to appear. Occluding each eye alternately on succeeding days (Hubel & Wiesel, 1965) results in the gradual disappearance of units that respond to more than a single eye. The same study showed that a wide disparity produced by surgery of eye muscles eliminated binocular units. Shlaer (1971) used prisms to control amounts of disparity. Binocular function adjusts to small amounts, such as up to 2° of vertical disparity and somewhat more in the lateral direction. Ten degrees is too wide a disparity for further refinement of fine tuning of stereoscopically sensitive units or even for their survival as binocular units.

A functional dependence for the refinement of orientation selectivity is well demonstrated in several recent studies. Units are present in normal kittens and cats that are relatively more responsive to a "preferred" orientation among all those possible in the frontal plane. Specificity of orientation increases with development under conditions of normal stimulation. If only certain contour orientations are available to the developing visual system, the cells that later are found to respond are restricted to those having sensitivities within a range of about 45° to that orientation or less (Hirsch & Spinelli, 1970, 1971; Blakemore & Cooper, 1970, 1971). Behaviorally, the animals appear to be seeing only the previously experienced sets of contours. As summarized by Blakemore and Cooper (1971), "the brain becomes specialized to detect the commonest features in its visual world [p. 366]."

Exposure of young kittens to spots of light in a visual environment without straight line contours (Pettigrew & Freeman, 1973) gave further evidence for the effects of early experience on the sensitivity of cortical neurons. Kittens were dark-reared to 28 days after birth. Then for 13 days they spent 3 hr daily in a planetariumlike sphere with spot sources of light, none of which was closer together than 3° of visual angle. A detailed study of single cells in two such kittens revealed many cells that were optimally stimulated by moving spots and only two cells that were clearly edge detectors. While the majority of cells were activated from both eyes there was an atypical absence of summation within each cell's receptive field. A control cat that was raised in the dark showed neurons with no clear preference for lines or spots although there was a weak directional preference for the stimulus sweep.

Motion and orientation selectivity of units in area 17 of 6-month-old kittens were markedly reduced (Table I) and a specialization of responsiveness to stroboscopic flash was developed in strobe-reared kittens (Cynader, Berman, & Hein, 1973). These alterations in the basic receptive field organization of the visual cortex can best be interpreted as a set of modifications imposed on a background of innately organized center–surround facilitative and inhibitory interconnections.

TABLE I

RECEPTIVE FIELD PROPERTIES OF CELLS IN THE VISUAL (STRIATE) CORTEX OF CATS REARED NORMALLY OR UNDER STROBOSCOPIC ILLUMINATION TO 6 MONTHS OF AGE. STROBE FLASHES OCCURRED AT 2-SEC. INTERVALS TO STOP MOVEMENT OF IMAGES ON THE RETINAS*

Number of Cells	Normally reared	Strobe reared
Directionally tested	230	84
Direction selective,%	83	38
Orientation tested	248	85
Orientation selective, %	97	15
Strobe tested	121	60
Strobe responsive, %	10	53

* From Cynader *et al.* (1973)

IV. Subcortical Effects, Brain Excitability

A. UNIT ACTIVITY IN THE SUPERIOR COLLICULUS

The effects of pattern deprivation on responses of units in the superior colliculus are in many respects parallel to those in the visual cortex. After MD, cells in both colliculi are driven almost exclusively by the normal eye, and they show motion selectivity (Wickelgren & Sterling, 1969). After BD the normal binocularity of collicular units is markedly reduced, and they no longer show directional selectivity (Wickelgren & Sterling, 1970), a change that resembles closely the effect of decortication in normally reared cats. Furthermore, as in decortication, the cells respond mostly to stimulation of the contralateral eye. A clear implication of these findings is that the unit activity of the superior colliculus in response to visual stimulation in the normally reared cat is strongly dependent upon input from the visual cortex (Wickelgren & Sterling, 1970; Rosenquist & Palmer, 1971). Sherman (1972) points out that the monocular segment of the superior colliculus, when it is studied, might be expected to give essentially normal responses following MD. This region would presumably be spared from the effects of "decortication" resulting from the monocular pattern deprivation.

B. Development of Seizure Thresholds

Long-Evans hooded rats reared under a 12-hr light and 12-hr dark cycle show a steady fall in current intensities required to produce a minimal seizure pattern to approximately 17 days of age, followed by slower but consistent rising threshold levels. Meisami and Timiras (1971) compared rats so reared with other groups, including one group reared in darkness. Somatic growth and hormonal status were compared. The dark-reared animals showed a significant shift in the developmental curve for seizure thresholds in which the threshold values generally and the inflection point were delayed approximately 8–10 days. The dark-reared animals remained more sensitive through the final days of the experiments, terminated at 42 days of age.

Meisami and Timiras conclude that their data are in agreement with reports by others of spontaneous seizures in cats and monkeys after prolonged dark-rearing. We may also relate these findings to those of EEG arousal (Section C).

C. EEG Arousal after Sensory Restriction

The hyperactivty of restricted animals upon first exposures to unfamiliar stimulation has received repeated documentation. Melzack and Burns (1965) sought to discover EEG correlates of these behavioral observations. Beagle dogs reared from 3 weeks of age to 1–2 years in well lighted but visually simplified and spatially limited environments were compared with littermates having a more open and enriched environment. Marked differences of EEG patterns were found from implanted electrodes both in the cortex and in the reticular formation. Novel cage environments or opening the cages for novel visual stimulation were found over a series of spaced trials to result in excessive arousal. The authors proposed that behavioral effects of sensory restriction may be directly related to such arousal and "a failure to filter out irrelevant information."

V. Human Findings and Implications

One deleterious human consequence of environmentally induced specialization in the cells of the visual brain may be traced to early uncorrected astigmatism. Differences in resolving power, even with corrections for astigmatic refractive errors, have been discovered in human subjects and must be ascribed to central neural assymetries in horizontal versus vertical edge detectors (Freeman, Mitchell, & Milledot, 1972). Even laser interference fringes imposed directly on the retina are poorly resolved in the orientation plane of the earlier partial visual contour deprivation.

A reduced total number or a diminished responsiveness of units that respond to contour may be the basis for human as well as animal data showing diminished amplitudes in the cortical evoked potentials to patterned light. In young children an esotropia (cross-eyed condition) is one symptom that is correlated with reduced acuity in the nonfixating eye. This is referred to as "suppression" without any implication that its mechanism is understood. Lombroso, Duffy, and Robb (1960) have shown that evoked potentials recorded over the visual areas of the brain are reduced in amplitude when the amblyopic eye is stimulated by patterned light relative to the response when the other eye is so stimulated. Although not a direct demonstration of mechanism, these results are what would be expected if the condition is associated with the reduced activity of "edge detector" cells in the occipital cortex.

VI. Evoked Potentials after Auditory Deprivation

Electrophysiological studies of sensory deprivation for other senses than vision are scarce. A beginning has been reported in which auditory evoked potentials were compared in two groups of rats, one reared for 8 months in a sound shielded room with ambient sound levels below 15 dB, and the other in which sounds fluctuated between 40 and 80 dB. The results (Batkin, Groth, & Watson, 1970) were expressed as audiograms obtained by determining threshold sound intensities for pure tones as required to elicit cortical evoked potentials. The animals reared under low-sound conditions had significantly reduced sensitivity in the range from 500 to 10,000 Hz. When these animals were brought into the room with louder sounds there was some recovery in some animals after 3 weeks of this noisier condition. Other studies of the effects of sound deprivation have dealt with behavioral measures (Chapter VII).

References

Barlow, H. B. & Pettigrew, J. D. Lack of specificity of neurons in the visual cortex of young kittens. *Journal of Physiology (London)*, 1971, **218**, 98P–100P.

Batkin, S., Groth, H., Watson J. R. & Ansberry, M. Effects of auditory deprivation on the development of auditory sensitivity in albino rats. *Electroencephalography and Clinical Neurophysiology*, 1970, **28**, 351–359.

Baxter, B. L. The effect of visual deprivation during postnatal maturation on the electrocorticogram of the cat. *Experimental Neurology,* 1966, **14**, 224–237.

Baxter, B. L. & Riesen, A. H. Electroretinogram of the visually deprived cat. *Science,* 1961, **134**, 1626–1627.

Bishop, P. O., Henry, G. H., & Smith, C. J. Binocular interaction fields of single units in the cat striate cortex. *Journal of Physiology,* 1971, **216**, 39–68.

Blakemore, C. & Cooper, G. Development of the brain depends on the visual environment. *Nature,* 1970, **228**, 477–478.

Blakemore, C. & Cooper, G. F. Modification of visual cortex by experience. *Brain Research,* 1971, **31**, 366. (EBBS Abstracts)

Bonaventure, N., Goswamy, S., & Karli, P. Electroretinogram and visually evoked responses in rabbits reared in total darkness or in continuous illumination. *Documenta Ophthalmologica,* 1971, **30**, 339–348.

Callison, D. A., & Spencer, J. W. Effect of chronic undernutrition and/or visual deprivation upon the visual evoked potential from the developing rat brain. *Developmental Psychobiology,* 1968, **1**, 196–204.

Chow, K. L. & Stewart, D. L. Reversal of structural and functional effects of long-term visual deprivation in cats. *Experimental Neurology,* 1972, **34**, 409–433.

Cornwell, A. C. & Sharpless, S. K. Electrophysiological retinal changes and visual deprivation. *Vision Research,* 1968, **8**, 389–401.

Cynader, M., Berman, N., & Hein, A. Cats reared in stroboscopic illumination: effects on receptive fields in visual cortex. *Proceedings of the National Academy of Sciences, USA,* 1973, **70**, 1353–1354.

Dzidzishvili, N. N. Electrocorticographical study after exclusion of sight function. *Gagra Symposia,* 1963, **4**, 203–224.

Eysel, U. Th., Flynn, J. T., & Gaedt, Chr. Spatial summation of excitation and inhibition in receptive fields of neurons in the lateral geniculate body of the cat and the influence of visual deprivation. *Pflügers Archiv-European Journal of Physiology,* 1971, **327**, 82–94.

Eysel, U. Th. & Gaedt, Chr. Maintained activity in the lateral geniculate body of the cat and the effects of visual deprivation. *Pflügers Archiv-European Journal of Physiology,* **327**, 1971, 68–81.

Fifková, E. Effect of light and visual deprivation on the retina. *Experimental Neurology,* 1972, **35**, 450–457.

Fourment, A. & Scherrer, J. Réponses électrocorticales du lapin élevé dans l'obscurité. *Journal de Physiologie* (*Paris*), 1961, **53**, 340–341.

Fox, M. W. *Integrative development of brain and behavior in the dog.* Chicago: University of Chicago Press, 1971.

Freeman, R. D., Mitchell, D. M., & Milledot, M. A neural effect of partial visual deprivation in humans. *Science,* 1972. **175**, 1384–1386.

Ganz, L., Fitch, M., & Satterberg, J. A. The selective effect of visual deprivation on receptive field shape determined neurophysiologically. *Experimental Neurology,* 1968, **22**, 614–637.

Ganz, L. & Haffner, M. E. Permanent perceptual and neurophysiological effects of visual deprivation in the cat. *Experimental Brain Research,* **21**, 1974, **20**, 67–87.

Glass, J. D. Photically evoked potentials in cat neocortex altered by visual pattern deprivation. *Brain Research,* 1971, **30**, 207–210.

Glass, J. D. Photically evoked potentials from cat neocortex before and after recovery from visual deprivation. *Experimental Neurology,* 1973, **39**, 123–139.

Goswamy, S., Bonaventure, N., & Karli, P. Sur l'origine des particularités de l'ERG observées chez le Lapin èlévé dans différentes conditions d'éclairement ambient. *Comptes Rendus des Séances de la Société de Biologie,* 1967, **161,** 2628–2631.

Guillery, R. W. Binocular competition in the control of geniculate cell growth. *Journal of Comparative Neurology,* 1972, **144**, 117–130.

Hamasaki, D. I. & Flynn, J. T. Depression of the ERG after patching. *A.M.A. Archives of Ophthalmology,* 1973, **89**, 472–475.

Hamasaki, D. I. & Pollack, J. G. Depression of the late receptor potential and the ERG by light deprivation in cats. *Vision Research,* 1972, **12**, 835–842.

Hamasaki, D. I., Rackensperger, W., and Vesper, J. Spatial organization of normal and visually deprived units in the lateral geniculate nucleus of the cat. *Vision Research,* 1972, **12**, 843–854.

Harter, M. R. & Suitt, C. D. Visually-evoked cortical responses and pattern vision in the infant: A longitudinal study. *Psychonomic Science,* 1970, **18**, 235–237.

Harter, M. R. & White, C. T. Effects of contour sharpness and check size on visually evoked cortical potentials. *Vision Research,* 1968, **8**, 701–711.

Hellström, B. & Zetterström, B. The effect of light on the manifestation of the electroretinogram and on histochemically demonstrable SH-groups in the retina. *Experimental Cell Research,* 1956, **10**, 248–251.

Hirsch, H. V. B., & Spinelli, D. Visual experience modifies distribution of horizontally and vertically oriented receptive fields in cats. *Science,* 1970, **168**, 869–871.

Hirsch, H. V. B., & Spinelli, D. Modification of receptive field orientation in cats by selective visual exposure during development. *Experimental Brain Research,* 1971, **12**, 509–527.

Hubel, D. H., & Wiesel, T. N. Receptive fields, binocular interaction and functional architecture in the cat's visual cortex. *Journal of Physiology,* 1962, **160,** 106–154.

Hubel, D. H., & Wiesel, T. N. Receptive fields of cells in striate cortex of very young, visually inexperienced kittens. *Journal of Neurophysiology,* 1963, **26**, 994–1002.

Hubel, D. H., & Wiesel, T. N. Binocular interaction in striate cortex of kittens reared with artificial squint. *Journal of Neurophysiology,* 1965, **28**, 1041–1059.

Hubel, D. H., & Wiesel, T. N. Stereoscopic vision in macaque monkey. *Nature (London),* 1970, **225**, 41–42. (a)

Hubel, D. H., & Wiesel, T. N. The period of susceptibility to the physiological effects of unilateral eye closure in kittens. *Journal of Physiology,* 1970, **206**, 419–436. (b)

Lindsley, D. B., Wendt, R. H., Lindsley, D. F., Fox, S. S., Howell, J., & Adey, W. R. Diurnal activity, behavior and EEG responses in visually deprived monkeys. *Annals of the New York Academy of Sciences,* 1964, **117**, 564–587.

Lombroso, C., Duffy, F., & Robb, R. Selective suppression of cerebral evoked potentials to patterned light in amblyopia ex anopsia. *Electroencephalography and Clinical Neurophysiology,* 1969, **27**, 238–247.

Marty, R. Development post-natal des réponses sensorielle du cortex cérébral chez la chat et le lapin. *Archives d' Anatomie Microscopique et de Morphologie Expérimentale,* 1962, **51**, 129–264.

Meisami, E. & Timiras, P. S. Influence of early visual input on development of brain excitability in the rat. *American Journal of Physiology,* 1971, **220**, 233–238.

Melzack, R. & Burns, S. K. Neurophysiological effects of early sensory restrictions. *Experimental Neurology,* 1965, **13**, 163–175.

Noell, W. K., Walker, V. S., Kang, B. S. & Berman, S. Retinal damage by light in rats. *Investigative Ophthalmology,* 1966, **5**, 450–473.

Pettigrew, J. D. The importance of early visual experience for neurons of the developing geniculostriate system. *Investigative Ophthalmology,* 1972, **11**, 386–394.

Pettigrew, J. D., & Freeman, R. D. Visual experience without lines: effect on developing cortical neurons. *Science,* 1973, **182**, 599–600.

Pettigrew, J. D., Nikara, T., & Bishop, P. O. Binocular interaction on single units in cat striate cortex: Simultaneous stimulation by single moving slit with receptive fields in correspondence. *Experimental Brain Research,* 1968, **6**, 391–410.

Reuter, J. H., Legein, C. P. J. J. M. M., Van der Mark, F., & Van Hof, M. W. The electroretinogram in normal and light deprived rabbits. *Documenta Ophthalmologica,* 1971, **30**, 349–361.

Riesen, A. H. Effects of early deprivation of photic stimulation. In S. F. Osler & R. E. Cooke (Eds.), *The biosocial basis of mental retardation.* Baltimore, Maryland: Johns Hopkins Press, 1965. Pp. 61–85.

Rose, G. H., & Ellingson, R. J. Ontogenesis of evoked potentials. In W. A. Himwich (Ed.), *Developmental neurobiology.* Springfield, Illinois: Charles C Thomas, 1970. Pp. 393–440.

Rosenquist, A. C. & Palmer, L. A. Visual receptive field properties of cells of the superior colliculus after cortical lesions in the cat. *Experimental Neurology,* 1971, **33**, 629–652.

Scherrer, J. & Fourment, A. Electrocortical effects of sensory deprivation during development. In W. A. Himwich and H. E. Himwich (Eds.), *Progress in brain research.* Vol. 9, *The developing brain.* Amsterdam: Elsevier, 1964. Pp. 103–112.

Sherman, S. M. Visual development in cats. *Investigative Ophthalmology,* 1972, **11**, 394–401.

Sherman, S. M., Hoffmann, K. P., & Stone, J. Loss of a specific cell type from dorsal lateral geniculate nucleus in visually deprived cats. *Journal of Neurophysiology,* 1972, **35**, 532–541.

Sherman, S. M. & Sanderson, K. J. Binocular interaction on cells of the dorsal lateral geniculate nucleus of visually deprived cats. *Brain Research,* 1972, **37**, 126–131.

Shlaer, R. Shift in binocular disparity causes compensating change in the cortical structure of kittens. *Science,* 1971, **173**, 638–641.

Siegel, J., Coleman, P., & Riesen, A. H. Deficient pattern evoked responses in pattern deprived cats. *Electroencephalography and Clinical Neurophysiology,* 1973, **35**, 569–573.

Spehlmann, R. The averaged electrical responses to diffuse and to patterned light in the human. *Electroencephalography and Clinical Neurophysiology,* 1965, **19**, 560–569.

von Noorden, G. K., Dowling, J. E., & Ferguson, D. C. Experimental amblyopia in monkeys. *Archives of Ophthalmology,* 1970, **84**, 206–214.

Wickelgren, B. G. & Sterling, P. Effect on the superior colliculus of cortical removal in visually deprived cats. *Nature,* 1969, **224**, 1032–1033.

Wickelgren, B. G. & Sterling, P. Function of the projection from the visual cortex to the superior colliculus. *Brain, Behavior, and Evolution,* 1970, **3**, 210–218.

Wendt, R. H., Lindsley, D. F., Adey, W. R., & Fox, S. S. Self-maintained stimulation in monkeys after long-term visual deprivation. *Science,* 1962, **139**, 336–338.

Wiesel, T. N. & Hubel, D. H. Effects of visual deprivation on morphology and physiology of cells in the cat's lateral geniculate body. *Journal of Neurophysiology,* 1963, **26**, 978–993. (a)

Wiesel, T. N. & Hubel, D. H. Single-cell responses in striate cortex of kittens deprived of vision in one eye. *Journal of Neurophysiology,* 1963, **26**, 1003–1017. (b)

Wiesel, T. N. & Hubel, D. H. Comparison of the effects of unilateral and bilateral eye closure on cortical unit responses in kittens. *Journal of Neurophysiology,* 1965, **28**, 1029–1040. (a)

Wiesel, T. N. & Hubel, D. H. Extent of recovery from the effects of visual deprivation in kittens. *Journal of Neurophysiology,* 1965, **28**, 1060–1072. (b)

Yinon, U. & Auerbach, E. Deprivation of pattern vision studied by visual evoked potentials in the rat cortex. *Experimental Neurology,* 1973, **38**, 231–251.

Zetterström, B. The effect of light on the appearance and development of the electroretinogram in newborn kittens. *Acta Physiologica Scandinavica,* 1955/56, **35**, 272–279.

CHAPTER VI

Orientation in Visual Space by Neonates and Its Modification by Visual Deprivation

Leo Ganz

Department of Psychology
Stanford University

An encyclopedia article on instinct cited by Spalding (1873) some hundred years ago reads:

> It is likewise said that the chick recognizes grains of corn at first sight, and can so direct its movements as to pick them up at once; being thus able to know the meaning of what it sees, to measure the distance of objects instinctively, and to graduate its movements to that knowledge—all which is, in the present state of our laws of mind, wholly incredible [p. 282].

At the time, the philosophical issue of nativism–empiricism had smoldered for three centuries (Hochberg, 1962), and yet there was still virtually no scientific knowledge regarding the innate competence of organisms to orient themselves in space nor any understanding into genetic mechanisms. Given such ignorance, it was reasonable to be skeptical. Soon thereafter, a visual deprivation experiment by Spalding (1873) yielded the first scientific evidence. He noted that newly hatched chicks were too helpless immediately upon hatching to provide a fair test of their perceptual abilities. Accordingly, just as the chicks began to break out of their eggs, he drew a hood over their head, close-fitting around their neck so that no normal patterned vision was possible. Some wore opaque hoods; others wore translucent hoods allowing homogeneous light but not patterned light. After 1–3 days, he removed the hood and noted their behavior immediately thereafter:

> To take, by way of example, the observations in a single case a little in detail:—A chicken that had been made the subject of experiments on hearing, was unhooded when nearly three days old. For six minutes it sat chirping and looking about it; at the end of that time it followed with its head and eyes the movements of a fly twelve inches distant; at ten minutes it made a peck at its own toes, and the next instant it made a vigorous dart at the fly, which had come within reach of its neck, and seized and swallowed it at the first stroke; for seven minutes more it sat calling and looking about it, when a hive-bee coming sufficiently near was seized at a dart and thrown some distance, much disabled. For twenty minutes it sat on the spot where its eyes had been unveiled without attempting to walk a step. It was then placed on rough ground within sight and call of a hen with a brood of its own age. After standing chirping for about a minute, it started off towards the hen, displaying as keen a perception of the qualities of the outer world as it was ever likely to possess in after life. It never required to knock its head against a stone to discover that there was "no road that way." It leaped over the smaller obstacles that lay in its path and ran around the larger, reaching the mother in as nearly a straight line as the nature of the ground would permit. This, let it be remembered, was the first time it had ever walked by sight. [Spalding, 1873, p. 284.]

Spalding recognized that while initially a philosophical issue, nativism–empiricism was more appropriately a question of fact: one to which the visual deprivation experiment could give an answer. His observations on 20 visually deprived chicks convinced him they had a sense of visual direction, could move their head in the direction of moving objects, could peck at small objects and, therefore, could both estimate distance and translate that estimate into appropriate action, and could direct themselves toward goals without hitting intervening obstacles, again demonstrating an innate competence for perceptual–motor coordination and depth estimation. We shall examine below whether further and more systematic experimentation has supported Spalding. (For a historical analysis of the nativism-empiricism issue, see Hochberg, 1962.)

We see then that visual deprivation studies address themselves principally to three psychological issues. First there is the classical problem of innate competence. Are there specific orienting behaviors or depth-related behaviors which organisms manifest prior to exposure to visual stimuli? Ideally, innate competence should be examined in neonates. Unfortunately, this proves unfeasible in organisms which are embryologically immature at birth. Visual deprivation is then used to postpone the critical first test until a level of neural maturity is reached which permits a fairer test of visual competence. A second issue deals with the question of sustenance and development: What is the essential visual-nurturing environment needed to maintain and perfect that initial competence? By removing one or another aspect from an organism's visual environment, one can determine the essential visual nurturants. The latter are then considered the basic visual–environmental determinants of the development of visual perception. Third, sensory deprivation experiments bear strongly on the question of structure–function relationships. Some visual deprivation treatments are known to induce highly selective atrophic effects in the structures of the visual system (Hubel & Wiesel, 1965; Wiesel & Hubel, 1965a; Ganz, Fitch, & Satterberg, 1968; Hirsch & Spinelli, 1970; Blakemore & Cooper, 1970; Chow & Stewart, 1972; Globus, Chapter II of this volume). Considering these atrophic effects within the logic of an ablation paradigm, one can then examine which visual functions disappear in association with which atrophied structures and, conversely, which structures and functions are dissociated.

In this chapter, we divide deprivation studies into three sections, proceeding from the most to the least severe treatments: (1) binocular pattern deprivation (BD), (2) monocular pattern deprivation (MD), (3) deprivation of visual–motor correlation (V–MCD). Within each section we consider visual–motor tests such as visual placing, visual cliff, and the optokinetic response under separate headings.

The effects of visual deprivation on object shape recognition have recently been reviewed elsewhere (Ganz, 1974); there is no need to cover the same material twice. Accordingly, the present chapter addresses itself to a quite different realm of phenomena: the effects of visual deprivation on behavior in space. For an excellent review of the animal literature of the general area of orientation in space, the reader's attention is directed to Walk (1965).

I. Binocular Pattern Deprivation

As the name implies, binocular pattern deprivation (BD) involves rearing an organism in a visually homogeneous environment devoid of the usual patterned heterogeneities. It is accomplished by either rearing in total darkness, or in diffuse light, or, as is often the case, in a combination of the two. By diffuse light, we mean a homogeneous, patternless light that is obtained by covering an animal with a close-fitting white cloth hood, or fitting it with transluscent contact lenses, or by suturing both its eyelids together surgically. We make no distinction between dark-rearing and diffuse light conditions because the behavioral results that we will consider do not warrant such a distinction. One exception to this general statement has been reported for visual placing (see p. 179). It is true that when dark-rearing has been continued from birth to as long as 24 months, a chimpanzee will show drastic morphological deterioration of the ganglion cell layer of the retina, and, hence, will show a total absence of orientation behavior (Chow, Riesen, & Newell, 1957; Riesen, 1958). In what follows, however, the experimental treatment is much less prolonged. As a result, degeneration of the eye is not present, or, at least, is considerably less serious (Rasch, Swift, Riesen, & Chow, 1961; Weiskrantz, 1958). Therefore, the changes of visual–motor behavior which ensue after shorter periods of deprivation are not attributable to structural changes in the eye. Perhaps the best two reasons for believing this to be true are: (1) dark-reared cats can be shown to have normal powers of resolution (Ganz & Fitch, 1968), and (2) all the deficiencies of visual–motor behavior which result from deprivation and which are described below have been found to return to normal under various postdeprivation environments.

A. Open Field Test

As Spalding (1973) had shown, perhaps one of the simplest tests that have been used to measure orientation in visual space is to place an animal in an environment with a variety of obstacles and observe whether or not the animal avoids them when moving about. Observers agree that a cat reared in total darkness (Riesen, Kurke, & Mellinger, 1953; Walk & Gibson, 1961; Baxter, 1966) or with both eyes sutured closed—a binocular diffuse light condition (Wiesel & Hubel, 1965b)—does not avoid obstacles successfully; it bumps into them. This holds equally true for dark-reared rhesus monkeys (Fantz, 1965; Wilson & Riesen, 1966). In addition, the character of the animal's gait is usually quite abnormal. Walk and Gibson (1961) observed that the dark-reared kitten's locomotion was slow and awkward, with the animal's stomach on the ground; it was really more like a crawl than a walk. Wiesel and Hubel (1963) characterized the gait as broad and hesitant. In the latter study it was also reported that during the actual deprivation treatment, these same kittens, with both their eyes sutured closed, locomoted quickly and unerringly and avoided obstacles well. In other words, with both eyes deprived of pattern vision, the animals adjust. They utilize auditory or other cues with great skill to orient themselves spatially. The initial exposure to visual patterns totally disrupts that adjustment.

Parenthetically, this last observation and others of a similar nature (Riesen *et al.*, 1953) suggest that the initial postdeprivation exposures are typically highly arousing to the deprived organism, so much so that it may be unable to perform tasks on which it has previously shown competence.

For example, in an open field situation a binocularly deprived kitten may locomote fairly rapidly and orient itself surprisingly well with both eyes closed—presumably utilizing nonvisual cues. When its eyes are opened, there is an initial period in which the animal "freezes," or moves about with reckless abandon bumping into many objects. Cataract patients have shown similar disorientations shortly after the cataract removal (von Senden, 1932). The conclusion that new sensory experience induces severe disrupting effects of an emotional nature must make us doubly cautious about concluding that there are deficiencies of competence from evidence consisting of performance failures during initial testing following deprivation.

The effects of binocular deprivation on orientation in an open-field are typically reversible. If exposure to a normal visual environment follows deprivation, recovery is the rule. For example, Baxter (1966) noted that cats reared from birth to about 1 year in total darkness, avoided objects successfully within 10 days if they were kept in a very active, stimulating, and responsive environment. In a typical laboratory cage, the same recovery required about 30 days, and more, sometimes not ever showing recovery.

Another factor regulating the amount of recovery is the length of deprivation. Fantz (1965) found that monkeys dark-reared for $\frac{1}{2}$–11 weeks were avoiding obstacles within 0–4 days after the end of the deprivation period, whereas monkeys kept in darkness for 16 or 20 weeks needed 21 and 30 days of patterned light experience to develop successful obstacle avoidance. In this test, an "obstacle field" was employed. It consisted of a square box with a patterned floor laced with 2-inch-square vertical rods at 9 intervals in one-half of the box. The monkey "demonstrated spatial orientation by repeatedly walking between and around posts without touching them, by following walks and corners, and by reaching for parts and walks." Two of his animals, one deprived for 2 weeks and one deprived for 5 weeks, mastered the task on the very first test. The successful negotiation of an obstacle field with such minimal visual experience is, of course, particularly interesting because it suggests that the monkeys have an innate ability to orient themselves relative to objects in their field of view. If monkeys have this innate competence, whereas monkeys dark-reared for a longer period of time are noticeably poorer (Fantz, 1965; Wilson & Riesen, 1966), then one must conclude that orientation in space is innate. In turn, this implies that visual deprivation suppresses the proper utilization of that innate competence. The fact that Fantz (1965) found that longer recovery time was needed for monkeys who were deprived longer is also consistent with the suppression hypothesis. It is not consistent with the strong empiricist hypothesis: namely, that no directed visual–motor coordination is possible without visual experience. The weaker empiricist hypothesis states that there is an innate framework which permits innate visual–motor coordination in accordance with the momentary details of limb length, muscle strength, etc. If experience is necessary for visual-motor coordination, an animal with short deprivation should be as naïve as an animal with longer deprivation. Hence, they should recover equally quickly. This is not what Fantz found, and, in conclusion, the strong empiricist hypothesis is suspect; the weak empiricist hypothesis, however, is still tenable.

B. Looming

An object that looms is one that approaches fairly quickly and whose retinal area increases in size accordingly. In a normal visual environment, looming signals an imminent collision. Many organisms blink their eyes, dodge their head, and show certain postural adjustments when presented with a looming object (Schiff, 1965). The effect can be simulated by a shadow caster; the critical cue is magnification of sufficient velocity. Crabs, frogs, turtles, kittens, and monkeys (Schiff, Caviness, & Gibson, 1962) all show the response. In man, White (1963) reported that the eye blink to a rapidly approaching object develops at about 2 months of age, but more recent work suggests the response appears earlier and, in fact, may be innate. Following an unpublished observation by T. G. R. Bower that infants respond to symmetrically looming shadows by a complex response that consists of an initial widening of the eyes, a head withdrawal, and a raising of the arms, Ball and Tronick (1971) submitted this observation to systematic scrutiny. Infants ranging in age from 2 to 11 weeks of age were shown the increasing shadow (which simulates approach) or decreasing shadow (which simulates withdrawal) of a necker cube (see Fig. 1). They used either a shadow that increased symmetrically, so that it appeared to an adult observer to be on a hit path toward the infants, or an asymmetrical growth that appeared on a miss path. The response to the hit path was significantly different from the miss path: the infants moved their head back, brought their arms up to their face, and "stiffened" their torso only to the hit path. The response was obtained even in the earliest age groups. No age effect was apparent.

The literature on binocular deprivation is in agreement that BD animals fail to blink to a rapidly approaching object when first tested (Walk & Gibson, 1961; Baxter, 1966; Wilson & Riesen, 1966). According to these reports, the response begins to appear after the animals have been in patterned light for 10–16 days.

C. Reaching for an Object

Does one have to learn to direct one's limbs so as to reach an object that one sees? In other words, is there an innate sense of visual direction for

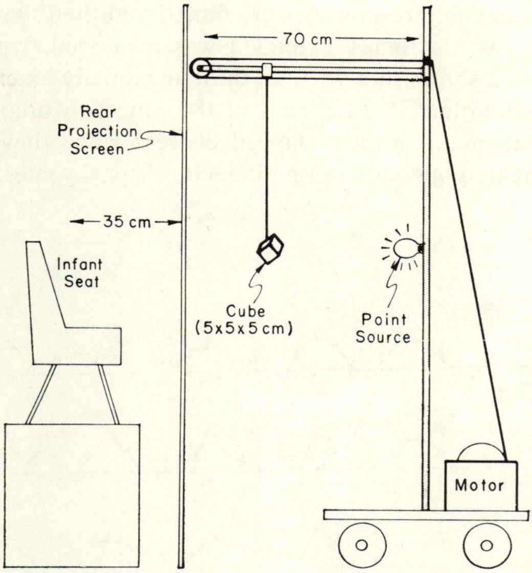

Fig. 1. Shadow-casting apparatus (Ball & Tronick, 1971) used to produce expanding shadows. As the cube moves toward the light source, the shadow thrown on the rear projection screen becomes larger. Such an expanding shadow appears to visually specify an approaching object, even to young infants, and arouse a predictable response.

limb movements? (We will discuss visual direction of the eyes and head in more detail later in the chapter). In an animal such as a cat, rat, or man, it is difficult to study the problem directly in neonates because their control of their limb movements is poor (White, Castle, & Held, 1964). The monkey, however, is far more precocious. For example, in their observations of an infant monkey born in the laboratory, Lashley and Watson (1913) note on day four, "He twice reached out toward Jim [a male monkey] with a quick out thrusting of the arm." More observations of reaching out toward objects, using mostly large limb muscles, were made on days eight, nine, and eleven. With a much larger group of neonates, Hines (1942) observed reaching for an object on day three. Fantz (1965) tested infant monkeys' ability to locate objects by presenting a bottle at different positions in the monkey's visual field and looking for repeated reaching with hand or mouth. Animals reared in the dark just a few days showed correctly directed reaching after a single day of visual experience.

In a recent study (Bower, Broughton, & Moore, 1970), a careful investigation of the reaching behavior of human neonates was carried out. Neonatal infants (all reportedly delivered without medication) between 6 and 11 days of age were presented a small orange ball, at a number of locations. Their reaching responses were filmed and then the angle of reach when the hand was maximally extended was measured from film by two observers. Figure 2 shows that 75% of these maximally extended responses were found to be within 5° (1.5 cm) of the object. Moreover, they were able to show that infants always showed distress when they reached for a virtual object, created optically using binocular disparity cues, a reach which

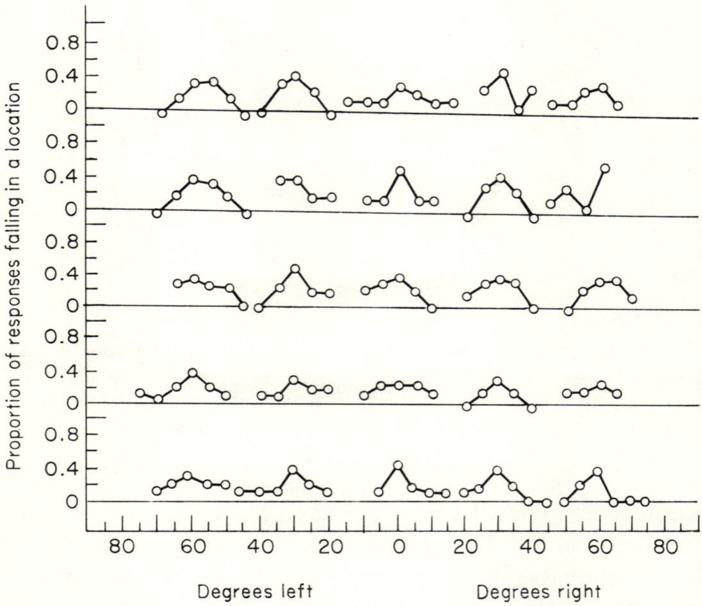

Fig. 2. Summary graph showing the frequency distribution of reaching responses of several infants. The responses were measured from cinematic records at the point when the limb was maximally extended. (From Bower *et al.*, 1970.)

could not satisfy its intention. This distress was interpreted to mean that the reach was a purposeful one.

Dark-reared animals typically will not reach toward an object (Fantz, 1965; Wilson & Riesen, 1966). If the deprivation is shorter than 5 weeks, fairly well-directed reaches are obtained after 1 day of visual experience (Fantz, 1965). With longer periods or deprivation, the amount of visual experience needed before correctly directed reaching is obtained becomes progressively greater.

In summary, the evidence is still somewhat sketchy. What there is suggests that either no experience is necessary, or at most something of the order of a day of visual experience is required to obtain appropriately directed, though not very accurate, movement of limbs in the direction of visually presented objects. This certainly suggests a genetically determined competence. The system subsequently gains considerable precision as a result of visual experience; conversely, that system of competences is made less accessible to the animal, that is, it is suppressed by the absence of visual experience. The amount of this suppression is apparently monotonically related to the amount of binocular deprivation. There is also a suggestion that this eye–limb system matures during the neonatal period, since Foley (1934, 1935), Hines (1942), Lashley and Watson (1913), and Tinklepaugh and Hartman (1932) only observed reaching after at least 3 days of postnatal visual–motor experience, whereas Fantz observed reaching after 1 day of visual experience in slightly older animals who had been given a very short dose of dark-rearing.

D. Visual Placing

If a cat that has had no visual deprivation is held by the torso with forelimbs free, and is brought slowly toward a horizontal surface, it will extend its paws in the direction of that surface, in a manner appropriate for an impending landing, as shown in Fig. 3 (lower right quadrant). Visual placing has been widely studied, systematic investigation starting probably with Rademaker (1931), and with Warkentin and Smith (1937). This response is not obtained in neonatal kittens, but does not depend on any experience with patterned light (Hein, Gower, & Diamond, 1970b). In their study, kittens were dark-reared to 6 weeks of age. When they were permitted to move freely in a lighted environment while wearing translucent plastic occluders over sclera and cornea, 4.5 and 16 hr of diffuse light, all kittens showed a visual placing response. Therefore, this response is innate.

The diffuse light treatment appears to be essential because cats reared from birth to 6 weeks of age in darkness do not show visual placement (Riesen & Aarons, 1959; Walk & Gibson, 1961). Other studies have reported similar results (Wiesel & Hubel, 1965; Baxter, 1966; Wilson & Riesen, 1966). Therefore, early diffuse light experience appears to either potentiate or sustain the genetically provided circuits through the postnatal period of neural maturation. Once dark-reared cats are placed in a normal patterned light environment, they develop visual placing in a few hours (Riesen, 1961b; Ganz & Fitch, 1968; Hein, 1970) after a short period of dark-rearing.

An interesting comparison can be made with Warkentin and Smith's (1937) study where it was reported that newborn normal kittens required 22–28 days before showing a visual placing response. Thus, the older but

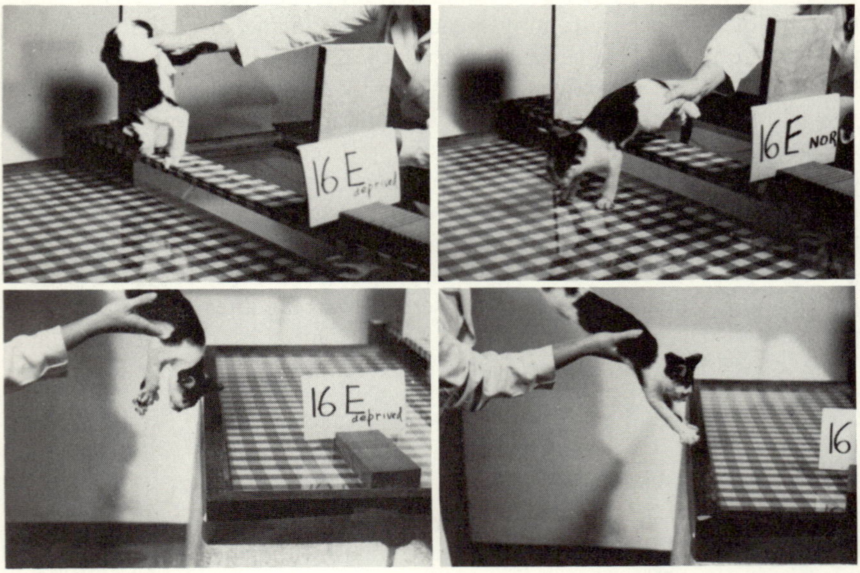

Fig. 3. A monocularly reared cat being tested for resistence to descent on the shallow-appearing side of the visual cliff (top panels) and for visual placing (bottom panels). Only the deprived eye is open in the left panels, and only the normal eye is open in the right panels. (From Ganz & Fitch, 1968.)

visually equally naïve dark-reared kittens visual-placed with much less visual experience than the normal neonates. We conclude, first, that there is a strong maturational component in the visual placing response which reaches completion at about 1 month of age. Once it is completed, small amounts of light exposure, even if simply diffuse light, seem sufficient to trigger the response.

Another observation which supports the notion of a maturational factor comes from Warkentin and Smith's data. Kittens that open their eyes at day three postnatally show their first visual placing response at the same time—namely, 22–28 days of age—as those that open their eyes on day fifteen. The additional 12 days of visual experience that the first group has, as compared to the second, makes no difference. This suggests that the visual placing response is not dependent on patterned visual experience prior to the completion of a specific maturational sequence. But the simplest and most direct proof comes from the Hein *et al.* (1970b) observation that visual placing is found in kittens after 4 weeks of diffuse light-rearing. Thus, the extensor response of the forelimbs to a rapidly expanding surface texture appear to be in large measure maturational. The one effect of dark-rearing seems to be negative, namely to cause a moderate delay in the appearance of the response. It becomes temporarily suppressed, but can be retrieved with 1 hr, or slightly more, of appropriate experience. In other words, visual deprivation suppresses performance, but not competence.

In recent years, a more demanding version of the visual placing response has been developed (Hein & Held, 1967). As shown in Fig. 4, the kitten is brought toward a serrated surface with one forelimb free. A successful

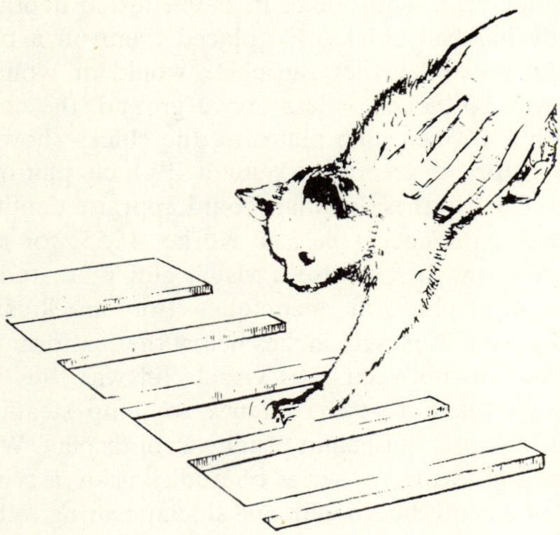

Fig. 4. A normal kitten showing a visual placing response on the serrated edge apparatus. (From Hein & Held, 1967.)

landing requires an accurate placement of that forelimb onto one of the protruding prongs. Diffuse light-reared kittens perform very poorly, whereas normals land almost invariably onto a prong. Thus, kittens deprived of pattern vision show simple visual placing but fail on the serrated edge test.[1]

[1] Hein and Held (1967) have shown that the two forms of visual placing responses can be dissociated: following diverse types of visual deprivation, kittens will show the classical visual placing response but fail on their serrated edge apparatus (see also Hein & Diamond, 1971b). On this basis they have concluded that the classical visual placing response is visually elicited, while the response to the serrated edge is visually guided. They have therefore termed the second response a visually guided placing response. We believe, however, that such terminology is premature and possibly misleading. The classical test involves visual guidance of the forelimbs on the basis of depth cues. In Fig. 4 (bottom, right panel) it can be noted how the forelimbs are

This appears to establish the fact that the development of precise perceptual–motor coordination requires visual experience. Later in the chapter we will analyze in greater detail the specific character of that visual experience.

E. Visual Cliff

Somewhat informally, but with elegant simplicity, Spalding (1873) noted that young pigs, reared with a blindfold, jumped off a small platform quite readily. In a similar vein, Thorndike, in 1899, tested depth discrimination ability of recently hatched chicks. He placed them on a pedestal of particular height and noted whether the chick would or would not descend. If the platform was 10 inches or less above ground, the chicks descended immediately; with a 16-inch high platform, the chicks showed a latency of several minutes before descending. With a 39-inch platform, the chicks never descended. Clearly these animals could appraise depths visually prior to extensive visual experience (see also Kurke, 1955, for similar results). Waugh (1910) was the first to use a visual cliff in a study on mice. He adapted Thorndike's platform technique. For an illusion of greater height he placed a pane of glass 4 inches below the platform and illuminated it so that the glass was not seen. The visual cliff was thus higher than the actual cliff. Waugh found that the latency to jump steadily increased in accordance with the apparent height of the visual display. Walk and Gibson (1961) performed an extensive series of studies using a type of visual cliff which consisted of a centerboard with one side appearing to be deep and the other shallow looking (see Fig. 5d). One of the measures they used was the proportion of descents on the shallow side. Many species were tested, and many visual parameters of the cliff were explored. It was clear, at the outset, that a very large number of species of various ages showed a strong aversion for the deep side of the cliff. This seemed to hold for all—chicks, goats, lambs, rats, cats, monkeys, humans—except certain species such as water turtles for which depths do not necessarily hold danger in their natural environment.

---

aimed at the approaching surface edge. Moreover, no double dissociation has yet been demonstrated. One would have to demonstrate an animal that guided its limbs on a left–right basis, but did not respond to the depth cues of the classical test, which appears implausible but not impossible. Without double dissociation, the difference between the two tests may simply be one of problem difficulty rather than a difference in the quality of visual guidance. Given these hesitations, we are loathe to call the response to the serrated edge a visually guided placing response, since this implies, falsely we believe, that the classical placing response is not visually guided. Therefore, we use here and recommend the adoption of more neutral terminology: *serrated edge test* and *visual placing on the serrated edge test.*

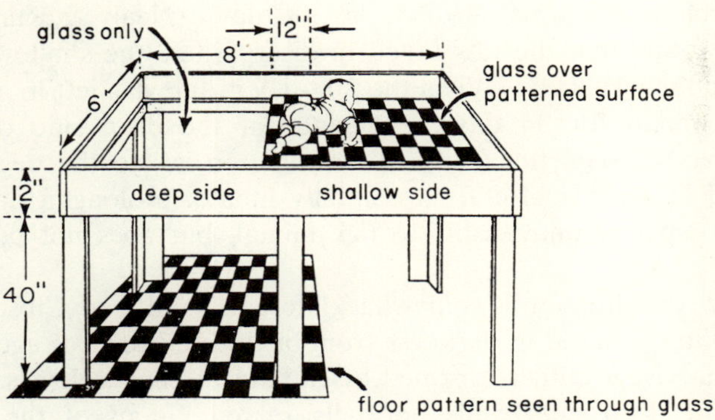

Fig. 5. Visual cliff apparatus. An infant is stepping off the centerboard toward the shallow-appearing side. (From Walk & Gibson, 1961.)

Is this aversion innate? With neonatal chicks, and a fairly coarse pattern under the glass, 76% of the descents were on the shallow side and 6% on the deep side (10 inches under the glass). It would seem that an innate appreciation of depths is an intrinsic part of the chicks' visual system. Similar observations were made on ungulates which are motorically precocious at birth, for example, goats and lambs. For them also, then depth perception is innate. It is not difficult to appreciate why a mountain goat, which can walk immediately after birth, must be able to appraise cliff depth without extensive trial and error pretraining.

With an animal such as a rat or cat—which is motorically immature at birth—testing on the visual cliff must be postponed until the animal can step off the centerboard without difficulty. Toward this end, animals have been dark-reared and then tested. Some basis for believing that rats have innate depth perception had existed since Lashley and Russell's study (1934). They had shown that rats on a jumping-stand gauge the force of a jump in accordance with the distance from the jumping stand to the landing area. Lashley and Russell then applied this fact to test a group of rats raised in darkness. They found that for a series of distances, force was nearly as accurately related to the gap distance as in light-reared rats. This seemed to establish an innate basis for depth perception in rats. Because the study had several possible flaws—food odor cues might have been present, pretraining on the jump stand was carried on in the light—a fresh experimental attack on the problem using the visual cliff apparatus was very welcome. Rats reared from birth to 90 days performed as well as normals on the visual cliff (Walk, Gibson, & Tighe, 1957; Walk & Gibson, 1961). This was later replicated (Nealy & Edwards, 1960). However, if dark-rearing was carried on for longer time periods, such as 140 days

(Walk, Trychin, & Karmel, 1965), or 300 days (Nealy & Riley, 1963), then it was found that the rats failed to discriminate the shallow from the deep side on the visual cliff. When the 300-day group was left in a patterned light environment for 34 days, avoidance of the deep side of the cliff returned. We see then that depth discrimination is—to the degree that it is measured by the visual cliff—essentially innate; prolonged dark-rearing makes that capacity unavailable to the animal, but does not permanently destroy it.

In the cat, the situation is somewhat different. Walk and Gibson (1961) found that kittens raised in darkness from birth to 27 days of age, and then tested on the visual cliff, performed essentially at chance levels. They did not avoid the deep side, while normally reared kittens of the same age stepped on to the shallow side 87% of the time, and not once onto the deep side. Subsequently, the kittens were maintained in darkness, but brought out only once each day for visual cliff testing. Avoidance of the deep side gradually improved until the animals were performing essentially perfectly after 7 days. One might at first conclude that the kittens were learning to avoid deep places as a result of their reinforcement history during the seven daily 10–15 min experience periods. But a moment's thought will show that just the reverse is true. Since the only visual experience the cats obtained was on the cliff itself, what they should have learned was that both sides of the centerboard are equally safe. Therefore, since the depth avoidance emerged counter to any reinforcement effects, we must assume the experience on the cliff did not train the kittens to avoid depths, but merely helped uncover an innate capacity that was there all along, but was either not potentiated or was even actively suppressed as a result of the dark-rearing. In other words, the postdeprivation experience affected performance, not knowledge. It is as if some general experience with visual patterns is necessary to activate, or prime, or release, the cat's depth-evaluation/depth-avoidance mechanism.

The same conclusion can be drawn from other deprivation studies (for example, Held and Hein, 1963). Cats were reared in darkness to 8 and 12 weeks of age. Some of the kittens—the so-called active group—were then brought out and given 3 hr of experience walking in a circular maze. While the active kitten had a great deal of patterned visual experience, it had essentially no experience in falling off edges. After being reared this way for an additional 3–21 days, they were tested on the visual cliff and all animals showed strong aversion to the deep side. Thus, with kittens, generalized active experience with visual patterns is sufficient to develop an aversion to depths.

The monkey responds to the visual cliff and to dark-rearing in a manner quite similar to the cat. In one study it was found that young monkeys of about 10 days of age stepped on to the deep side of the cliff (Walk & Gibson, 1961), but seemed to locomote abnormally while doing so. Another study on neonatal monkeys found that they discriminated depth at least at 3 days of age (Rosenblum & Cross, 1963). In the youngest group tested (3 days of age), 62% of the descents were on the shallow side and only 10% were on the deep side. The behavior of the monkeys also differed when placed on the deep rather than on the shallow side of the visual cliff: they were observed to give many more signs of distress when on the glass overlying the deep side; this behavior was not manifested when they were placed on the shallow part. After periods of dark-rearing ranging from 3 days to 20 weeks, all but 2 monkeys failed to discriminate shallow from deep (Fantz, 1965; Wilson & Riesen, 1966). The two exceptions in Fantz' study are most interesting since they discriminated deep from shallow on the very first tests after being removed from the dark. In other words, they discriminated depth innately. Fantz found that recovery of the aversion to the deep side in a ½–3-week deprived group requires 0–4 days of patterned light; a 5–8-week deprived group required 19–27 days (Wilson & Riesen obtained comparable recovery values); a group deprived 11–20 weeks did not recover within the observation period. In other words, the longer the dark-rearing, the more the capacity is suppressed, and the longer the recovery period needed to regain the function. Again, this monotonic relationship supports the notion of an innate competence. The alternative does not make sense. One would have to conclude that long-term dark-rearing could cause the animals to not know depth more profoundly than short-term dark-rearing. It seems intuitively clear that total ignorance cannot take a variety of values and be more or less profound.

The conclusions we draw from visual cliff experiments are the following. First, an innate aversion to visually presented depth is present in a wide variety of species. This, in turn, depends on the animal's ability to estimate depth in space. Walk and Gibson (1961) have shown that the most probable mechanism underlying such depth estimations is a monocular mechanism, more specifically motion parallax. To use the motion parallax cue, the organism must notice, as it moves its head while locomoting on the centerboard, that the centerboard is in motion relative to a stable background. In addition, such relative motion must be innately associated with avoidance and escape behavior. On the "near" side, there is no such relative motion; both centerboard and background move nearly together. Therefore, the fact that neonates discriminate near from far means they can make relative velocity judgments, and attach meaning to those judgments. It is of some interest, in this regard, that motion-sensitive and orientation selective cortical neurons have been found in neonatal and visually naïve kittens (Hubel & Wiesel, 1963; Pettigrew & Freeman, 1973).

The second conclusion we can draw is that extended dark-rearing appears to hamper effective performance on the cliff. It does not destroy the capacity of the organism to appraise depth and avoid it. We conclude this from results during recovery from dark-rearing that show an organism does not need experience in seeing an edge, then falling off from that edge, and the like to gradually build up a fear of heights. General pattern experience is sufficient. We would conclude, then, that in cats, visual pattern experience of a nonspecific kind is necessary to maintain the innate structures that mediate depth avoidance, but is not necessary to develop those structures.

F. Head and Ocular Pursuit Movements

The question analyzed here is, first, whether visual direction is so well coordinated with the extra-ocular muscle control system and the system controlling the head that pursuit movements are present innately. Second, we shall inquire into the effect of dark-rearing on this system. The requirements of such a system are far from trivial. If an infant fixates an object, and that object moves to the right, a correct pursuit movement depends on generating a compensatory saccade which will take the eye to where the object will be expected to be shortly thereafter. This, in turn, depends on at least three judgments: (1) the direction in which the object has moved, (2) the speed of its motion, (3) whether the movement was self-generated (reafferent) or externally generated (exafferent). For example, when the eyes are accurately pursuing a set of stripes, there is little motion on the retina. This must be interpreted as equivalent to real motion of the distal environment. In turn, this interpreted motion must be used to continue the commands to the eyes so as to maintain them in motion.

When a large, slowly moving field of large stripes is presented (see Fig. 6), one can obtain pursuant movements of the eyes and head, the so-called optokinetic response. This effect was first reported by Bárány (1908). It consists of a slow pursuit phase in which the eyes deviate in the direction of the moving stripes followed by a rapid jerk in the opposite direction, the so-called saccadic return. With newborn kittens, observations of head nystagmus in an optokinetic drum have been made on the first day after eye opening (Warkentin & Smith, 1937). It is true however, that thinner lines are often not pursued until after a month of maturation has elapsed. Electrically recorded optokinetic responses obtained from a naïve and an experienced eye are shown in Fig. 7. The response comprises a saccade, which appears in the records as an abrupt departure from the ongoing base line, followed, threafter, by a tracking movement, which appears as a smooth decay toward the base line. The reader should note particularly that an eye exposed only several hours to patterned light will show smooth tracking.

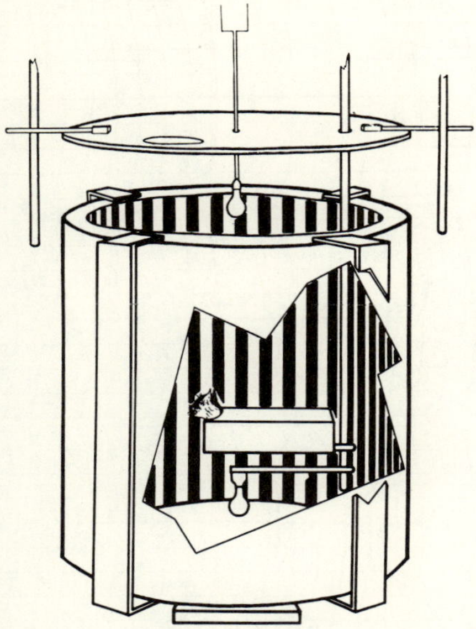

Fig. 6. A cat in an optokinetic drum. (From Smith, 1937.)

Rock, Tauber, and Heller (1965), presented a large, moving array of horizontally moving vertical stripes to a school of guppies as they dropped out of the mother at birth or soon thereafter. The newborn fish pursued the moving stripes immediately. Ordy, Massopust, and Wolin (1962) observed eye movements in rhesus infants on the day of birth to stripes 36 min of arc. These were found in all four rhesus monkeys tested, even though the authors used a very conservative estimate of optokinetic response. The eye movements were characterized as "prompt, sustained, rhythmic, and properly directed ocular responses [p. 375]." Acuity improved steadily over the next 30 days until, at the end, strong responses were obtained by a 4-min of arc line. McGinnis (1930) carried out a similar study in human newborn infants and also reported pursuit movements. He used an optokinetic drum virtually covering the infant's entire visual field. With such an apparatus, nystagmus of the head and eyes occurs as early as a few hours after birth. A response is always obtained if the infant is awake and not distressed. These same infants pursue a moving object during the next 2 weeks, but these pursuit movements are often interspersed with movements in the opposite direction.

Moving a single object in the visual field is a much less potent instigator of pursuit movements. But here, too, innate pursuit movements are observed. (McGinnis gives an excellent review of the literature prior to 1930.)

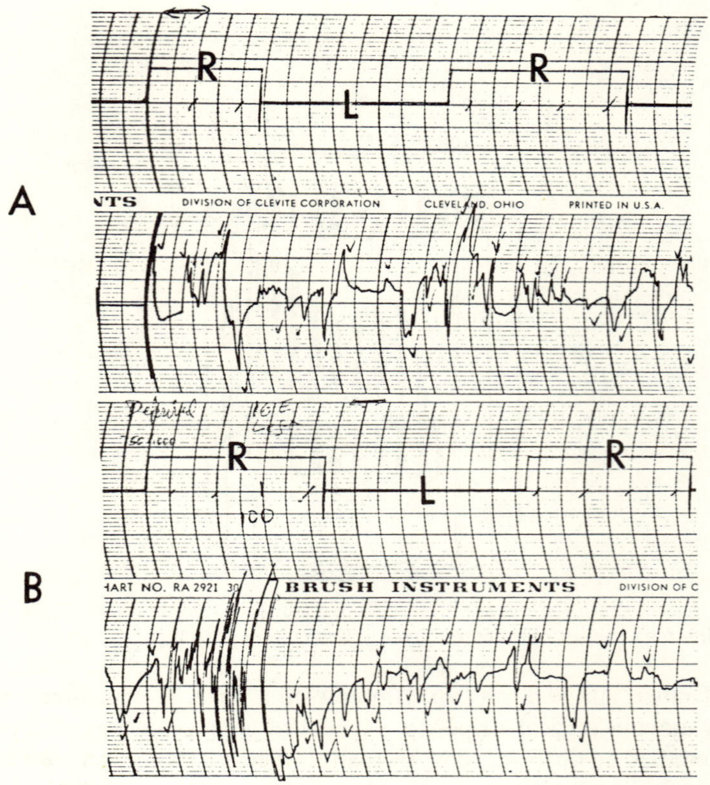

Fig. 7. Optokinetic response recorded from a monocularly reared kitten on the first trial, following deprivation. Eye movements were recorded using the electrical technique. The top record was taken while only the normal eye was open; the bottom record was recorded while only the deprived eye was open, several hours after that eye was opened (Ganz & Fitch, 1968). The stimulus artifact denotes the direction of movement of the optokinetic drum. The stripes were 2° 23′ in width, and the radius of the drum was 50 cm, with the cat's eyes at the center of rotation. The drum was rotated slowly to and fro by hand, at a velocity of 1–2 rpm. The vertical arcs on the record denote 1-sec divisions. **R** and **L** refer to the directions of motion of the moving drum. The check marks denote saccade-tracing pairs of eye-movements. Time constant of the amplifiers: 10 sec. Note should be taken that the deprived eye shows saccades followed by smooth tracking movements, shown here by the smooth return to the base line.

Infant rhesus monkeys 4 days old will follow, with their eyes, an object about 4 in away which is moved slowly across their visual field (Mowbray & Cadell, 1962). A few days later, appropriate head movements are added as part of the response. Human infants have been observed to pursue visually an object moving horizontally in their visual field soon after birth (White *et al.*, 1964). The pursuit movements often consist of a series of jerky refixations and tend to be large. When the direction of the moving object is changed, the latency period before the eye movements change direction is comparatively long. These characteristics give the pursuit movements a jerky quality. During the next 6 weeks the movements become more refined, pursuit can be carried for a longer duration, and the latency of response to a change in direction is reduced. In humans, smooth tracking is reported to occur at about 1 month of age (White *et al.,* 1964). As the infant matures, an increasing number of head-movement responses are added.

Gorman, Cogan, and Gellis (1957) obtained visual data on 100 human newborn infants using the optokinetic response. They obtained acuity estimates in the range of 11–33 min of arc.

What are the effects of binocular deprivation? After early dark-rearing, pursuit movements in an optokinetic drum are less readily obtained (Riesen, 1958: chimpanzee, 28 weeks of dark-rearing plus 1½ hr diffuse light per day). The pursuit of small objects is often missing when first tested (Riesen, 1958; Walk & Gibson, 1961; Baxter, 1966; Wilson & Riesen, 1966). Typically, these responses return after 4–15 days in patterned light. In one study, neonatal monkeys were given either 3 or 9 weeks of patterned-light deprivation and then were tested in an optokinetic drum (Riesen, Ramsey, & Wilson, 1964). The animals showed pursuit movements in the optokinetic drum immediately. There were acuity losses, but these had disappeared by the second day of testing.

The pattern that emerges, then, is of a system which is genetically determined. Pursuit movements of the head and eye are essentially present at birth. This, in turn, implies that organisms can evaluate visual direction and velocity, and can compensate for reafferently generated motion. During the early days of life, the system undergoes a maturational progression in which the organism becomes capable of following smaller objects and of following more smoothly, in general. The jerky pursuit movements of the neonate probably reflect the operation of a cruder system, one requiring a larger error signal before a correctional eye movement is made. Dark-rearing or binocular diffuse light rearing seems to suppress the oculomotor system, but recovery is typically quite rapid.

G. Conclusions

Many mammals are born with an innate competence to orient themselves in space by means of visual cues. At the moment, there is no reason not to believe that all mammalian species with adequate visual resolving powers possess this innate competence. Some, such as cat and man, may require postnatal maturation, but not visual experience. Neonatal organisms have been shown to orient their eyes so as to follow moving grids, avoid obstacles, reach for objects in roughly the right direction, and to visually place and avoid depths. In analyzing these accomplishments, we have concluded that the neonates must be capable of analyzing, at the very least, visual direction, have the capacity to orient the eyes and limbs with respect to a given visual direction, evaluate visual motions as to both direction and velocity judgments, attach avoidance responses to certain relative velocity situations, and discount self-produced motion (i.e., compensate for reafferent motion). Visual-motor experience probably enhances the performance precision of many of these competences. Conversely, these capacities can all be suppressed by early dark-rearing or diffuse-light rearing. By suppression we mean that some knowledge or capacity that the organism has is, for a particular period, inaccessible to it, even though that knowledge or capacity can be shown not to have been abolished. After it is removed from the depriving environment, recovery ensues. However, longer visual deprivation invariably deepens the degree of suppression. With deeper suppression, recovery is slower and requires a more active interaction with the environment.

II. Monocular Pattern Deprivation

There have been at least two main reasons for rearing animals with visual experience in one eye and no patterned-light experience in the other eye. The first stems from early criticisms directed at deprivation experiments. Since sensory deprivation admittedly created excitable, overwrought animals, animals who had difficulty habituating to irrelevent stimuli (Thompson & Heron, 1954; Riesen, 1961; Melzack, 1962), conclusions about sensory deficits would be hazardous if such animals failed to perform in mazes, failed to form differentiated conditioned reflexes, and the like. The ideal control seemingly would be the animal itself. If it failed to perform using its deprived eye, but remained successful when using its normal eye, then one could not invoke characterological explanations involving general emotional, motivational, intellectual, or disposition states; with such results, one could justifiably conclude that the deprived-eye sensory–motor system suffered a disadvantage—for whatever reason—when compared to its experienced-eye counterpart. The second reason (Chow & Nissen, 1955; cf. Riesen *et al.*, 1953) was related to a theoretical question regarding empiristic versus nativistic theories of perception. If shape recognition depended on neural Gestalten generated in the central nervous system by the stimulus —as, for example, Lashley's interference waves—it seemed reasonable to expect that a discrimination learned through an experienced eye would transfer interocularly to the deprived eye. An empiristic theory (for example, Hebb, 1949), on the other hand, would predict that such interocular transfer depended on prior experience, specifically the simultaneous use of the two eyes in a patterned-light environment. This question has been resolved. Interocular transfer occurs from an experienced to a deprived eye (Meyers & McCleary, 1964). Apart from the methodological considerations and the specific issue of interocular equivalence, the monocular deprivation experiments have generated some new and interesting observations, to which we turn.

A. Open Field Test

If we rear a cat with one eye open and one eye closed, and then test it with his deprived eye in an open field with a variety of obstacles, it invariably bumps into obstructions and locomotes hesitantly, with its feet broad based (Riesen & Mellinger, 1956; Wiesel & Hubel, 1963; Wiesel & Hubel, 1965b; Ganz & Fitch, 1968; Dews & Wiesel, 1970). In this regard, certainly on first testing, the results are not much different from those obtained with binocularly deprived animals.

One possible difference that emerges is that the monocular animals require a longer period of time to recover than the binocularly deprived. For example, in their first report on the effects of deprivation in cats, Wiesel and Hubel (1963) observed very little recovery. In a later report (1965b) some recovery was found after 2–3 weeks of experience. With their deprived eye, the kittens started avoiding large objects, but not small ones. Ganz and Fitch (1968) tested some MD subjects 14 days after the deprived eye was opened. There was virtually no improvement in the open field behavior. After the animals had been given 3–5 months of binocular patterned light, they began to avoid obstacles when tested only with their deprived eye. But, even then, their behavior was most peculiar. Frequently, for example, they would approach an object up to a distance of about 5–8 in, slow down, and jump back, as if startled, when their vibrissae contacted the object. The startle suggested poor depth perception and poor recognition abilities. The only monocular animals that recovered full or nearly full visual–motor competence were those given a reverse-suture treatment: the experienced eye was sutured closed and the deprived eye was left open for a period of time comparable to the initial deprivation treatment. After such a treatment, the more active cats jumped across gaps, estimated depth accurately, approached objects with confidence, and showed other signs of recovery described later in this chapter (see Dews & Wiesel, 1970). The less active, more fearful animals showed little recovery, even with reverse-suture treatment.

Monocularly reared cats fail both the classical VP and serrated edge tests with their deprived eye when first tested (Riesen & Mellinger, 1956; Ganz &

Fitch, 1968; Dews & Wiesel, 1970). As an illustration, we see in Fig. 4 (bottom, left panel) an MD cat brought toward the surface edge. It lies relaxed, even limp in the experimenter's hands, showing no response. A moment later, when this cat's vibrissae touched the edge of the table, the tactual stimulation then elicited a prompt and strong extensor response. Therefore, the deprived animal shows tactual placing but not visual placing.

Recovery on the VP_1 test is typically rapid, occurring within the first 2 weeks in every animal tested (Ganz & Fitch, 1968). This includes animals raised as long as 6 months with monocular deprivation. Recovery on the serrated edge test depends on the length of the deprivation period (Dews & Wiesel, 1970). If the deprivation period is 4½–6 weeks long, recovery is fairly rapid, requiring only simple binocular pattern experience. When the monocular deprivation is much longer, 12–16 weeks, then binocular pattern exposure during the recovery period, no matter how long, is insufficient to develop performance on the serrated edge test. After long monocular deprivation, one must apply the reverse-suture procedure for several months before recovery occurs.

B. Visual Cliff Test

Monocularly reared cats do very poorly on other tasks requiring depth estimation. A very simple test of this deficiency involves placing the MD cat on a small platform ten cm or so above the table (Riesen & Mellinger, 1956; Wiesel & Hubel, 1963; Ganz & Fitch, 1968). With only its experienced eye open, the cat often steps off the platform immediately, walking forwards, placing one forelimb and then the next one down onto the table without hesitation. With only its deprived eye open, the cat will show a much longer latency before stepping off—sometimes staying 20–30 min immobilized and frightened—and then slowly back off, placing one hind limb slowly back until the table is touched, and then the next, and so on. Some animals are much less inhibited; those can be observed to walk off a table surface into thin air (Wiesel & Hubel, 1963). On the visual cliff test they fail to discriminate the two sides (Ganz & Fitch, 1968). As might be expected, they tend not to descend from the centerboard on either side. The visual cliff test can be modified to determine the animal's passive avoidance of the two sides of the cliff. The animal is held by the hind limbs and directed toward one or the other side. The animals' resistance is then estimated by a magnitude estimation procedure. In Fig. 4 (top, left panel), a cat is shown with his deprived eye open, being pushed toward the shallow side of the cliff. It resists strongly. The adjoining photograph shows the same cat with its experienced eye; it does not resist. The measure we have used is the difference in estimated resistance—resistance toward the deep side and resistance toward the shallow side. It has proved a more sensitive test with deprived animals than the spontaneous descent procedure. The results indicate that MD cats do not show greater passive avoidance of the deep than of the shallow side (Ganz & Fitch, 1968).

What recovery of function do we obtain in monocularly deprived animals on the visual cliff? The version of the test involving spontaneous descents of the animal from the centerboard shows improvement after 14 days of binocular experience, particularly in the short-deprivation groups. The animals now descend twice as often on the visually shallow side than on the visually deep side. On the forced descent version of the test, again 14 days after the monocular suture is opened, resistance to being pushed on the deep side was three to four times as great as resistance toward the shallow side. Again, the animals with shorter deprivation periods showed greater recovery (Ganz & Fitch, 1968). Eventually, all animals tested showed strong avoidance of the deep side of the cliff (Ganz & Fitch, 1968, Table 6). Recovery occurred even without a reverse-suture treatment. Thus, the passive avoidance of cliffs, and the appreciation of depth based on monocular cues, on which this response depends, appears to be temporarily suppressed by dark-rearing—whether monocular or binocular—but recovery occurs fairly readily. Recovery is slower when deprivation is longer, as in the BD studies (Fantz, 1965; Walk *et al.*, 1965).

We can compare the speed of recovery in a binocular and a monocular experiment, both involving animals that were usually deprived for 4 weeks. In Walk and Gibson's study (1961), when the deprivation period was over the binocular kittens were brought out of the dark for a few minutes each day. This was a period just long enough to test them on the cliff. The animals initially descended equally frequently on the deep and on the shallow side of the cliff. By the end of the seventh day, they were performing perfectly, descending onto the shallow side on every trial. Thus, they required a total of about 1 hr of visual experience. The monocular kittens (Ganz & Fitch, 1968), after 2 weeks of continuous patterned light experience, were descending onto the shallow side about two thirds of the time. We see, then, that recovery of depth fear on the visual cliff is much slower in the monocular group.

C. Head and Ocular Pursuit Movements

Monocularly reared animals often show weak pursuit movements of head and eyes (Chow & Nissen, 1955; Riesen & Mellinger, 1956; Wiesel & Hubel, 1963; Wiesel & Hubel, 1965; Ganz & Fitch, 1968). Large objects, or very bright ones, are sometimes pursued intermittently; small objects often are not pursued at all. In an optokinetic drum (see Fig. 6), which can provide

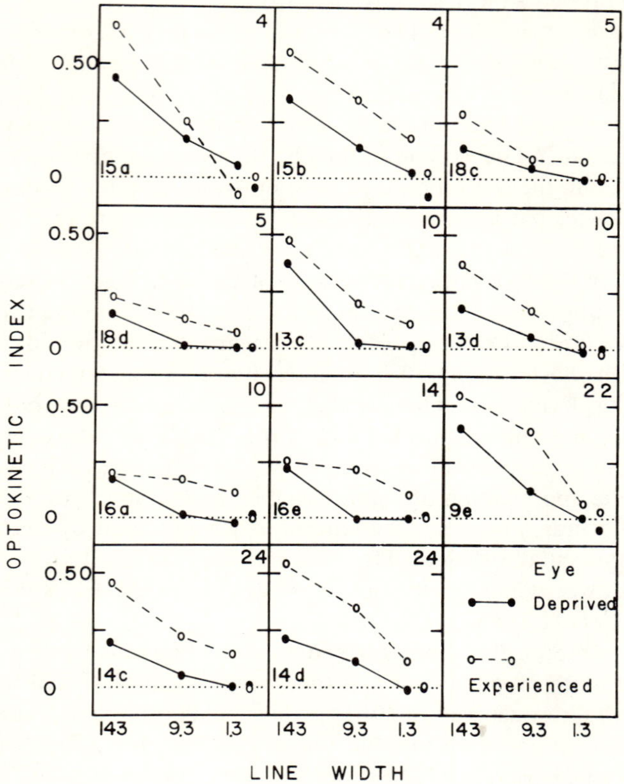

Fig. 8. Visual acuity in the monocularly reared cat as measured by the optokinetic response. Each frame represents the results of a single animal. The number in the upper right refers to the period of deprivation in weeks. The number in the lower left corner identifies the animal. The abcissa depicts the various line widths employed. The ordinate is a measure of the eye-tracking tendency of the eye (see Ganz & Fitch, 1968, for details).

very powerful cues for pursuit motions of the eyes, we have observed correctly directed and smooth ocular pursuit in all monocularly reared animals on the first day of testing. One such EOG record is shown in Fig. 7. These tests started immediately after the termination of the deprivation treatment. The fact that smooth tracking movements are found even on the very first tests indicates, we believe, an innate basis for these pursuit movements.

Nevertheless, it was found that all monocularly reared animals showed a greater disposition toward following moving lines with their experienced eye than with their deprived eye. The optokinetic index (for details, see Ganz &

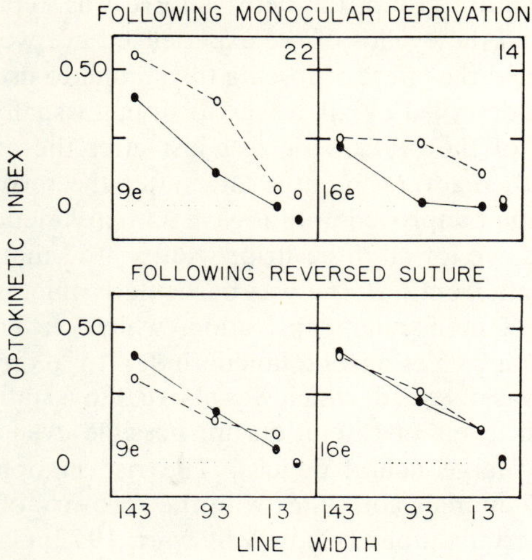

Fig. 9 The effect of a cross-suture treatment on the optokinetic response of a monocularly deprived eye. The solid line represents data taken from stimulation of the initially deprived eye; the dashed line represents experienced-eye data. Note that the deprived eye improves after cross-suture treatment. (From Ganz & Fitch, 1968.)

Fitch, 1968) of 11 monocularly reared cats is shown in Fig. 8. A high index is an indication of a high ratio of tracking movements in the direction of stripe motion. The index of 0 indicates a total absence of tracking. We see quite clearly that the index is higher when the cats use their experienced eye than when they use their deprived eye (all testing was monocular). This holds true for all the different line widths. The cats are less disposed to follow even supra-threshold stimuli, such as 143 min of arc stripes with their deprived eye. We interpret this finding to mean that visual stimuli are less able to elicit arousal and orienting when presented to the deprived eye, even when there are no problems of resolution. This suggests the optokinetic index may be a good indicator of the amblyopic character of the deprived eye. The animal in effect neglects stimuli, even those which are clearly suprathreshold, presented to the deprived eye. If this is true, then it becomes interesting to inquire into the effects of various exposure conditions on the optokinetic index during the recovery period following deprivation. One recovery group was left with both its eyes open for several months, and then retested with each eye separately. There was essentially no recovery. The optokinetic index of the deprived eye was still noticeably weaker in its disposition to track moving lines than that of the experienced one (for details, see Ganz & Fitch, 1968).

In the reverse-suture group, the deprived eye was kept open during the recovery period and the eyelids of the experienced eye were sutured closed. Presumably, this had the effect of forcing the animal to use visual cues coming in through its deprived eye if it was to orient visually at all. Figure 9 shows the results of the optokinetic test just after the original monocular deprivation, and then several months later after the reverse-suture period. The deprived eye had improved until it gave an optokinetic index equivalent to the experienced eye for all three stripe widths: 143 min, 9.3 min, and 1.3 min of arc. The data from Cat 16e was particularly interesting. This cat received 4 months of monocular deprivation, which we know induces very severe neural changes. Yet an optokinetic index to a very fine line of 1.3 min of arc width was obtained, which was above 0 to a statistically significant extent. Thus, high levels of resolution are possible even after the animals suffer surprisingly large neural deficits. The rise in optokinetic index in cross-sutured MD animals correlates with the recovery of some abilities to perform shape discriminations (Chow & Stewart, 1972; Ganz, 1972; Ganz & Hafner, 1974).

We do not have adequate data with which to compare the effects of monocular and binocular treatments on the optokinetic response. It is noteworthy, however, that binocularly deprived monkeys showed essentially normal optokinetic performance levels several days after the termination of the deprivation treatment (Riesen *et al.*, 1964), whereas monocular cats, without reverse-suture treatments, show a permanent reduction in performance. It has been shown that MD cats have a very small percentage of cells remaining in their visual cortex which are highly selective to motion and contour orientation (Wiesel & Hubel, 1963, 1965a; Ganz *et al.*, 1968). Binocularly deprived cats show moderate losses. There is, therefore, a reasonable correlation between the behavioral and neurophysiological deficits.

III. Deprivation of Visual–Motor Correlations

We have seen the many ways in which the visual environment elicits appropriate behaviors, often with minimal practice. The placing response is elicited by a surface expanding and gradually superimposing itself over another surface; depth avoidance responses of various kinds are elicited in the presence of texture gradients moving at different velocities on the retina; an object moving relative to its background elicits an appropriately directed reaching response, and so forth. In each of these situations, a predictable response repertoire emerges, given the right eliciting environment, either innately or after a small amount of priming experience. Dark-rearing generally suppresses these responses. We now turn to a more subtle deprivation treatment. What would be the effect of preventing the customary response repertoire from occurring in the presence of an eliciting stimulus? In this type of deprivation treatment, we allow the animal to emit the response repertoires; at other times we allow it to experience patterned stimuli; but we prevent the concurrence of a subset of stimuli with a subset of responses. Let us call it visual–motor correlation deprivation (V-MCD).

First, we will discuss the results of this treatment on discrimination behavior. Then we will return to our main topic of orientation in space. In the first experiment of this sort (Riesen, 1958), an infant chimpanzee was reared in darkness and then exposed to light for 1 hr and a half a day while held supine on a horizontal surface. The subject could see the ceiling, walls, light source, and moving persons in the laboratory, but was unable to see much of its body, particularly not its limbs. In the dark, the animal could move freely. Thus, neither afferent stimulation nor motor activity were totally deprived. Each was experienced, but experienced in isolation, never the two together. The deprivation thus involved only certain concurrences; the animal could see many objects but not its limbs; it could move, but not see its movements. Other movement–sensory concurrences, such as eye and head movements correlated with vision, were permitted during the deprivation period. In other words, the chimp was deprived only of experiencing a subclass of visual–motor correlations. The treatment was carried to 7 months of age. Other experimental animals were either kept in total darkness without interruption or given only diffuse light during the $1\frac{1}{2}$-hr period. A control animal was reared in darkness and given pattern light experience under conditions of free mobility. The results revealed that on some aspects of orientation in space, the visuo–motor deprived chimp did as well as the control animals and was superior to the animals who were totally deprived of pattern vision; it showed a strong optokinetic response to moving stripes; it pursued a single moving object with eyes and head; it fixated a person; and showed a startle response to a looming figure. This of course, is not surprising, since all of these activities could be exercised by the animal during its supine experience period. They all involved tasks whose visuo-motor correlations the chimp had experienced. But, interestingly, it proved deficient on some tasks. For example, learning to discriminate visually a milk bottle from other objects of similar size but different shape and color was deficient. This was an interesting finding because the sheer sensory contents of the experimental and control animals were not very different. The distinguishing treatment consisted in the control animal receiving visual stimulation while it was moving about, while the experimental animal did not. Therefore, a discrimination deficit seemed to be attributable to an absence of visual–

motor concomitance. A later experiment by Riesen and Aarons (1959) confirmed this result. Kittens were raised in total darkness to 6 weeks of age. At that age, their dark-rearing was interrupted once each day by 1 hr of visual experience. A form deprived group (BD) was given diffuse light; a visuo–motor-correlation deprived group (V-MCD) was given normal pattern vision; the latter was held in a stocklike arrangement and could see normal stationary and moving objects, such as moving laboratory personnel. The cats could move their heads, eyes, limbs, and torsos, but could not see their limbs or torsos, nor could they touch the objects that they were seeing. An unrestricted pattern vision group was given normal visual pattern experiences while locomoting freely in an exercise pen. At the end of the deprivation period they were presented with a fairly difficult movement discrimination task. Neither the V-MCD nor the BD group could solve it within 3700 trials. The control group learned the problem within 640–1709 trials. The severity of the loss of discrimination ability was surprising. This was especially so because all the experimental animals had learned an intensity discrimination in the same apparatus as quickly as the controls; they, therefore, had no difficulty with orientation in space. This entire study was repeated and extended (Riesen, 1965), and the basic findings replicated. We see once again that on a relatively simple problem, such as an intensity

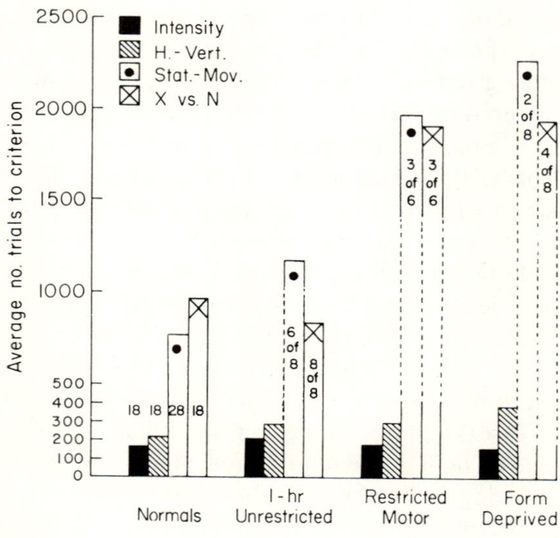

Fig. 10. Visual discrimination learning by cats after four rearing conditions (training limit, 1000 trials). The restricted motor group was deprived only of specific visual–motor concomitances. (From Riesen, 1965.)

difference between two windows, all groups are roughly comparable. In other words, the lack of visual–motor correlation does not induce disorientation in space permanent enough to affect the learning of a discrimination in a Yerkes alley. The same holds true for a simple form orientation problem (horizontal versus vertical stripes, Fig. 11). For such problems as a discrimination between a moving versus stationary dot, or a discrimination between an X and an N, the form deprived group and the visual–motor correlation deprivation group were severely deficient, both groups equally deficient. It is perhaps not so surprising that a group totally deprived of form vision should be deficient in discriminating forms. What is surprising is that the V-MCD group is equally poor. Their deficit in form discrimination caused by lack of visual–motor correlation, is independent of the capacity to orient in space and, as will be seen below, outlasts disorientation effects. The two effects are quite distinguishable. It has been suggested, with much evidence to support it, that many of the effects of visual deprivation are attributable to visuo–motor coordination deficiencies (Meyers & McCleary, 1964; Held, 1968). However, it appears equally true, judging from the studies just cited, that deprivation treatments induce form discrimination deficits independent of such coordination deficits. (This issue is analyzed elsewhere in greater detail; see Ganz, 1974.)

The experiments of Riesen and his associates established an important point, namely that the deprivation of concurrences between sensory input and motor outflow is sufficient to induce temporary deficits in orientation in space and more permanent deficits in shape discrimination. This occurs even though sensory input per se is normal enough. In analyzing just what it is of which the animals are deprived, two possibilities suggest themselves. Let us consider first the stimulus–response suppression hypothesis: the kittens are deprived of reinforcement for responses in the presence of their visual eliciting stimuli. The animals' locomotion in space is drastically reduced in the presence of visual stimuli. As an illustration, we can visualize a kitten seeing a mouse scurrying about; the kitten trys to move toward the prey, but its legs hit the restraints of the box in which it is held. Thus, this particular response tendency tends to extinguish for lack of a rewarding environment. Approaching, crouching, pouncing, reaching, orienting, attending, with respect to visual stimuli, all fail to be followed by consummatory acts. In fact, most of these actions are impossible under the conditions of restraint. These movements are therefore expected to extinguish in the presence of visual stimuli. In other words, visual stimuli lose their effectiveness in controlling the animal's behavior because of a deprivation of S–R contiguities. In a sense, the animals become binocularly amblyopic. This explanation is merely a simple application of learning theory: stimuli presented contiguously with no responding become associated with no responding.

A slightly different but by no means incompatible model is the reafference hypothesis: the kitten is deprived of a particular source of reafferent stimulation, the sight of its moving limbs and torso. Other reafferent stimulation—for example, movement of the visual field following movement of the head and eyes—are still present. In a series of important experiments, Held and Hein (Held & Hein, 1963; Hein & Held, 1967; Hein, Held, & Gower, 1970a; Hein, Gower, & Diamond, 1970b; Hein & Diamond, 1971a, b) have attempted to extract the limb–reafference-deprivation component and examine its effects. They believe that the reafferent perception of a moving part of the body is essential for the development of coordination between that body part and the sensory organ receiving the reafferent input. In one experiment (Hein & Held, 1967) 6 kittens were reared in darkness until 4 weeks of age. Then they were brought out for 6 hr a day and allowed to move freely while wearing a lightweight opaque collar (see Fig. 11). The collar did not

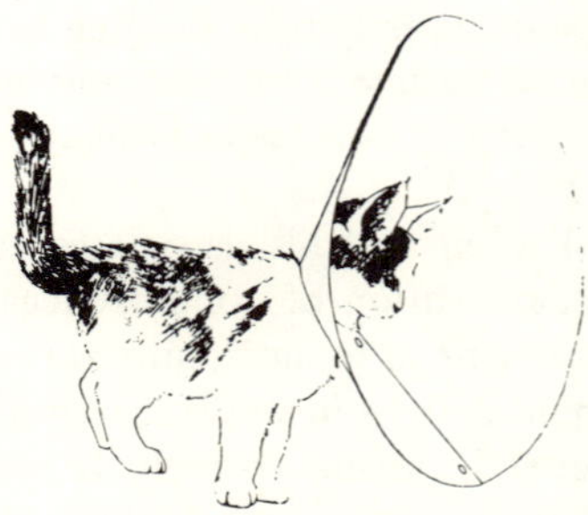

Fig. 11. Kitten wearing a collar that prevents sight of limbs and torso. (From Hein & Held, 1967.)

interfere with locomotion but prevented sight of the limbs and torso. The remaining hours were spent in the dark. After 12 days, the kittens were tested on the classical visual placing test and all of them showed the extension response. However they all failed on the serrated edge test. Hein and Held observed that the cats made a stereotyped response, some repeatedly positioning the paw in front of the nose, others in front of the shoulder joint, etc. As the animals were carried downward, the extended limb fell just as frequently through the empty cutout in the serrated edge as it landed on a prong. Therefore, they concluded, the kittens who were deprived of concurrences between sight of their limbs and movement of their limbs suffered deficiencies in visually mediated guidance of those limbs. In another test of eye–paw coordination, a ball was dangled in front of a cat. The collar-reared kittens showed normal head and eye orientation, but were unable to strike the ball as accurately as the normally reared kittens. In other words, the kittens whose exposure to light had previously been coupled with the opaque collar showed deficiencies in eye–paw coordination.

In a recent series of analytic experiments, Hein and his colleagues have shown that the effects of visual–motor correlation deprivation can be astonishingly specific. In one experiment (Hein *et al.*, 1970a), the two eyes were dissociated (their Experiment 3; Condition A). Kittens were reared in darkness for 5–12 weeks of age, then given special visual exposure. For 3 hr/day the V-MCD kitten could walk freely about a room while wearing an opaque collar (as shown in Fig. 11) which prevented it from seeing its limbs and torso; the remaining time was spent in darkness. Control kittens were treated identically, except that they wore transparent collars so that they could see their body during self-produced movement. After such experience, the V-MCD kittens showed the simple placing response to an approaching edge, but failed on the more demanding serrated edge. Several variations of this basic experiment were conducted. For example, in Condition B, both eyes were exposed together while the opaque collar was worn, but only one eye was exposed when the transparent collar was worn. The same results were obtained. Therefore, these authors conclude that the deprivation of correlations between self-initiated movement and visual stimulation, specifically of the organism's own limbs and torso, prevents the normal development of visuomotor coordination. Each eye must receive its own set of correlated visual feedback.

In a further series of experiments (Hein & Diamond, 1971a), it has been shown that if the visual–motor correlation exposure period is in dim light, there is no transfer to bright light. Furthermore, visually guided experience with one forelimb does not transfer to the other limb (Hein & Diamond, 1971b); animals that had seen a binocular view of one limb during the exposure period were able to guide that limb to the prongs on the serrated edge, but when tested with a limb not viewed prior to testing, they performed at chance levels. These results suggest that the role of correlated visual feedback is highly specific. But it cannot settle the question whether the deprivation has induced a highly specific loss of or prevented the development of highly specific visual–motor connections. When one notes that the period of visual exposure in the Hein *et al.* experiments is given at 5–12 weeks of age, a period during which as little as 6 hr is sufficient to induce a measurable deterioration in the pattern of neural connectivity (Hubel & Wiesel, 1970), then it is not implausible to consider that specific losses may be induced by the deprivation treatment. Since decorrelated visual input has been shown to be detrimental to capacities, such as visually guided extension responses (Hein *et al.*, 1970a), there is in effect no difference between the two positions: a loss in neural connections or a change as a result of decorrelated experience. The only remaining empirical question involves an estimate of the degree of innate capacity. Parenthetically, it might be noted that the absence of interocular transfer is puzzling, when one recalls that: (1) visually naïve cats show interocular transfer of form discriminations (Meyers & McCleary, 1964), (2) adult humans invariably show interocular transfer of visuo–motor adjustment to prism-induced displacements of the visual field (Harris, 1965), (3) visual cortex neurons of visually naive cats are preponderantly binocular in their connections (Wiesel & Hubel, 1963).

One aspect of the V-MCD experiments that is worthy of note is that recovery has been very rapid: performance on the serrated edge improved markedly in one study (Hein & Held, 1967) after only 18 hr of patterned light experienced without hood. Even faster recovery was present in another experiment (Hein, 1970). In this study, neonatal kittens were wearing opaque collars whenever they received visual exposure. On the thirty-sixth day, they were given several hours of monocular exposure with a transparent collar with one eye open. Then they were tested for visual placing (VP_2 test). When using the eye which had viewed through the transparent collar, the animal could guide its limbs to the prongs of the interrupted surface and to the swinging balls. When the other eye was used—the one that did not benefit from these several hours of experience—the animal failed to reach accurately either for the prongs or the ball. The second eye acquired the capacity within as little as an hour.

There are two aspects of Hein's collar experiments which are of great interest concerning the question of the development of visually guided behavior. The first has to do with the extremely fast appearance of visual placing on the serrated edge test following deprivation.

It will be recalled that there are two theoretical positions on which the visual–motor deprivation experiments bear: the empiristic, and the nativistic model.

First, the empiristic theory of the development of visual–motor coordination of Held and his colleagues (Hein & Held, 1962; Held & Freedman, 1963) can be described as follows: when an observer moves with respect to the various objects in his everyday world, his view of them changes. Their images move on his retinas in a manner highly correlated with his movements. Thus, any one of his movements tends to cause a characteristic sensory feedback. The central nervous system retains information concerning the correlation between the output signals which originate the movements and the sensory input dependent in part on that movement (reafferent stimulation). The retention of this correlational information is thought to be essential for maintaining accurate sensory–motor control. Evidence comes in part from studies on adaptation to wearing displacing prisms. These studies show that full compensation is achieved only where the subject is actively moving his limbs while wearing the prisms (for a review of these findings, see Held & Freedman, 1963). It is an essential aspect of the theory that each limb movement in each direction of visual space for every position of the eyes, and, separately, for each position of the head entails a specific set of values that the nervous system must keep track of to permit eye–limb coordination (Held & Freedman, 1963). It is important to realize that according to this position, for accurate visuo–motor coordination an animal must match every position of the head and eyes with some visual feedback of where the hand was after a particular movement. Therefore, thousands of correlations are required for each limb separately. Held and Hein have extended this theory to apply equally to the development of visual–motor coordination. Very simply, they do not believe that an organism is born with correlated information about the position of his limb in his visual field after a particular efferent pattern is sent downstream, given some particular position of head and eyes. Thus, the thousands upon thousands of correlations must be gradually built up through experience seeing the limb while it is moved. Every part of the visual field must be separately calibrated for every separate direction of the head and eyes. Two tests of the empiristic theory become (1) speed of learning and (2) breadth of transfer from training to test. If this theory is correct, we expect slow learning of visual–motor coordination and a narrow transfer.

Second, a more nativistic model (that is, a weak empiristic position) simply asserts that many species are born with a nervous system which permits the evaluation of visual direction and permits to a first approximation the mapping of visual directions onto reaching and locomotor movements. After maturation is completed, which, in the cat, requires about 30 days, movements will be elicited in correct directions, but with poor accuracy. Modifications and refinements of the basic S–R linkages occur every time an organism intends a movement (that is, perhaps an active, voluntary movement) and receives feedback information of a discrepancy between intent and result. (For a recent learning theory formulation of the plasticity underlying visual–motor coordination, see, for example, Taub, 1968.) When an animal is exposed to a visual–motor correlation deprivation—because he is faced with an extinction situation—he learns to suppress most limb movements in the presence of a visual environment. The suppression then accounts for the poor performance on the VPG Test and in reaching for a ball. A few hours with a clear collar give the animal some reinforced responses toward visual goals. For example, the kitten sees a step through the transparent ruff, intends to step up onto it, and succeeds. Such reinforcing experiences reduce the general suppression of limb movements, and allow the animal to show what he knew all along. That the kitten has knowledge of where to point his limbs is indicated by two facts in Hein's results. First, the rapidity of the learning. If a kitten really does not know how to aim its limbs so as to reach objects seen visually, it appears unlikely that the kitten can learn all the necessary correlations of limb reafference on one hand with every visual direction and every position of torso and head, in a few hours. Those who disagree cannot have spent much time teaching a kitten a simple visual–motor association. How can kittens acquire what must constitute thousands of separate motor–sensory feedback correlations in a few hours? It seems implausible. It is equally implausible that monkeys learn visually guided reaching by 3 days of age, when directionally correct (if crude) reaching movements are shown. Therefore, they must have had much of this knowledge to begin with. Second, we note that in Hein's experiment there is extensive transfer of learning. The kittens with transparent ruffs were locomoting on the floor. Yet, they transfer to very different combinations of torso and head involved when the kitten is brought toward the serrated edge in the visual placing test, or when the kitten is standing on three legs, its head raised, and its arm swatting a moving ball. Certainly, there must have been one kitten who did not experience its limb in some visual direction, with its head and eyes oriented just in the way it holds them on the visual placing test or while swatting the ball. Yet, Hein does not report any failures. The very fast recovery and broad generalization mean we must either give up the theory that each reafferent experience makes its specific contribution to the motor–sensory correlation pool, a theory with a good deal of support from human prism adaptation studies, or we must choose the nativistic model plus the S–R suppression notion of the effects of visual–motor deprivation. This model would state that cats, monkeys, and many other animals have an innate mapping of visual direction on the motor metric of limb movement. This initial mapping then undergoes normal learning changes as a result of particular S–R contiguities. There appears to be a sensitive period in early life of heightened sensitivities to these contiguities.

In a related V-MCD study (Held & Bauer, 1967), infant monkeys were raised from birth in an apparatus (see Fig. 12) that provided physical support, and permitted a wide range of limb activity. A cloth bib pinned around the neck prevented sight of the limbs. During the rearing period the infants were trained as follows. A milk bottle was presented to the animal's view:

> . . . if the monkey oriented head and eyes to the bottle and extended its unrestrained limb horizontally, the nipple was brought to its mouth for a few seconds. . . . when we first presented the bottle, the monkey made flailing responses with the free arm. In the course of daily testing the conditioned extension became stereotyped and unrelated to the direction in which the bottle appeared. By the end of the conditioning period, presentation of the bottle elicited head and eye orientation to it and a token extension of the arm and shoulder level [Held & Bower, 1967, p. 719].

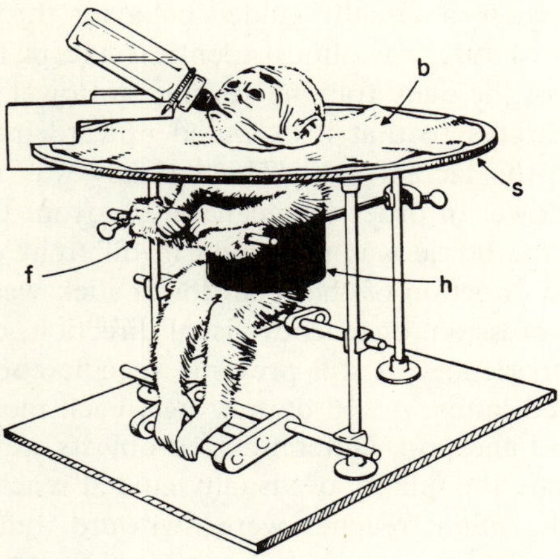

Fig. 12. Apparatus used by Held and Bauer (1967) to rear infant monkeys without sight of their limbs and torso.

Following 35 days of such rearing, the bib was removed so that the animal could view its limbs, and a small object was presented within reaching distance. Although objects elicited extension, the reaching motion stopped as soon as the hand entered the field of view. The animal appeared totally captivated by a fascination with its hand. As this hand watching diminished, during a period of 1 hr, visually guided reaching could be observed and was found to be poor. During the next 20 days, such exposure periods were given daily and reaching and anticipatory grasping gradually increased and became more like that of a normal animal. (This recovery did not immediately transfer to the other limb, which required its own recovery period, though there was roughly a 50% savings). The authors conclude that visually guided movement of a limb requires a specific experience in viewing that actively moved limb.

The S–R suppression interpretation can also be applied to the Held and Bauer experiment (Walk & Bond, 1971). The monkey, if he does reach out for visible objects with his hand beneath the bib, would soon extinguish this response tendency. In fact, the training which the experimenters administered would further suppress any visually guided reaching. In other words, according to this explanation, the training extinguished a variety of responses to a visible object; instead, the experiment reinforced a stereotyped nonvisually guided response. The S–R suppression hypothesis obtains some support from an experiment by Walk and Bond (1971). They addressed themselves, like Held and Bauer, specifically to the question of the neonatal deprivation of the sight of the hand and its effects on visually guided orientation of the limbs. At the same time, however, they attempted to avoid the suppression of visually guided behavior through lack of reinforcement. Their procedure was almost identical except for one important change: the nature of the daily training session. A dowel stick was held up in front of the apparatus so that it extended upward into the visual field and downward into the tactual field. The monkey was required to reach out and grasp the dowel in order to receive a sip from the feeding bottle. From trial to trial, the bottle was presented in different directions. Therefore, reaching in the direction of the seen dowel stick was reinforced. This avoids response suppression, or teaches visual direction, or both. Although it provides these experiences, it still prevents specific correlations between seen and commanded limbs. At 36 days of age, each monkey was allowed to view its right hand and arm. Different sized objects were presented to its visual field to evaluate the quality of visually guided reaching and grasping. They report that the initial reaches were awkward, but that fairly large objects could be reached on the first day of testing. More delicate tasks, such as grasping small objects from the experimenter's fingers, required more practice. It was not the visual direction that presented difficulties, but the intricacies of fine grasping. In contrast to Held and Bauer (1967), the reaching acts were not interrupted by hand watching, either on the first test session, or subsequently. The Walk and Bond experiment indicates that deprivation of the sight of the hand (that is, hand and limb reafference) is not detrimental to the development of gross eye-hand coordination if the animals are given reinforcement for appropriate visually guided responses. Further support for this position comes from a series of fascinating experiments showing that monkeys can acquire moderately complicated behavior repertoires when vision and proprioception are both eliminated (for a recent review, see Taub & Berman, 1968).

Phrased slightly differently, Walk and Bond demonstrate that S–R suppression—the main effect of V-MCD—is not due to the absence of reafferent stimulation. It is due to a factor usually confounded with reafference deprivation, namely the absence of differential reinforcement of limb movements in the presence of visual stimuli. This lack of reinforcement brings about the extinction of responses to visual stimuli from approaching edges, moving objects, and the like. If, as in the Walk and Bond experiment, the animal is deprived of certain visual–motor correlations, but not of differential reinforcement of limb movement in the direction of visual stimuli, appropriate visually guided reaching can still be obtained after the deprivation period.

Having examined the effects of visuo–motor deprivation, we can now turn to a study of rearing under conditions of visuo–motor decorrelation

(Held & Hein, 1963). Experimental conditions are so arranged that the normal one-to-one relationship between a voluntary movement and the resultant sensory input is not absent but randomized. Kittens were raised in the dark until 8 to 12 weeks of age. Beginning at that age they were exposed in pairs to 3 daily hours of visual experience in a gondola apparatus illustrated in Fig. 13. The active kitten (A) was free to move in the circular alley in any direction. Its motions were transmitted via various

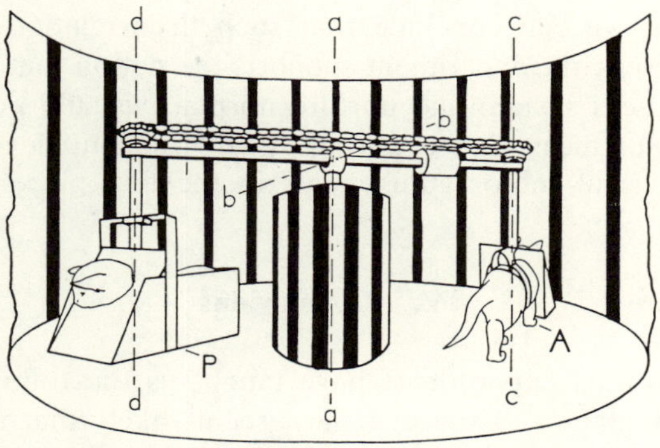

Fig. 13. The gondola apparatus used to present decorrelated visual–motor experience. (From Held & Hein, 1963.)

linkages to the passive kitten in the gondola (P). When the active kitten rotated about a vertical axis, the gondola carrying the passive kitten was similarly rotated, and so on for the three dimensions of space. Except for the exposure period in the gondola apparatus, the animals were in darkness. The kittens were tested six times each day for visual paw placing. When one of the active–passive pair showed the response, both were then tested on the visual cliff, for a response to a looming object, and for visual pursuit of a moving object. The results showed that once the active kitten showed visual placing, it also blinked to a looming stimulus and avoided the deep side of the cliff. The passive kitten at the same age invariably failed to show visual placing, failed to blink to an approaching object, and failed to discriminate the deep from the shallow sides of the visual cliff. Although the deficiencies were quite dramatic, recovery was equally dramatic. Within 48 hr after being given a period of free locomotion in an illuminated room, all P kittens showed visual placing and avoided the deep side of the cliff.

The results of the gondola experiment were initially interpreted to provide further evidence that reafference of the limbs is essential for the normal development of perceptual–motor coordination of those limbs. But we now know that visual placing is innate in kittens, requiring only diffuse light to prime a genetic endowment (Hein *et al.,* 1970b). It has also been shown that kittens given passive experience in the gondola require a longer mean exposure of normal, active experience before showing the visual placing response (41 hr) than a group with no previous light experience (30 hr) (Hein *et al.,* 1970a). Therefore, for the passive kitten, the gondola experience disrupts abilities present at birth. The gondola provides the passive kitten visual stimulation decorrelated from movements of the head and eyes. Therefore, we can conclude that such decorrelation is clearly disruptive. Conversely, the experiment supports the notion that normal visual–motor concurrences sustain and nurture normal, visually guided behavior. But that does not mean that a nurturant environment develops the basic framework of visual–motor adjustments in the first place.

IV. Conclusions

Visual deprivation experiments have taught us the following about the ontogeny of orientation to space. It now seems likely that rats, cats, monkeys, and, we would venture to guess, man, all have an innate competence to perform comparatively simple behavioral orientations in space, such as those represented by visually paw placing or avoidance of deep cliffs. The absence of normal visual–motor concurrences must induce a suppression or an extinction of orienting behavior that was innately provided for. Conversely, normal visual–motor concomitances sustain and increase the precision of the basic network of visual–motor response competence that is innately provided.

References

Ball, W., & Tronick, E. Infant responses to impending collision: optical and real. *Science,* 1971, **171**, 818–820.

Bárány, R. Die Untersuchung der optischen und vestibularen reflektorischen Augenbewebungen in einem Falle von einseitiger Blicklahmung. *Monatsschrift für Ohrenkrankheit,* 1908, **42**, 109–113.

Baxter, B. L. Effect of visual deprivation during postnatal maturation on the electroencephalogram of the cat. *Experimental Neurology,* 1966, **14**, 224–237.

Blakemore, C., & Cooper, G. F. Development of the brain depends on the visual environment. *Nature,* 1970, **228**, 477–478.

Bower, T. G. R., Broughton, J. M., & Moore, M. K. Demonstration of intention in the reaching behaviour of neonate humans. *Nature,* 1970, **228**, 679–681.

Chow, K. L., & Nissen, H. W. Interocular transfer of learning in visually naive and experienced infant chimpanzees. *Journal of Comparative Physiological Psychology,* 1955, **48**, 229–237.

Chow, K. L., Riesen, A. H., & Newell, F. W. Degeneration of retinal ganglion cells in infant chimpanzees reared in darkness. *Journal of Comparative Neurology,* 1957, **107**, 27–42.

Chow, K. L., & Steward, D. L. Reversal of structural and functional effects of long-term visual deprivation in cats. *Experimental Neurology,* 1972, **34**, 409–433.

Dews, P. B., & Wiesel, T. N. Consequences of monocular deprivation on visual behavior in kittens. *Journal of Physiology,* 1970, **206**, 437–455.

Fantz, R. L. Ontogeny of perception. In A. M. Schrier, H. F. Harlow, & F. Stollnitz (Eds.), *Behavior of non human primates: modern research trends,* Vol. II. New York: Academic Press, 1965.

Foley, J. P., Jr. First year development of a rhesus monkey (*Macaca mulatta*) reared in isolation during the first 18 months. *Journal of Genetic Psychology,* 1934, **45**, 34–105.

Foley, J. P., Jr. Two year development of a rhesus monkey (*Macaca mulatta*) reared in isolation. *Journal of Genetic Psychology,* 1935, **47**, 73–97.

Ganz, L. Sensory deprivation and visual discrimination. In H. Lukas-Teuber (Ed.), *Handbook of sensory physiology,* Vol. VIII. Berlin and New York: Springer-Verlag, 1974, in press.

Ganz, L., & Fitch, M. The effect of visual deprivation on perceptual behavior. *Experimental Neurology,* 1968, **22**, 638–660.

Ganz, L. & Hafner, M. E. Permanent perceptual and neurophysiological effects of visual deprivation in the cat. *Experimental Brain Research,* 1974, **20,** 67–87.

Ganz, L., Fitch, M., & Satterberg, J. A. The selective effect of visual deprivation on receptive field shape determined neurophysiologically. *Experimental Neurology,* 1968, **22**, 614–637.

Gorman, J. J., Cogan, D. G., & Gellis, S. S. An apparatus for grading visual acuity of infants on the basis of optokinetic nystagmus. *Pediatrics,* 1957, **19**, 1088–1092.

Harris, C. S. Perceptual adaptation to inverted, and displaced vision. *Psychological Review,* 1965, **72**, 419–444.

Hebb, D. O. *The organization of behavior.* New York: Wiley, 1949.

Hein, A. Recovering spatial motor coordination after visual cortex lesions. In D. Hamburg (Ed.), *Perception and its disorders.* Research Publications of the Association for Research in Nervous Mental Disease, Vol. 48. Baltimore: Williams & Wilkins, 1970.

Hein, A., & Diamond, R. M. Independence of cat's scotopic and photopic systems in acquiring control of visually guided behavior. *Journal of Comparative and Physiological Psychology,* 1971, **76**, 31–38. (a)

Hein, A., & Diamond, R. M. Contrasting development of visually triggered and guided movements in kittens with respect to interocular and interlimb equivalence. *Journal of Comparative and Physiological Psychology,* 1971, **76**, 219–224. (b)

Hein A., Gower, E. C., & Diamond, R. M. Exposure requirements for developing the triggered component of the visual-placing response. *Journal of Comparative and Physiological Psychology,* 1970, **73**, 188–192.

Hein, A., & Held, R. A neural model for labile sensorimotor coordinations. *Biological Prototypes and Synthetic Systems,* 1962, **1**, 71–74.

Hein, A., & Held, R. Dissociation of the visual placing response into elicited and guided components. *Science,* 1967, **158**, 390–391.

Hein, A., Held, R., & Gower, E. C. Development and segmentation of visually controlled movement by selective exposure during rearing. *Journal of Comparative and Physiological Psychology,* 1970, **73**, 181–187.

Held, R. Dissociation of visual functions by deprivation and rearrangement. *Psychologische Forschung,* 1968, **31**, 338–348.

Held, R., & Bauer, J. A. Visually guided reaching in infant monkeys after restricted rearing. *Science,* 1967, **155**, 718–720.

Held, R., & Freedman, S. J. Plasticity in human sensorimotor control. *Science,* 1963, **142**, 455–462.

Held, R., & Hein, A. Movement-produced stimulation in the development of visually guided behavior. *Journal of Comparative and Physiological Psychology,* 1963, **56**, 872–876.

Hines, M. The development and regression of reflexes, postures, and progression in the young macaque. *Contributions in Embryology, Carnegie Institute, Washington, D.C.,* 1942, **30**, 153–209.

Hirsch, H. V. B., & Spinelli, D. N. Visual experience modifies distribution of horizontally and vertically oriented receptive fields in cats. *Science,* 1970, **168**, 869–871.

Hochberg, J. E. Nativism and empiricism in psychology. In L. Postman (Ed.), *Psychology in the making.* New York: Knopf, 1962. Pp. 255–330.

Hubel, D. H., & Wiesel, T. N. Receptive fields of cells in striate cortex of very young, visually inexperienced kittens. *Journal of Neurophysiology,* 1963, **26**, 994–1002.

Hubel, D. H., & Wiesel, T. N. Binocular interaction in striate cortex in kittens reared with artificial squint. *Journal of Neurophysiology,* 1965, **28**, 1041–1059.

Hubel, D. H., & Wiesel, T. N. The period of susceptibility to the physiological effects of unilateral eye closure in kittens. *Journal of Physiology,* 1970, **206**, 419–436.

Kurke, M. I. The role of motor experience in the visual discrimination of depth in the chick. *Journal of Genetic Psychology,* 1955, **86**, 191–196.

Lashley, K. S., & Russell, J. T. The mechanism of vision. XI. A preliminary test of innate organization. *Journal of Genetic Psychology,* 1934, **45**, 136–144.

Lashley, K. S., & Watson, J. B. Notes of the development of a young monkey. *Journal of Animal Behavior,* 1913, **30**, 114–139.

McGinnis, J. M. Eye-movements and optic nystagmus in early infancy. *Genetic Psychological Monographs,* 1930, **8**, 321–430.

Melzack, R. Effects of early perceptual restriction on simple visual discrimination. *Science,* 1962, **137**, 978–979.

Meyers, B., & McCleary, R. Interocular transfer of a pattern discrimination in pattern deprived cats. *Journal of Comparative and Physiological Psychology,* 1964, **57**, 16–21.

Mowbray, J. B., & Cadell, T. E. Early behavior patterns in rhesus monkeys. *Journal of Comparative and Physiological Psychology,* 1962, **55**, 350–357.

Nealy, S. M., & Edwards, B. J. "Depth perception" in rats without pattern vision experience. *Journal of Comparative and Physiological Psychology,* 1960, **53**, 468–469.

Nealy, S. M., & Riley, D. Loss and recovery of discrimination of visual depth in dark-reared rats. *American Journal of Psychology,* 1963, **76**, 329–332.

Ordy, J. M., Massopust, L. C., & Wolin, L. R. Postnatal development of the retina, ERG, and acuity in the rhesus monkey. *Experimental Neurology,* 1962, **5**, 364–382.

Pettigrew, J. D., & Freeman, R. D. Visual experience without lines: Effect on developing cortical neurons. *Science,* 1973, **182**, 599–601.

Rademaker, G. G. J. *Das Stehen.* Berlin and New York: Springer-Verlag, 1931.

Rasch, E., Swift, H., Riesen, A. H., & Chow, K. L. Altered structure and composition of retinal cells in dark-reared mammals. *Experimental Cell Research,* 1961, **25**, 348–363.

Riesen, A. H. Plasticity of behavior: Psychological aspects. In H. F. Harlow & C. N. Woolsey (Eds.), *Biological and biochemical bases of behavior.* Madison, Wisconsin: University of Wisconsin Press, 1958.

Riesen, A. H. Excessive arousal effects of stimulation after early sensory deprivation. In P. Solomon, P. E. Kubzansky, P. H. Liederman, J. H. Mendelson, R. Trumbull, & D. Wexler (Eds.), *Sensory deprivation.* Cambridge, Massachusetts: Harvard University Press, 1961. Pp. 34–40. (a)

Riesen, A. H. Studying perceptual development using the technique of sensory deprivation. *Journal of Nervous and Mental Diseases,* 1961, **132**, 21–25. (b)

Riesen, A. H. Effects of early deprivation of photic stimulation. In S. F. Osler, & R. E. Cooke (Eds.), *The biosocial basis of mental retardation.* Baltimore, Maryland: Johns Hopkins Press, 1965.

Riesen, A. H., & Aarons, L. Visual movement and intensity discrimination in cats after early deprivation of pattern vision. *Journal of Comparative and Physiological Psychology,* 1959, **52**, 142–149.

Riesen, A. H., Kurke, M. I., & Mellinger, J. C. Interocular transfer of habits learned monocularly in visually naive and visually experienced cats. *Journal of Comparative and Physiological Psychology,* 1953, **46**, 166–172.

Riesen, A. H., & Mellinger, J. C. Interocular transfer of habits in cats after alternating monocular visual experience. *Journal of Comparative and Physiological Psychology,* 1956, **49**, 516–520.

Riesen, A. H., Ramsey, R. L., & Wilson, P. D. Development of visual acuity in Rhesus monkeys deprived of patterned light during early infancy. *Psychonomic Science,* 1964, **1**, 33–34.

Rock, I., Tauber, E. S., & Heller, D. P. Perception of stroboscopic movement: Evidence for its innate basis. *Science,* 1965, **147**, 1050–1052.

Rosenblum, L. A., & Cross, H. A. Performance of neonatal monkeys in the visual cliff situation. *American Journal of Psychology,* 1963, **76**, 318–320.

Schiff, W., The perception of impending collision: a study of visually directed avoidance behavior. *Psychological Monographs,* 1965, **79**, Whole No. 604.

Schiff, W., Caviness, J. A., & Gibson, J. J. Persistent fear responses in rhesus monkeys on the optical stimulus of "looming." *Science,* 1962, **136**, 982–983.

Senden, M. von. *Raum-und Gestalt-auffassung bei operierten Blindgeborenen vor und nach der Operation.* Leipzig: Barth, 1932.

Smith, K. U. The effects of removal of the striate cortex upon certain unlearned visually controlled reactions in the cat. *Journal of Genetic Psychology,* 1937, **50**, 137–156.

Spalding, D. A. Instinct with original observations on young animals. *Macmillan's Magazine,* 1873, **27**, 282–293. [Reprinted in *British Journal of Animal Behavior,* **2**, 2–11.]

Taub, E. Prism compensation as a learning phenomenon: A phylogenetic comparison. In S. J. Freedman (Ed.), *The neuropsychology of spatially oriented behavior.* Homewood, Illinois: Dorsey Press, 1968. Pp. 77–106.

Taub, E., & Berman, A. J. Movement and learning in the absence of sensory feedback. In S. J. Freedman (Ed.), *The neuropsychology of spatially oriented behavior.* Homewood, Illinois: Dorsey Press, 1968. Pp. 173–192.

Thompson, W. R., & Heron, W. The effects of restricting early experience on the problem-solving capacity of dogs. *Canadian Journal of Psychology,* 1954, **8,** 17–31.

Thorndike, E. The instinctive reactions of young chicks. *Psychological Review,* 1899, **6,** 282–291.

Tinklepaugh, O. L., & Hartman, C. G. Behavior and maternal care of the newborn monkey (*Macaca mulatta*). *Journal of Genetic Psychology,* 1932, **40,** 257–286.

Walk, R. The study of visual depth and distance perception in animals. *Recent Advances in the Study of Behavior,* 1965, **1,** 99–154.

Walk, R. D., & Bond, E. K. The development of visually guided reaching in monkeys reared without sight of the hands. *Psychonomic Science,* 1971, **23,** 115–116.

Walk, R. D., & Gibson, E. J. A comparative and analytic study of visual depth perception. *Psychological Monographs,* 1961, **75,** Whole No. 519.

Walk, R. D., Gibson, E. J., & Tighe, T. J. Behavior of light- and dark-reared rats on a visual cliff. *Science,* 1957, **126,** 80–81.

Walk, R. D., Trychin, S., & Karmel, B. Z. Depth perception in the dark-reared rat as a function of time in the dark. *Psychonomic Science,* 1965, **3,** 9–10.

Warkentin, J., & Smith, K. U. The development of visual acuity in the cat. *Journal of Genetic Psychology,* 1937, **50,** 371–399.

Waugh, K. T. The role of vision in the mental life of the mouse. *Journal of Comparative and Neurological Psychology,* 1910, **20,** 549–599.

Weiskrantz, L. Sensory deprivation and the cat's optic nervous system. *Nature,* 1958, **181,** 1047–1050.

White, B. L. The development of perception during the first six months of life. Paper presented at the meeting of the American Association for the Advancement of Science, Cleveland, December, 1963.

White, B. L., Castle, P., & Held, R. Observations on the development of visually-directed reaching. *Child Development,* 1964, **35,** 349–364.

Wiesel, T. N., & Hubel, D. H. Single-cell responses in striate cortex of kittens deprived of vision in one eye. *Journal of Neurophysiology,* 1963, **26,** 1003–1007.

Wiesel, T. N., & Hubel, D. H. Comparison of the effects of unilateral and bilateral eye closure on cortical unit responses in kittens. *Journal of Neurophysiology,* 1965, **28,** 1029–1040. (a)

Wiesel, T. N., & Hubel, D. H. Extent of recovery from the effects of visual deprivation in kittens. *Journal of Neurophysiology,* 1965, **28,** 1060–1072. (b)

Wilson, P. D., & Riesen, A. H. Visual development in Rhesus monkeys neonatally deprived of patterned light. *Journal of Comparative and Physiological Psychology,* 1966, **61,** 87–95.

Wolff, P. H., & White, B. L. Visual pursuit and attention in young infants. *Journal of the American Academy of Child Psychiatry,* 1965, **4,** 473–484.

CHAPTER VII

Behavioral Consequences of Variations in Early Sensory Environments

Austin H. Riesen

Department of Psychology
University of California, Riverside

Dale E. Zilbert

Division of Adult Services,
Clark Institute of Psychiatry
Toronto, Canada

I. The Scope of Behavioral Studies

A. Environmental Variables in Sensory Deprivation Studies

Early studies of the effects of variations in sensory environments reflected a concern that unless stimulations within a given modality were eliminated or, at least, drastically reduced, no later behavioral consequences would be found. While this approach was useful in demonstrating some innately organized behaviors (see Chapter VI), as in the example of visual cliff discriminations and in the demonstration of innate stimulus preferences, it failed to identify effects of qualitative variations in the early environment. After 1950, the need for studies with less extreme forms of environmental control was recognized. Elimination of certain components and combinations of environmental stimuli provided data that were more valuable in providing an understanding of behavioral and physiological principles of development. Dark-rearing had widespread effects. Interpretations could be couched primarily in terms of concepts such as neural atrophy or physiological disorganization. When pattern deprivation or hue impoverishment or low intensity sound was substituted, more definitive answers to questions became possible. The value of less extreme experimental manipulations has been verified repeatedly in studies employing simplified visual, auditory, somatosensory, and social environments.

Qualitative environmental enrichment studies were soon added to the spectrum and found also to produce significant effects. These served to soften the bite of criticisms by ethologists that the integrity of organisms was severely jeopardized in the early studies, and only abnormal behavior patterns resulted. These criticisms did not destroy discoveries of some fundamental neurophysiological processes which have been reviewed in earlier chapters of the present volume.

One of the important areas of research that developed from moderate approaches was that of the "novelty-enhancement" studies that are the subject of Chapter VIII. Another important advance has come from studies of crude responses that reflect innate organization of spatial behaviors and the conditions needed for their improved accuracy and for the maintenance of high levels of sensory–motor skills. By restricting input to one eye and by controlling motor behaviors during visual exposure, the contributions of sensory–motor and binocular versus monocular experience are being discovered. The crucial roles of eye movements are being investigated. Impressive are the findings that specific kinds of stimulation are required for neuropsychological development, and that organisms seek stimulation that has been in short supply.

B. Measures of Behavior

1. *Emotional Behavior*

To obtain measures that promptly reveal consequences of sensory restriction, innate emotional responses have obvious advantages over learned discrimination behaviors. The arousal that moderately unusual stimulation produces has been an important contributory variable from the outset of this work. Cautious locomotion, fear and avoidance of novel stimuli, and enhanced orienting responses have helped to reveal what deprived organisms could or could not do. These measures will be seen to enter into many of the experiments of this and the next chapter.

2. *Exploratory Behavior, Preference Responding, Motivation*

Stimulus seeking behavior and the closely related two-choice preference measures made familiar by Fantz' studies with monkeys, apes, and human infants are proving to be of outstanding importance in the study of early perceptual development under varying opportunities for early interactions with the sensory environment. Not only are innate perceptual preferences revealed in such studies, but the modifiability of these in accordance with response contingencies are being investigated both by intergroup comparisons and by longitudinal studies of the same individuals. The pre- and posttesting research design principles of Lessac and Solomon (1969) are particularly suited for studies that utilize these measures. The motivational variable requires careful scrutiny in these studies if they are to be correctly interpreted.

3. *Discriminative and Problem-Solving Behavior*

When limits of performance are investigated following sensory deprivation, the use of learning and problem solving behavior may be the necessary if laborious method of choice. A rather prolonged training period is sometimes required. This may confound the interpretation of the results, since immediate postdeprivation data cannot be obtained. In effects that persist for months, as in the studies of monocular form deprivation (Dews & Wiesel, 1970), this problem is minimized. The procedure has worked best when responses called for have been simplified as far as possible, and when graded series of problems have been used. The graded series should include dicriminations that permit successful performance on the easier problems of the series. This assures the investigator that the method is effective, and when appropriately mixed into the series supports the motivation of the subject in problem solving behavior.

II. Studies of Visual Deprivation

Experiments with neonatal animals allow manipulation of the initial visual environment, permitting the identification of those variables that are critical for the development of accurately guided behavior and of capacities for discriminating along selected dimensions of the sensory cues. The use of long-term dark-rearing in primates proved to result eventually in atrophic changes in the retina and optic nerve, with loss of retinal ganglion cells and other local morphochemical changes (Chow, Riesen, & Newell, 1957; Rasch, Swift, Riesen, & Chow, 1961; Riesen, 1950; Winsburg & Riesen, 1966). This was one of the first findings that resulted in experiments with less severe visual restriction. The several variations in type of deprivation produce important differences in the resulting visual behaviors.

A. Light Deprivation

Depriving animals of light from birth severely retards the development of visual abilities, and such animals appear blind in tests of obstacle avoidance and on other response indicators upon their first exposure to a normally patterned visual environment. Riesen (1947) has described the extreme visual incompetence of two young chimpanzees when they were first removed from their darkroom after being reared for 16 months in the dark. Some basic visual capacities were present in these dark-reared animals immediately upon exposure to light but, in general, their visual–motor abilities were markedly impaired. Responses present from the beginning of visual testing included constriction of the pupil to light, startle responses to sudden changes in illumination, and jerky visual pursuit of a moving light source. Optokinetic responses were present, but visually guided behavior was extremely inept and visual acuity, the resolving capacity of the eye, was deficient. There was no evidence of visual recognition and no visual startle response; if an object was brought slowly toward the face, the first response was a startled jump when tactual contact occurred. No sustained visual fixation of either stationary or moving objects could be elicited in any of the early tests. Not all of the deficits present initially proved permanent. Normal recognition of objects, blinking in response to visual threat, smooth pursuit of moving objects, the coordination of the two eyes, and the ability to use visual cues to guide locomotion developed, but only gradually, after many months in a normal visual environment. Shorter periods of deprivation had less severe effects, although the acquisition of visually mediated responses also proceeded slowly in chimpanzees after rearing for 7, or even 3 months in the dark (Riesen, 1950).

The normal stimulus generalization gradient to hue does not require visual experience, but, rather, it develops innately without light stimulation. Ganz and Riesen (1962) compared generalization gradients to hue in dark-reared and normally reared macaques. Beginning at 10 weeks of age, the monkeys were trained, using operant conditioning techniques, to press a key for liquid reinforcement during the presentation of a monochromatic light stimulus, and not to respond in darkness. Generalization was measured using seven other hues at intervals along the spectral continuum between 450 and 630 μm presented under extinction. On the first test day, both groups responded with a broad generalization gradient, but with subsequent testing the slope for the hue naïve group steepened, and, over the 7-day testing period, exceeded that of the experienced group which displayed a more moderate gradient that did not change substantially over the testing period.

Fantz (1965) studied the effects of rearing monkeys in darkness from birth for periods varying from 1 to 11 weeks. Monkeys kept in the dark for a short period of time usually exhibited competent visually guided behavior after several hours or days in patterned light, but those animals sustaining longer periods of deprivation generally displayed poor spatial orientation and were impaired in recognizing objects. The effects of different durations of dark-rearing upon pattern preferences were examined using a procedure developed by Fantz (1956). Visual fixation was used as an index of visual discrimination by comparing the duration of fixation of different targets exposed systematically in a test chamber. Tests of fixation preference revealed that those monkeys maintained in the dark for 6 weeks or less subsequently displayed an obvious preference for solid patterns over plain surfaces and a weaker, but reliable, preference for solid over flat objects. With longer periods of deprivation, animals displayed abnormal preferences, showing little or no preference for patterned or solid objects, but rather an increasing tendency to respond to stimuli differentially on the basis of color, size, or brightness.

Experiments with other species have confirmed the observation that light deprivation during the early postnatal weeks has significant effects upon the development of visually dependent abilities. Kittens reared entirely in the dark displayed pupillary constriction and lid closure to light stimulation (Riesen & Aarons, 1959; Held & Hein, 1963) and exhibited placing responses to tactual stimulation (Held & Hein, 1963; Ganz & Fitch, 1968) upon removal from the darkroom; however, neither visual placing to an edge or a surface (Ganz & Fitch, 1968; Hein & Diamond, 1971; Held & Hein, 1963; Riesen & Aarons, 1959) nor accurate guided reaching to an interrupted surface (Hein & Diamond, 1971) could be elicited. Most of these abilities did develop after many hours in illuminated surroundings. Depth perception, as measured using the visual cliff, was impaired in visually naive kittens when they were tested initially after 26 days in the dark, but discriminative responding did develop with subsequent light experience and by the seventh day of patterned light experience all kittens descended reliably to the shallow side of the visual cliff (Walk & Gibson, 1961). Held and Hein (1963) have studied the development of visual abilities in kittens reared in total darkness from birth until 8–12 weeks of age. The animals did not show visual placing and accurate depth discrimination on the visual cliff when first tested under normal illumination, but these responses did appear after the kittens had received an average of 30 hr of normal light experience. A preliminary report (van Hof-van Duin, & Kobayashi, 1972) has indicated that cats reared in complete darkness for 7 months do display normal placing reactions and jumping, a crude measure of depth perception, after 8–10 weeks in a normally illuminated environment. Baxter (1966) found such recovery after even longer dark-rearing.

Complete light deprivation does not retard the ability of kittens to learn a visual intensity discrimination. Kittens reared in total darkness from birth to age 16 weeks learned a light–dark discrimination at the same rate as normally reared animals (Aarons, Halasz, & Riesen, 1963). Riesen, Kurke, and Mellinger (1953) compared form discrimination learning in dark-reared and normally reared kittens. The experimental animals were reared in the dark from birth. Beginning at 14 weeks of age they were brought into the light for 30 min daily and given diffused light stimulation in one eye and patterned light in the other until the age of 17 or 20 weeks. Discrimination learning then was assessed using a modified Yerkes–Watson box. Dark-reared animals were markedly impaired compared to normally reared animals in learning to discriminate between horizontal and vertical striations and between a triangle and a circle. A recent report has indicated that pattern vision in kittens may be relatively insensitive to the effects of light deprivation. Kittens deprived of light from birth until 7 months of age subsequently were able to learn to discriminate striated patterns of different orientations at the same rate as normally reared cats (van Hof *et al.*, 1972).

Goodman (1932) has described the characteristic posture of the dark-reared rabbit: forelegs widely spread and head held so that its snout nearly touched the floor, as if attempting to maximize somesthetic and olfactory cues. This gait was still detectable as different from normal even 2 months after the animal was transferred into the light. Although visual behavior was severely retarded in an albino rabbit reared in the dark from birth until 5 months of age, some visual reflexes still were present, including eye blink to light and the pupillary reflex. There was a rapid improvement in guided behavior during the first 10 days of exposure to light, and by the end of the first month the rabbit displayed visual pursuit and eye blink to approaching objects. Van Hof (1971) has confirmed Goodman's behavioral observations, noting the peculiar posture of Dutch rabbits deprived of light for 7 months after birth and that behavior in the first few weeks after removal from the darkroom differed from that of normal rabbits. Visual acuity in rabbits is disrupted by light deprivation. Visual resolution, determined by changing the width of black and white striations, was better in normally reared than in light-deprived rabbits (van Hof, 1971). Pattern vision in rabbits is extremely resistant to the effects of deprivation. Rabbits deprived of light for 7 months after birth subsequently learned to discriminate horizontal (90°) versus vertical (0°) striations, and 45 versus 135° striations in a two-choice discrimination box at the same rate as normal rabbits. Furthermore, angular threshold values, representing the ability to detect small oblique angle difference (25, 15, 10, and 5°) from vertical, were approximately equal for light-deprived and normally reared rabbits (van Hof, 1971). Dark-reared rabbits were able to learn a series of pattern discriminations (upright versus inverted triangle, triangle versus square, and circle versus square), and their rate of learning did not differ from control rabbits (Kobayashi & van Hof, 1970). This result with geometric forms may place rabbits in a unique category.

Rats are resistant to the effects of total visual deprivation. Depth discrimination, as measured by the visual cliff, remained intact in rats after 90 days of light deprivation (Walk, Gibson, & Tighe, 1957), but it was disrupted when the discrimination was made more difficult by decreasing the apparent visual depth to be discriminated from 10 to 4 inches. The resulting deficit persisted even after 2 weeks in the light (Walk & Bond, 1968). Longer periods of deprivation were studied by Nealey and Riley (1963). They determined that after dark-rearing for 140 days or longer, discrimination of depth was lost, but with subsequent visual experience rats recovered after even 300 days of dark-rearing from birth. Dark-rearing does not impair the ability of rats to discriminate between stimuli on the basis of intensity (Tees, 1968a). A subsequent study revealed that luminance cues were used much more by light-reared than by dark-reared rats in the solution of such intensity discriminations (Tees, 1971). Dark-reared rats learn simple pattern discriminations at the same rate as light-reared rats, but have greater difficulty in learning to discriminate complex forms. Tees (1968b) reported that hooded rats deprived of light from birth to 90 days of age learned horizontal–vertical, then vertical–oblique, and oblique–oblique discriminations as rapidly as light-reared animals, but were impaired in learning to discriminate X versus N. Heller (1968) found that rearing in darkness prevented size constancy discriminations, whereas depth on the visual cliff and retinal size discriminations were apparently no different from those of light-reared controls. The dark-reared animals developed size constancy within 10 days after living under normal illumination.

Two studies from eastern European laboratories have confirmed the findings of retarded behavioral modification in dark-reared rabbits (Volokhov & Shiljagina, 1972) and rats (Chaloupka, 1971). Both studies used rates of formation of conditioned responses as measures. Extinction of the conditioned avoidance reactions was even more retarded than their acquisition. Altered latencies and amplitudes of cortical evoked responses were also reported.

Chickens reared in total darkness from hatching until 10 weeks of age were inferior to normally reared chickens in learning a triangle versus circle discrimination (Tucker, 1957), although a study by Fantz (1957) has revealed that in a form preference test, discrimination of triangle from circle is possible in 2-day-old, dark-reared chicks.

B. Pattern Deprivation

The studies reviewed above illustrate that the normal development of visual abilities does not proceed when neonatal animals are reared in total darkness. That animals reared with only the opportunity for diffused light stimulation exhibit similar kinds of visual retardation supports the notion that light by itself is not a sufficient condition for visual development.

The visual abilities of chimpanzees raised to age 7 months in darkness, with $1\frac{1}{2}$ hr of daily exposure to diffused light, were examined upon their removal to daylight surroundings (Riesen, 1950, 1958). Visual reflexes were present from the beginning of behavioral testing. Smooth visual tracking and fixation responses developed within the first month of patterned visual experience. Acuity in these animals was not grossly defective; they displayed a visual resolution of 3 min of arc, but their ability to discriminate visual patterns developed very slowly. The chimpanzees were conditioned to utilize a visual cue to avoid shock and then were trained to discriminate this stimulus from other neutral stimuli differing from it in color, size, orientation or shape. Discriminations of size, color, and orientation were acquired quite readily, while the form discrimination was learned only after extensive training.

There is good evidence that stimulation by visual patterns is essential if animals are to develop the normal complement of visually dependent abilities. One and one half hours of patterned light daily, over 7 months, was sufficient to support the development of visual behavior in an otherwise totally dark-reared chimpanzee (Riesen, 1950). When moved to normal daylight surroundings, its visual performance was indistinguishable from normally reared chimpanzees, with the exceptions that it failed to display avoidance of strange objects or a preference for familiar persons.

Deficits in visually dependent abilities have been reported in monkeys reared with the opportunity for diffused light experience. Wilson and Riesen (1966) reared rhesus monkeys in the dark with 2.4 hr of diffused light exposure daily. At 20 or 60 days of age, the monkeys began receiving 2.5 hr of daily patterned light experience. The monkeys showed well-developed pupillary responses and occulomotor orientation to brightness contrasts when first brought into patterned light. Other visually guided responses appeared with subsequent visual experience. Visual regard and pursuit of objects developed after an average of 8 days (20 hr), visual placing within 9 days, avoidance of apparent depth on the visual cliff by 20 days, and the development of accurate eye–hand coordination in visually guided reaching appeared after an average of 21 days. No animal responded with an eye blink to visual threat within 30 days of patterned light exposure. The development of visual acuity in these diffused light-reared macaques was examined in a study by Riesen, Ramsey and Wilson (1964). The results demonstrated a systematic improvement in visual acuity with patterned light stimulation. Beginning on the first day of patterned light exposure, visual acuity was tested daily using the optokinetic drum. Movements of the animal's eyes in tracking rotating stripes of different widths provided an index of visual resolution. Acuity was poor initially, but improved promptly with experience in patterned light at a rate comparable to the development of acuity in normally reared monkeys (Ordy, Massopust, & Wolin, 1962). All animals eventually displayed a visual resolution of 4 min of arc, but those animals reared for 20 days in diffused light developed this acuity with fewer hours of patterned light experience than monkeys reared in diffused light for 60 days.

Diffused light-reared monkeys readily learn to discriminate stimuli on the basis of differences in intensity. Wilson and Riesen (1966) reported that monkeys reared 20 or 60 days with diffused light-stimulation learned a brightness discrimination in a two-choice Yerkes–Watson box at the same rate as had previously been reported for young, normally reared monkeys (Zimmerman, 1961). After training on the brightness discrimination was completed, differences between target brightnesses were reduced by steps, and the monkeys were tested at each level of difficulty to obtain a measure of brightness difference thresholds. It was found that the brightness threshold dropped systematically with increasing visual experience. Form discriminations are more difficult for pattern deprived monkeys to acquire. Although monkeys reared for 60 days with only diffused light stimulation did not differ from those reared for only 20 days in the number of trials they required to learn to discriminate horizontal versus vertical striations and triangle versus circle, these tasks were significantly more difficult for these visually naive monkeys than for normally reared monkeys.

Monkeys (*Macaca mulatta*) reared with translucent occluders to 18 months of age were behaviorally blind and showed only slight recovery, varying somewhat with individual animals over the period of 6 weeks following removal of the occluders (Berger & Meier, 1968). Spontaneous nystagmoid eye movements interfered with fixation and pursuit movements in the waking monkeys, and abnormal rates and amplitudes of eye movements during REM sleep developed during the period of visual pattern deprivation.

Cats deprived of patterned visual stimulation from birth exhibit pupillary light reflexes upon first testing in patterned light (Hubel & Wiesel, 1963), although the pupillary reflex has been described as sluggish with prolonged deprivation (Chow & Stewart, 1972). Poor visual guidance of behavior has been reported consistently for pattern deprived cats. These animals have difficulty using visual cues to direct locomotion in an open field, their gait is broad based and hesitant, and they frequently bump into obstacles (Chow & Stewart, 1972; Ganz & Fitch, 1968; Rizzolatti & Tradardi, 1971; Wiesel & Hubel, 1963, 1965). Although all diffused light-reared kittens displayed tactual placing, most investigators report that they fail to show visual placing with forelimbs to a solid opaque or highly textured surface when first tested after removal into normal surroundings (Wiesel & Hubel, 1963, 1965; Ganz & Fitch, 1968). Hein, Gower, and Diamond (1970) reared kittens in total darkness from birth. At age 6 weeks they were fitted with translucent occluders and permitted to locomote freely in a normal environment. Visual-placing responses were examined after varying periods of diffused light stimulation. All kittens first exhibited visually triggered extension after between 4.5 and 16 hr of diffused light stimulation. These authors distinguish triggered extension and guided visual placing responses. Extension responding may develop without patterned light experience.

Hein and Diamond (1971) report interocular transfer of the visually triggered extension. Kittens were maintained in total darkness until age 5–8 weeks. They were then exposed for 3 hr each day in a normal light environment with one eye occluded with a black vinyl contact and the other eye receiving diffused light stimulation through a translucent vinyl diffuser. After 9–15 hr of this experience, the kittens all displayed visually triggered extension using the eye which had received diffused light stimulation. Moreover, when they were then tested while using their totally light-deprived eye, all animals exhibited the forelimb triggered extension. Visually guided placing requires evidence for localizing a prong of a series of prongs separated by wider gaps (much like black keys on a piano keyboard). Monocular patterned light experience permits this development, but only with the one eye that is practiced. Such absence of interocular transfer as well as the initial requirement for several hours of simultaneous viewing of the paw and the textured visual environment distinguishes guided placing from triggered extension (Experiment 2 in Hein & Diamond, 1971).

Pattern deprived cats do not show evidence of depth perception, as measured by their accuracy in jumping down from heights (Rizzolatti & Tradardi, 1971; Wiesel & Hubel, 1963), their spontaneous performance on the visual cliff (Ganz & Fitch, 1968), or their relative resistance to being pushed toward the shallow or the deep side of the cliff (Ganz & Fitch, 1968). Fine visually guided responses are impaired. They show persisting failures in guided reaching to an interrupted (Ganz & Fitch, 1968) or a discrete surface (Dews & Wiesel, 1970). Initially form deprived cats failed to follow a moving light and did not exhibit the blink response to a rapidly approaching visual stimulus (Chow & Stewart, 1972; Ganz & Fitch, 1968; Wiesel & Hubel, 1963, 1965).

That visually guided behavior improves markedly with experience in patterned light has been well established. The ability of pattern deprived cats to guide themselves through an open field using visual cues improved slowly over 3–4 months, and with extensive recovery periods they could not be discriminated from normally reared animals on the basis of their visual–motor abilities (Chow & Stewart, 1972; Ganz & Fitch, 1968; Rizzolatti & Tradardi, 1971).

Riesen (1961a, b) presents data from an experiment by Munro and Riesen examining the development of visual placing as a function of visual experience. The kittens used as subjects in this study were reared in the usual laboratory environment from birth until 18 days of age. They then were placed in the darkroom for 23 hr each day and during the other hour they were in the light, either without visual restriction or while wearing hoods of fine percale which diffused the light. The unhooded kittens were tested daily for visual placing, first giving responses to visually perceived surfaces at 27 days. On the day following the appearance of the placing response in an unhooded kitten, its previously hooded littermates were left unhooded during the hour of light, and testing continued. No experimental animal showed the placing response when the hoods were first removed. Instead, all animals gave their first response after 5 hr in patterned light. Kittens reared from birth with the eyelids of one eye sutured shut were tested 1–6 months later, immediately after the eyelids had been surgically opened, and then were retested after the previously deprived eye had been open for 14 days (Ganz & Fitch, 1968). The ability of the deprived eye to elicit visual placing developed in both short- and long-term deprived cats in the interval between the first and second testings. At this time both spontaneous visual cliff discrimination and resistance of the cats to a push to the deep side indicated that these animals were capable of discriminative responding to differences in depth. Every animal developed reliable depth discrimination with extended visual experience. Another report indicates that in some cases deprivation can abolish the visual placing response. Wiesel and Hubel (1965) noted that kittens deprived of pattern vision by binocular or monocular lid suturing during the first 3 months of life were severely handicapped in the use of visual cues, and the visual placing response never appeared even with subsequent patterned light experience.

Guided paw placement to a discrete surface became excellent in animals deprived from birth for less than 7 weeks, but with prolonged deprivation animals showed permanent impairment (Dews & Wiesel, 1970). Visually guided reaching to a serrated surface did not develop, even with extensive visual experience after prolonged rearing in diffused light (Ganz & Fitch, 1968).

Kittens deprived of pattern vision from birth exhibit losses in detail vision. Ganz and Fitch (1968) reared kittens from birth for 1–6 months with the eyelids of one eye sutured together. Visual acuity, assessed in an optokinetic drum, was better with the experienced than with the naive eye. Although cats could track 1.3 min of arc stripes using their experienced eye, most could only track stripes of 143 min, or 9.3 min of arc using their deprived eye. After 4 months of binocular visual experience, resolution using the deprived eye still was consistently inferior. Reverse suturing, closing the sound eye and forcing the cat to use visual cues through the previously deprived eye, was found effective in producing marked improvements in acuity, resulting in nearly equivalent optokinetic indices for the two eyes (1.3 min of arc). Dews and Wiesel (1970) examined the effects of varying periods of deprivation upon visual acuity. Cats monocularly deprived of patterned light stimulation by lid suture for varying periods of time from birth were trained monocularly to discriminate continuous from interrupted horizontal striations. Cats deprived for the first 4–6 weeks after birth could discriminate gaps of 1.5 mm using their pattern-deprived eye, although they were more reliably accurate when using their experienced eye. Seven weeks of deprivation lowered acuity, so that the cats were not able to discriminate 1.5-mm gaps. Further extension of the deprivation period through the first 16 weeks had a more severe effect: testing with the deprived eye using a gap of 30 mm continued for as long as 2 years without improvement. Fitch (1971) determined acuity thresholds optokinetically for deprived (whether MD or BD) eyes of cats to lie between 2 and 10 min of arc following 12–16 weeks of rearing with lids sutured. Optokinetic responding, which survives cortical ablation, indicates that resolving power is less affected in subcortical vision than in vision that functions in form discrimination learning, as used by Dews and Wiesel (1970).

Intensity discrimination in cats, as in primates, is not affected by pattern deprivation. Riesen (1965) has reported that form-deprived cats learn an intensity discrimination in a Yerkes alley at about the same rate as normally reared controls. Cats reared with monocular or binocular lid suture for varying periods from birth all were able to discriminate luminosity differences (Dews & Wiesel, 1970) and to learn a light versus dark discrimination (Chow & Stewart, 1972; Rizzolatti & Tradardi, 1971).

Confirming studies with primates, deficits in diffused light-reared cats are in the discrimination of complex visual patterns. Discrimination of the orientation of multiple striations are learned most readily, possibly because the distinguishing cues are replicated reliably over the visual field (Riesen, 1958). Riesen (1965) has reported that the discrimination of horizontal from vertical striations was learned at about the same rate by kittens reared with only 1 hr of diffused light stimulation daily, and normally reared animals. Chow and Stewart (1972) studied the discrimination of horizontal from vertical orientation of black and white striations in long-term visually deprived cats. These animals had their eyelids sutured from birth, either monocularly or binocularly, until 16–24 months of age. Then recovery due to forced usage of the previously deprived eye was assessed using a go–no-go runway task. Orientation discriminations were learned by both monocularly and binocularly deprived cats. In contrast to these results, Ganz and Fitch (1968) reported that kittens reared for 1–6 months with monocular diffused light stimulation were unable to learn to discriminate a horizontal from a vertical grid of lines in a Yerkes Watson box. Chow and Stewart (1972) attribute differences in their findings to differences in procedure, suggesting that their paradigm maximized accurate performance by eliminating spatial complexities in the testing situation and by using a procedure which minimized errors by beginning discrimination training with an easy problem and reintroducing previously mastered tasks when the animals began to make errors.

There is good agreement that more complex patterns are not discriminated readily by diffused light-reared felines. Riesen (1965) has noted that binocularly pattern-deprived cats are retarded compared to normally reared animals in learning to discriminate X from N. Meyers and McCleary (1964) explored the possibility that the deficits in form discrimination observed in pattern deprived animals might be, in fact, a reflection of faulty visual–motor abilities. Kittens were reared with only diffused light from birth. Beginning at 30–35 weeks of age, the kittens were restrained in a holder and trained to discriminate between a cross and a circle using a discriminatory response, leg flexion, which did not require visual guidance. The deprived cats required about twice as many trials as normally reared animals to learn the pattern discrimination, thus confirming the importance of patterned visual experience in the development of form discrimination. Rizzolatti and Tradardi (1971) examined visual pattern discrimination in a two-choice discrimination box. The subjects in this study were kittens reared from 10 days to 5 months of age with one eye sutured shut. The training procedure employed by these investigators is notable because although on the initial training trials all animals were rewarded for a correct choice with food, after 500 trials, errors were punished with mild shock to the paws. The authors attribute the acquisition of the discriminations while using the previously deprived eye to the use of punishment, suggesting that it was effective in eliminating strong position habits and forced the animals to "pay attention." All cats were trained to criterion on the first problem using their normal eye; five overtraining trials were given and the animals then were trained using their deprived eyes. For all subsequent tasks, the eye to be trained first was selected in a mixed counterbalanced order. Although the cats required significantly more trials to learn the discriminations using their deprived than their experienced eyes, all animals were able to learn to discriminate between a triangle and an open square, a cross and a circle, an upright and an inverted N, and between a circle and a triangle.

C. Limited Pattern Exposure

The studies surveyed above affirm the importance of visual pattern experience for the development and maintenance of competent visual behavior. There has been little systematic work as yet to determine the specific limits of variation in visual pattern which are sufficient to support the development of visual abilities. It is clear from several preliminary studies, however, that early pattern exposure history is of critical importance. Providing pattern-deprived animals with the opportunity for visual fixation may be of value in minimizing the behavioral effects of visual deprivation. Riesen (1958) reared a chimpanzee in a dark room with the opportunity to look at a pair of blinking stars, each on for 2 sec, off for 1 sec. This animal also received 90 min each day of diffused light experience in a Plexiglas dome where it could view a black target that intermittently approached and receded. The chimpanzee still was avisual when first removed from the darkroom, but visual convergence subsequently developed more rapidly than in totally diffused light-reared animals, indicating some advantage over them in the development of visual fixation skills.

Cool (1966) has demonstrated the critical importance of early experience with specific patterns for the development of accurate form perception. Albino rats were reared in total darkness until 21 days of age and then were placed individually for 50 days in one of two specialized visual environments: angular or nonangular. The angular environments were rectangular, translucent cages with angles of various sizes painted on the walls in a random arrangement. The nonangular environments were large translucent light globes; curved lines of various lengths were painted on the sides of the globes. The rats reared in an angular environment learned to discriminate visual patterns, square versus triangle and circle from ellipse, in a Grice box at the same rate as normally reared rats. The other animals, deprived of early experience with angles, never learned the discriminations. This finding of an advantage of early visual exposure to angles has been replicated several times by independent investigators (see McCall & Lester, 1969), with some reporting associated evidence that nonangular figures as well as angular are subsequently more rapidly recognized.

The importance of the specific stimulus configurations available in the early visual environment has been dramatically confirmed in a study examining the visual abilities of kittens reared with normal binocular vision in an environment consisting entirely of vertical or horizontal stripes (Blakemore & Cooper, 1970). The kittens were housed from birth in total darkness. From the age of 2 weeks they were placed individually, for 5 hr each day, in a special cylindrical apparatus while wearing an opaque collar which prevented them from viewing their own bodies. The entire inner surface of the cylinder was covered with horizontally or vertically oriented high contrast black and white stripes. Beginning at 5 months, the kittens were removed from their dark cage for several hours each week for observation of their visual abilities. The kittens exhibited normal pupillary reflexes but their visually guided behavior was poor. The visual placing response and good visual depth discrimination were not present initially, but these did develop with about 10 hr of normal pattern stimulation. Some defects persisted even with pattern experience, for these kittens were unable to follow moving objects with a smooth sustained pursuit and they were effectively blind for patterns of lines perpendicular to the orientation they had experienced from birth. They failed to show a startle response to the approach of a stimulus covered with stripes of the inappropriate orientation and refused to visually place when lowered toward such a pattern. When tested with a long black or white rod that was held vertically and shaken, a kitten reared in a vertical environment would follow the rod and run and play with it; if the same rod was held horizontally, however, the kitten totally ignored it, whereas horizontally reared kittens were attracted.

Two types of evidence from human subjects suggest that visual acuity as a function of line orientation may be permanently established by differential early experience. Results such as those obtained with kittens inspired the search for such effects. Early uncorrected astigmatism (Mitchell, Freeman, Millidot & Haegerstrom, 1973) or differences in the human visual ecology (Annis & Frost, 1973) are correlated with small but significant differences in acuity scores for different edge orientations. The assumed neural substrates for such differences have been presented in Chapter V, Section III,C.

D. Pattern Vision without Eye Movements

That the visual deficits of diffused, light-reared animals might not be due exclusively to the lack of visual pattern stimulation is supported by the results of studies providing animals with the opportunity to look at patterns while preventing the usual normal scanning of stimulus contours. Animals reared with visual access to a patterned environment but without the opportunity for contouring eye movements have significant defects in their visual–motor abilities which are quite similar to those reported for animals reared with only the opportunity for diffused light stimulation. Orbach and Miller (1969) reared monkeys from birth in a stroboscopic environment which was illuminated once every 2 sec for .08 sec at a time. The flash duration was sufficient to permit normal patterned light stimulation, but it was much too brief to permit the monkeys to move their eyes to a new fixation point within the period of a given flash. After 8 months in this environment, the monkeys were transferred to normally illuminated surroundings and their visual abilities were assessed. Visual guided behavior was extremely inept, and these animals were unable to track moving objects smoothly. Form discrimination also was impaired; the discrimination of a stereometric cross and ring in a Wisconsin General Test Apparatus was learned more slowly by monkeys raised in intermittent illumination than by normally reared animals. Visual abilities improved systematically with increasing experience in a normally illuminated environment.

Rearing kittens in an intermittently illuminated environment also results in defects in visually dependent abilities (Hein, Gower, & Diamond, 1970). The animals in this experiment were dark-reared from birth to 3–6 weeks. For the next 7 or 14 days they were maintained in a stroboscopic environment where flashes of light lasting 9 μsec were presented every .5 sec. Visual abilities were then assessed under normal illumination. All kittens displayed visually triggered extension to a continuous surface, but were impaired in guided reaching to a serrated surface and did not show discrimination of visual depth when tested on the visual cliff. Seeing the paws and the textured environment only intermittently failed to provide the essential sensory–motor feedback.

Contouring eye movements are not essential for the generalization of a form discrimination in primates. Ganz and Wilson (1967) compared the generalization gradients to linear stimuli for normally reared monkeys and monkeys given pattern experience without the opportunity for visual scanning. The experimental animals used in this study were dark-reared from birth and given 2 hr of diffused light stimulation each day. The monkeys subsequently were trained, using operant conditioning techniques, to discriminate a horizontal from a vertical line while held in a primate chair with their heads firmly restrained. The stabilized image technique was used to present the discriminanda and effectively prevented the monkeys from following the stimulus contours with eye movements. Generalization then was tested to fragmented lines, smaller figures, and figures with altered figure–ground relationships. Preventing contouring eye movements did not result in any abnormalities in form generalization; both normally reared and eye movement restricted animals generalized in the same way.

E. Pattern Vision with Motor Restriction

All of the studies examined thus far have involved active, freely moving animals capable of locomotion in their visual environment. That exposure to patterned light during development does not by itself ensure the normal complement of visual abilities is indicated by studies permitting animals visual access to a patterned environment while restraining mobility. Riesen and Aarons (1959) reared kittens in total darkness from birth. At 6 weeks of age they began to receive either diffused or patterned light stimulation for 1 hr daily while held in a restraining holder. After 8–12 weeks of this experience, they were trained, in a modified Yerkes Watson box, on either an intensity or a movement discrimination. Both motor-restrained and normally reared cats learned the intensity discrimination, but the restrained cats never were able to learn a movement discrimination between a stationary and a slowly rotating cross. A subsequent study found that motor deprived cats also were impaired in discriminating between a stationary and a moving dot, requiring nearly four times as many trials as normally reared animals to learn this discrimination (Riesen, 1965). These results suggest that active movement of the animal and its limbs during perceptual development is critical if the animal is to be able to differentiate between self-initiated and externally produced movements across the visual field. Restraining animals during behavioral testing eliminates this confounding and permits the direct analysis of the ability of movement-restrained animals to discriminate between stationary and moving stimuli. Meyers (1964) reared cats in the dark from before the time that their eyes opened. At 7 weeks of age they began receiving binocular visual experience for 1 hr each day while held individually in restraining boxes. At 29 or 30 weeks of age the kittens were restrained in a holder and trained to discriminate between a stationary and a slowly rotating cross using a discriminatory response, a leg flexion, which did not require appreciable movement in visual space. The movement-restricted animals reached criterion as rapidly as normally reared animals.

Kittens reared with binocular visual experience, but with only monocular visual–motor experience, have deficits in using visual cues to guide locomotion through a series of barriers (Fish & Robinson, 1971). Kittens were reared in the dark from birth. At 6–8 weeks of age they were given binocular exposure in a normally illuminated environment for 1 hr each day while restrained in a holder. The experimental animals also were permitted unrestricted movement in an open field using one eye, the experienced eye, while the other eye, the visual–motor deprived eye, was occluded. At 18 months of age visual–motor abilities were assessed monocularly in an apparatus which required the cats to precisely negotiate a series of barriers. Compared to normally reared animals, the experimental animals had difficulty in traversing the apparatus. This result held whether the animals were tested using their visual–motor deprived eye or their experienced eye, although performance using the experienced eye was always significantly better.

Held and Hein, and their colleagues, have thoroughly investigated the notion that the deficits in visually dependent abilities of movement-deprived animals result from the lack of visual feedback accompanying self-produced movements in a normal environment. In an initial study, they compared the development of visual abilities in kittens that were free to locomote in patterned light and kittens that were passively transported through the same environment (Held & Hein, 1963). After several days in the apparatus the actively moving animals showed visual placing, accurate discrimination of visual depth, as measured using the visual cliff and eyeblink to rapidly approaching visual targets. Passively transported animals had received equivalent visual stimulation but never displayed good visual–motor coordination when first tested. Spatiomotor abilities did develop following 48 hr of freedom in a normally illuminated room. In a subsequent experiment, by exposing one eye during passive transport and the other during active locomotion, they demonstrated that the two eyes can independently acquire control of movement (Hein, Held, & Gower, 1970).

Deficits in finely guided visual abilities also result when an animal is deprived specifically of visual information of limb movement. Hein and Held (1967) dark-reared kittens until 6 weeks of age. They were then given 6 hr each day of free movement in a normally illuminated room while wearing light-weight opaque collars which prevented their viewing their limbs and torso. When tested after 12 days of this experience, all kittens displayed visual placing to a continuous surface, but not guided placing to an interrupted surface. Although head and eye orientation to a ball dangling at the end of a string appeared normal, striking responses of a paw were quite inaccurate. The kittens required an average of 15 hr of freedom in a normal environment before they displayed accurate guided reaching. A related study with infant monkeys revealed a similar dependence upon the sight of the limbs for the development of guided reaching (Held & Bauer, 1967). Infant monkeys were reared from birth to 34 days in a chair which prevented sight of their bodies. Between days 16 and 34, each monkey was conditioned to orient its head and eyes to extend its limbs horizontally upon presentation of the feeding bottle. At 35 days, one arm was exposed to view and the testing of visually guided reaching was begun. Normally reared monkeys reach for and manipulate objects before 30 days of age. The 35-day-old experimental monkeys were initially quite fascinated with viewing their newly exposed limbs. With increasing visual experience, the hand watching gradually abated and there was a concommitant improvement in the accuracy and precison of visually guided reaching. Testing was then begun with the previously unexposed limb; again there was prolonged hand watching initially, and guided reaching was poor at first, although it improved rapidly with subsequent visual experience.

Decorrelated visual–motor feedback is perhaps more damaging than simply no feedback at all. Dark-reared kittens were given 2–26 days of patterned light exposure while restrained in a holder, beginning at 4 weeks of age (Hein, et al., 1970), and with limbs and torso immobilized. In contrast to the results previously reported for passively transported animals (Held & Hein, 1963), these kittens displayed the triggered extension response to a broad surface. A further indication of the disruptive effects of decorrelated feedback is the observation that the acquisition of the visual placing response following free locomotion in a normally patterned visual environment develops more rapidly in dark-reared kittens than in kittens with prior visual experience acquired while being passively transported through the environment (Hein *et al.,* 1970).

F. Monocular versus Binocular Deprivation

Evidence has appeared consistently and repeatedly in Chapters II–VI that points to differences in the effects of monocular and binocular deprivation. On some measures the monocular deprivation procedure results in greater changes. When applied during a critical age range between 4 and 12 weeks after birth in cats, or during the first 6 months in monkeys, a persistent and almost irreversible amblyopia ex anopsia develops (Dews & Wiesel, 1970; von Noorden, Dowling, & Ferguson, 1970). This monocular "blindness" may be more resistant to forced usage than are the visual deficits that binocular pattern deprivation produces.

A study examining visual resolution in diffused light-reared monkeys reported severe acuity deficits without recovery (von Noorden *et al.,* 1970). In this study monkeys were deprived of patterned light by surgical closure of the right eye beginning during the first 4 weeks of life and lasting for periods varying between 11 and 28 months. The monkeys then were trained, using operant conditioning techniques, on an oddity discrimination involving Landolt rings in different positions. All animals displayed excellent acuity when tested with their normal eye. After acuity thresholds were established for the nondeprived eye, it was surgically closed and the acuity of the deprived eye was measured. The diffused light-stimulated eye had a large acuity loss. Using this eye, the monkeys were unable to discriminate the largest Landolt ring used (270 min of arc). This deficit did not recover even with extensive light experience. Retesting one monkey 56 months after closure of the sound eye failed to indicate any improvement in acuity. The deficit ascribed to these animals might be due in part to the training paradigm used. The authors noted that the monkeys were generally uncooperative and unwilling to perform in the apparatus when using their deprived eye because random responding failed to result in reinforcement. Observations by Chow and Stewart (1972) have indicated that the determination of discrimination abilities in deprived cats requires the use of training procedures which minimize errors, for if deprived animals make several errors in succession they are unwilling to perform.

Following monocular deprivation there is typically no savings (no interocular transfer) after the animal learns a discrimination task or an orienting response with one eye (Ganz & Fitch, 1968). Even the light intensity discrimination that transfers readily in dark-reared (Aarons *et al.*, 1963) or diffused light-reared cats (Riesen & Aarons, 1959) fails to show transfer after monocular pattern deprivation (Ganz, 1970; Ganz & Haffner, 1974). Pattern discriminations transfer readily after binocular diffused light stimulation during rearing (Ganz, 1970; Meyers & McCleary, 1964).

Fitch (1971) used a series of measures of visually guided behavior in kittens following eyelid suturing of one or both eyes. With the deprived eyes opened after 3 months, the animals performed poorly whether deprivation had been binocular or monocular, but improvement over 30 hr of testing was significantly greater in the binocularly deprived. However, with longer initial periods of deprivation (Sherman, 1973) the result may change. In Sherman's study, after 4–12 months of MD or BD it was the BD group that failed to orient "for several days after eye-opening," whereas the MD cats began almost immediately and improved their responding in a few days to objects presented in the monocular segment. This result is clearly in accord with what the data on changes in the lateral geniculate nucleus of monocularly deprived cats would lead us to expect. Sherman's study of visual field defects following deprivation will require reinterpretation of some of the earlier behavioral data. Sparing of Y cells in the monocular segments of the cat lateral geniculate nucleus (Sherman, Hoffman, & Stone, 1972) after monocular lid suturing may be peculiar to certain nonprimate mammals, but looking for a counterpart in a higher primate should be worth a search. Theory and practice in amblyopia treatment could be advanced by comparative studies.

Binocular pattern deprivation interferes less with binocular vision (and cells responsive to both eyes) than does MD, and possibly even than does misalignment of the two eyes after rectus muscle surgery or the wearing of prism lenses. In a review of his recent work, Sherman (1972b) reports that binocularly deprived cats had a fairly normal binocular visual field. Longer periods of binocular deprivation (Sherman, 1972a) do result consistently in a marked divergent squint (after 6–12 months of lid suture). Similar effects have been reported for primates (Riesen, 1958, p. 440). Recovery of binocular convergence and fixation is not impossible, as seen in both cats (Baxter, 1966) and chimpanzees (Riesen, 1958, p. 441 and Table 41).

Studies reviewed above illustrate that if both eyes have had the same visual experience, interocular transfer of visual discriminations proceeds readily. Other studies provide evidence that it is not necessary that both eyes have the same experience simultaneously. Riesen and Mellinger (1956) reared cats until 1–2 months of age in darkness. These animals then were given 2 hr of daily alternating monocular pattern experience. These animals were subsequently trained monocularly to discriminate a triangle from a circle. When they then were tested for interocular transfer, with some animals the discrimination transferred from the trained to the untrained eye. In a related study, Chow and Nissen (1955) reared a chimpanzee with monocular patterned light experience to each eye separately. This animal later displayed interocular transfer of discriminations of color and orientation of lines.

Although simultaneous binocular pattern experience is not critical for interocular transfer, without prior balanced input to the two eyes good interocular transfer does not occur. Riesen, Kurke, and Mellinger (1953) reared kittens in the dark for 14 weeks and then gave diffused light stimulation to one eye and patterned light stimulation to the other. At 17–20 weeks the cats were trained using their pattern exposed eye on a form discrimination. When subsequently tested for transfer, these animals failed to exhibit any evidence of interocular transfer to the naive eye.

Sherman (1971) compared interocular transfer in normally reared cats and in cats deprived of normal binocular vision by cutting the medial rectus muscle of one eye. The results confirm the importance of symmetry of visual input in the development of neural substrate, which provides the basis for good interocular transfer. None of the normally reared cats displayed any deficit in the transfer of either intensity or pattern discriminations from the trained to the untrained eye, whereas every experimental cat had some deficit.

Working with monkeys, von Noorden and Dowling (1970) simulated the human condition of squint (strabismus) by using surgery and traction sutures on medial and lateral rectus muscles. Esotropia produced in the first week of life resulted in marked losses of acuity (tested behaviorally with a graded series of Landolt rings) in the nonfixating eye. When this amblyopic eye was forced into use by closure of the fixating eye, slowly improving acuity developed over an eight-month period. Two exotropic monkeys showed no such prolonged deficits, as would be expected from the typical exotropic human child with alternating strabismus. Esotropia started in another monkey at 17 months produced no loss in acuity. These results with five young monkeys emphasize again the need for behavioral use of visual information during an early critical period. Passive stimulation is insufficient when pitted against active use of conflicting sensory input. Using "suppression" or "inhibition" concepts in an effort to explain these data serves primarily to point out the need to identify more precisely what happens neurophysiologically.

III. Studies of Auditory Deprivation

Although vision has been by far the most intensively studied of the senses, the results of other experiments on differential stimulation have indicated that alterations of auditory abilities also occur as a consequence of experience. In an early study (Wolf, 1943), one group of albino rats was deprived of auditory stimulation by sealing the ears with cotton and paraffin on the tenth day after birth, while another group was deprived of visual stimulation by enclosing the head in a paraffin cast 12–15 days after birth. Both deprivation conditions were terminated 25 days after birth. These rats subsequently were conditioned to approach for food upon presentation of a flashing light. Rats reared in darkness in infancy lost more often when placed in competition for the food with rats deprived of hearing. When a buzzer was substituted as the starting signal, auditory deprived animals were less successful, and the visually deprived animals won more often.

Gauron and Becker (1959) subsequently confirmed that limitations of auditory abilities do occur as a consequence of deprivation. Rats were reared under conditions similar to those used by Wolf, but the ear plugs used to effect the auditory deprivation were changed every 5 days as a precaution against possible infection. Tees (1967) used ear plugs with a sound-attenuation chamber to reduce auditory input. After deprivation from birth to 60 days, rats were retarded in learning sound patterns, tonal sequences, but not in responding to a change in pitch of one full octave.

Gottlieb (1971) investigated the effects of auditory deprivation and enrichment upon the development of aurally mediated responses in duck embryos. Embryos deprived of the opportunity to hear their own vocalizations and the vocalizations of sibs during development show a 24-hr delay in the usual ability to distingiush the maternal call of their own species from that of other species after hatching. Furthermore, precocious exposure to the vocalization of sibs accelerated the developmental changes in the overt response to the maternal call; such changes in response then occurred one day earlier than usual, indicating that a more advanced aurally mediated response had been brought about by prior stimulation.

IV. Studies of Tactual, Motor, and Somatosensory Deprivation

Experiments with several sensory modalities have confirmed the observation that restriction of stimulation during the early postnatal weeks has significant effects upon adult abilities and that early experience is critical for the achievement of well-coordinated responses to stimulation.

Nissen, Chow, and Semmes (1951) studied a male chimpanzee reared from 1 to 31 months of age under conditions where sensory stimulation from the limbs was radically reduced by the placement of cardboard mailing tubes over all four extremities, and where manipulative experience using the limbs was made physically impossible. Observations of general behavior during the rearing period indicated that the gross amount of body activity displayed by this animal was not markedly different from that displayed by normal infants. Standing and walking postures, when tested first at 14 and again at 31 months, were normal. The chimpanzee did, however, have an abnormal sitting posture, failed to climb, and did not cling or grasp the attendants. In general, coordination was poor; the animal failed to display precise guidance in using the fingers to poke at objects and to pick up pieces of food from the floor with its lips. When the fingers were forcibly curled about an object, the chimpanzee had difficulty letting go, a response similar to the forced grasping observed in newborn chimpanzees. The animal did not groom and failed to display the limb movement and sounds considered part of the normal grooming pattern.

Although the chimpanzee did respond to strong tactual stimulation by withdrawal of the limb or by scratching the affected part of the body, these movements were generally slower than in normals and were not accurately guided. Furthermore, these responses occurred only when there was the opportunity for visual guidance, for when vision was excluded as a cue by covering the eyes, the same tactual stimulation elicited only generalized body movement or squirming.

No determination of sensory thresholds was attempted in this study, but it was noted that the chimpanzee was severely handicapped in learning to discriminate two widely separated points of tactual stimulation.

Following termination of the restriction, there were some slow and gradual changes in behavior. Grasping, climbing, and clinging responses did develop, but grooming did not appear and the unusual sitting posture persisted.

A transitory motor deficit has been observed in juvenile rhesus monkeys placed in total body casts which permitted movements of only the hands, feet, and head for a period of 48 hr (Draper & Bernstein, 1963). The motor impairment was observed in the monkeys immediately after release, but was not noticeable after 15 min.

Interruption of normal afferent input to the nervous system during development also results in defects in motor abilities. Zalis, Zalis, Barron, and Oester (1965) compared the effects of interrupting the mixed sciatic nerve by section and nerve crush in albino rabbits within 48 hr after birth, or later, at 2 or 6 months of age. Although all animals displayed an initial period of paralysis immediately following surgery, and 9 months after surgery, the animals operated as adults and those operated at 2 months of age completely recovered motor function. Only the gait of those rabbits operated at birth was significantly impaired. In contrast to these behavioral effects, almost all of the animals showed evidence of physiological recovery, and even though some of the animals displayed a gait defect, symmetrical tonic and clonic contractions of all four limbs were observed under pentylenetetrazol induced convulsions. Thus, despite the ultimate restoration of nerve continuity, the absence of normal stimulation during early development could not be replaced in later life. Although motor recovery was better in those rabbits operated upon later in life, there was no difference in gross sensory recovery; most animals displayed nociceptive responses to pin prick and forceps pinching, indicating the return of some type of sensation.

Appropriate responses to painful stimulation also develop as a consequence of appropriate experiences in infancy. Thompson and Melzack (1956) examined responses to painful stimuli in Scotch terriers reared from birth in sensory isolation, protected from any painful experiences such as scratches, knocks, or blows. The dogs were exposed to a normal environment at between 7 and 10 months of age. Restricted dogs were impaired, compared to their normally reared littermates, in learning to avoid painful stimuli. Normally reared dogs learned to avoid such stimulation but the restricted dogs behaved wildly and aimlessly, when bitten by other dogs in play they neither flinched nor drew away. These animals responded with curiosity to a burning candle, sniffing the flame and thus burning their muzzles.

Findings reported by Lore (1969) suggest that the examination of the response of restriction-reared animals to painful stimuli can be confounded by their increased emotional reactivity to the novelty of the test situation. Pain avoidance behavior was compared in rats reared in a restricted or an enriched environment from 21 days of age until testing began at 77–81 days of age. During testing, the rats were exposed to a lighted candle for 5 min, both in their home cage and in a novel test cage. All rats investigated the lighted candle, but the restriction-reared rats made significantly more nose-flame contacts in the novel cage than in the home cage. In the home cage test the behavior of the experientially deprived rats was comparable to that of the rats reared in a richer environment.

V. Studies of Multisensory Enrichment and Deprivation

A. Emotionality, Exploratory and Stereotyped Behavior

Appropriate sensory experience is essential for the development of adaptive emotional responses. In general, early environmental restriction results in an increased tendency toward emotionality or fearfulness, whereas environmental enrichment reduces emotionality. Apparently these effects are longlasting. They are also less dependent upon specific sense modality used in either rearing or testing than are the perceptual–cognitive effects that are the major subject matter of this chapter. Early handling, cold stress, and multisensory stimulation are each effective environmental manipulations for reducing emotionality, increasing exploratory behavior, and reducing repetitive or stereotyped behavior such as swaying, self-grooming, and wall seeking. A major review of the studies in this area is that by Denenberg (1967), who himself contributed much impetus to research on early experience effects.

A consequence of multisensory stimulation includes subsequent facilitation of problem solving. This support may come from either motivational or perceptual learning, or both functioning in concert. Recent work is leading to the conclusion that older animals are benefitted by multisensory enrichment procedures, and we may conclude that the emphasis on early experience should be reexamined.

Riege (1971) has reported that year-old rats are as susceptible to some environmental influences as are weanling rats. Male rats were reared in standard colony cages and then at between 290 and 310 days of age they were placed for 50 days in enriched, impoverished, or in standard colony conditions (see Rosenzweig, Bennett, Diamond, 1972). Agility scores, as determined by stepdown latencies from a 12-cm platform, the time of clinging to a free suspended bar, and the number of boundary lines crossed during a free exploration period, all were significantly higher for rats reared in enriched rather than impoverished environments.

Rearing cats in restricted environments produces adults which are unusually susceptible to the impact of novel stimuli. Konrad and Bagshaw (1970) observed the responses of cats, reared in experience restricted or enriched environments from 1–2 days of age for 7½ months, in three testing situations involving novel behavior. These investigators reported that the restrictively reared cats were much more hesitant in approaching and exploring a novel room and its contents and that, in general, they explored less than did the enriched animals. Furthermore, they noted that these restricted animals displayed play behavior much later than the enriched animals. When the magnitudes of various autonomic orienting responses were measured in response to the presentation of simple novel stimuli, the restricted cats emitted much larger GSRs and displayed much larger respiratory disruptions. It was further noted that the restricted cats never struggled when placed under restraint while the control animals always did.

Monosevitz (1970) measured emotional behavior in random bred mice reared in an enriched environment from birth to 35 days of age and in standard laboratory-reared controls. Animals reared in enriched environments were significantly less emotional than controls during observations in an open field, but were significantly more active both in terms of number of squares crossed in an open field and in their activity in a running wheel.

Wood, Ruckelshaus, and Bowling (1960) compared exploratory behavior and emotionality in male and female rats reared in free or restricted environments from 21 days of age to 90 or 100 days. Restricted females explored much more than members of any other group. The other groups did not differ in amount of exploratory activity. Restricted males were significantly more emotional, as measured by counting the number of urinations and defecations, than either rats reared in a free environment or restriction-reared females.

Dogs raised in experience restricted environments also were highly responsive to novel stimuli. Thompson and Melzack (1956) examined the behavior of 7–10-month-old Scotch terriers raised from birth in sensory isolation. These restricted dogs became highly agitated and excited when exposed to a variety of novel stimuli including an opening umbrella and a slowly swelling balloon. The diffused undirected activity displayed by these animals was in striking contrast to the purposeful pattern of avoidance displayed by normally reared dogs.

Melzack (1968) has noted that dogs reared in restricted environments developed stereotyped response patterns, including tail chasing, whirling behavior, and other such self-directed activities.

Several studies have emphasized genetic differences in susceptibility to the effects of isolation. Melzack (1968) has compared the effects of restricted rearing upon the behavior of two different dog breeds—Scotch terriers and beagles. Both species displayed a high level of behavioral arousal when tested in novel situations, but Melzack observed that the beagle activity never reached the frenetic pitch of the Scotties. Although both breeds had difficulty responding selectively to novel stimuli, the Scotties had much more difficulty than the beagles in response to noxious stimuli.

Fuller (1967) assessed the effects of isolation on beagles and wire-haired terriers in an arena situation where differential responses to toys, humans, or to other puppies could be observed. Isolates made few responses to any of these stimuli. Fuller noted that isolation apparently magnified the usual differences in activity seen when dogs of these breeds were reared in the standard fashion. Beagles are characteristically less active and aggressive than terriers. Beagles reared in isolation were consistently less active than the terriers to the arena situation, although the behavior of pet-reared terriers and beagles did not differ in the arena situation.

Fuller further noted that the effects of isolation-rearing could be counteracted through a program of biweekly exposures in the arena during the rearing period or by rearing the puppies with additional visual stimulation, for example, by having a window cut into the wall of the isolation cage and permitting the isolates to look out into a busy laboratory. Rearing the puppies with toys or with a companion were not helpful in offsetting the effects of the isolation.

Lessac and Solomon (1969) compared the responses to novel stimuli of pure bred beagles placed in enriched or restricted environments for 1 year, beginning at 12 weeks of age. They reported that the behavior of the restricted dogs, upon release from isolation, was characterized by a high level of diffused and disorganized activity, and that there was no indication of adaptation to novel stimuli.

Observations of mongrel dogs raised in restricted environments for 1 week, beginning at 4 weeks of age (Fox & Stelzner, 1966; Agrawal, Fox, & Himwitch, 1967), revealed that puppies isolated even for very brief periods of time behaved similarly to puppies reared in social isolation for much longer periods of time by other investigators. The isolation-reared puppies engaged in frequent self directed activity, they were hyperactive, and they displayed a high level of diffused random activity. In contrast, the enriched environment animals were highly exploratory. They were very sociable, readily approached humans, and engaged in play with other puppies.

Stereotyped self-directed motor responses also have been observed in rhesus monkeys reared under conditions of environmental restriction (Mason, 1970). Monkeys reared under such restriction display an increased tendency toward fearfulness and/or increased emotionality toward novel stimuli or change.

Harlow, Dodsworth, and Harlow (1965) compared the effects of rearing monkeys from a few hours after birth until 3, 6, or 12 months of age in individual stainless chambers (total social isolation) or in bare wire cages with the opportunity to view, but not touch, other monkeys (partial social isolation). With increasing isolation, they found increasing interference with social behavior. Wtih long-term isolation, the primary social response was fear.

Angermeier and Phelps (1971) determined the limit of noxious stimulation required for effective responding using a shock avoidance or escape paradigm for both normally reared monkeys and monkeys reared in a restricted environment from 3 months to 12–16 months of age. They reported that the isolation reared group required significantly less shock for effective performance than did the monkeys reared in a normal environment.

Davenport and his colleageus (Davenport & Menzel, 1963; Beckett, Frohman, Davenport, Rogers, & Gottlieb, 1963; Davenport & Rogers, 1968, 1970) have carefully examined the functional relationship between early environment and later adult behavior in the chimpanzee. In all of these studies, chimpanzees were reared from birth until 2 years of age in conditions of social isolation, or the same isolation situation with either additional visual, social, or manipulative experience. All of the animals developed several stereotyped responses during the rearing period, including gross rhythmical body movements such as rocking and swaying; repetitive movements of body parts such as thumb or toe sucking, or hand clapping; and posturing. There were no reliable differences in the age of onset of these behaviors or the pattern of their development in the different rearing conditions. These stereotyped movements are not unique to conditions of extreme restriction, but also have been observed in all chimpanzees separated early from their mothers and raised in artificial conditions (Nissen, 1956). Social–sexual behaviors were markedly impaired in adult chimpanzees after restricted social experience during infancy (Riesen, 1971).

B. Learning and Memory in Sensory Deprivation Studies

The effect of sensory deprivation upon learning and memory has recently received wide attention; for instance, see reviews of effects of early experience on problem solving behavior by Mason (1970), Meyers (1971), and Gluck and Harlow (1971). Assessment of problem solving ability has been compared in animals reared in environments designed to reduce complexity of perceptual and motor stimulation or in environments which markedly enriched their total sensory and motor experience.

1. Rodents

Work with rodents has confirmed Hebb's (1949) observation that rats reared in a rich home environment were more successful problem solvers than rats reared in the usual laboratory cages.

Replications by other experimenters under more carefully controlled conditions have clearly demonstrated that performance on a series of detour problems in the Hebb Williams maze was enhanced in rats reared in a complex environment and impaired in rats reared in restricted environments. Hymovitch (1952) reared rats from 27–79 days of age under four different environmental conditions: in an enriched environment, in constraining metal cylinders, in standard mesh laboratory cages, or in solid opaque cages equipped with activity wheels. When tested at maturity, those rats reared in the enriched environment and those reared in mesh cages were clearly superior in problem solving ability as measured by the Hebb–Williams maze, to those animals reared in restricted environments. In a subsequent experiment, Forgays and Forgays (1952) confirmed the importance of the early environment. Rats reared in a free environment with "playthings" were better problem solvers than rats reared under other conditions, and restricted rats were inferior to the rats in all other rearing conditions. Woods, Ruckelshaus and Bowling (1960) compared performance on the Hebb–Williams maze in enriched and restricted rats. The male and female rats used as subjects in this study were reared in differential environments from 21 days of age to 90 or 100 days. When tested as adults on the Hebb–Williams maze, it was found that restricted females made significantly more errors than enriched females, and that performance of enriched males was superior to that of the restricted males. That the difference in the performance of the enriched and deprived rats can be attributed to their specific experiences in their rearing environments is confirmed by the observation that with added experience in the Hebb–Williams maze differences between enriched and restricted rats disappear. Sturgeon and Reid (1971) reared hooded rats in enriched or impoverished environments from 21 to 81 days of age. These animals were subsequently tested in the Hebb–Williams maze at 110 and 190 days of age. There were large differences between the groups on the first battery of tests with the animals from the enriched environment being superior problem solvers. There was little variation in the performance of the two groups on the second battery of tests; the impoverished animals were now indistinguishable from the enriched animals.

Superior performance of animals reared in enriched environments also was found when these animals were tested on tasks in other mazes. Bennett, Rosenzweig, and Diamond (1970) reported that rats weaned at 25 days of age and then placed in enriched rearing conditions for 30 days were better performers on the Lashley III and Dashiell checkerboard mazes than were rats reared for a similar period in a restricted environment. Further investigation has revealed that the enrichment and deprivation effects observed are independent of handling effects. Greenough, Madden, and Fleischmann (1972) assessed the effects of handling upon performance in otherwise isolated rats on a Lashley III maze and found that handling for 2 min daily for 30 days after weaning had no significant effect upon the ability of the rats to learn the maze.

The effects of selective deprivation and enrichment also have been de-demonstarted in adult animals. Riege (1971) reared rats in standard colony cages until they were between 290 and 310 days old and then placed them for 50 days in enriched, impoverished, or in standard colony conditions, and examined the effects of these differing environments upon maze learning. The enriched animals learned and ran the Lashley III maze concider-ably faster and with fewer errors than did their impoverished age mates. On reversal training, however, the performance of the enriched and the impoverished animals did not differ, suggesting the possibility that the initial advantage of the enriched animals might be due to their prior experience with barriers and obstacles rather than due to some unspecified nonspecific effect on the enrichment experience.

Krech, Rosenzweig, and Bennett (1962) have reported that when littermate rats were put into differential environments at 25 days of age and were left there for 1 month, those animals reared under conditions of environmental enrichment were significantly better in the solution of visual reversal discriminations based upon brightness. Further investigation, (Bennett *et al.*, 1970) using ordinary colony-reared rats as the baseline standard, has revealed that the basis for this difference in performance can be attributed to the severe impairment of function which occurs as a consequence of early restriction of experience rather than from any improvement in abilities developing as a result of enrichment of experience.

Furthermore, Bennett, *et al.* (1970) and Rosenzweig (1971) reported differential effects depending upon the age at which the selective rearing procedures are instituted. Rats were placed in enriched or impoverished environments at 30, 60, or 90 days of age, and maintained in these differential conditions for 30, 80, or 160 days. Animals were then trained on a series of visual reversal discrimination problems. In general, the enriched animals made fewer errors than their deprived littermates, but as the starting age is moved from 30, to 60, to 90 days, the performance of the enriched falls, and when the differential treatment was begun at 90 days, no reliable difference could be detected between the two groups.

A study by Cooper and Zubek (1958) has indicated that the rearing environment has differential effects depending upon the genetic characteristics of the animals used. These investigators maintained McGill maze bright and maze dull strains of rats in specialized environments from 25–65 days of age when testing in the Hebb–Williams maze was begun. They found that an enriched environment can considerably improve the learning ability of dull animals while having little effect on that of bright animals. Dull rats were not affected by their restricted environment while bright rats were significantly impaired in learning ability. After their enrichment experience, the dull enriched rats became equal in learning ability to the bright enriched animals, and after a period of early impoverishment the bright animals showed no better learning ability than the dull animals.

2. *Cats*

Wilson, Warren and Abbott (1965) investigated the effects of environmental enrichment upon the behavior of cats. Some cats were reared normally, others were handled 5 min each day from birth to 45 days of age; another group was given control experience from birth to 45 days and then was exposed on days 46–90 in a large playroom with playthings and other kittens; another group was given both handling and playroom experience. Behavioral observations at 4–7 months of age indicated that the kittens reared in a free environment explored more than control animals. These kittens made significantly fewer errors in the Hebb–Williams maze. Exposure to environmental complexity, however, did not facilitate discrimination or reversal learning by cats. Enrichment resulted in superior performance only when the task required precise spatial orientation in complex environments similar to the rearing situation.

3. *Dogs*

Melzack (1962) studied the effects of early perceptual restriction on later discrimination of visual stimuli in dogs. Pure bred beagles were maintained in cages that restricted their visual experience beginning at 3 weeks until they were 9 months of age. These restricted animals subsequently had greater difficulty in learning a black/white discrimination and its reversal than did their normally reared littermates (greater difficulty in learning a simple visual discrimination and utilizing it during reversal training). When these animals subsequently were trained to discriminate a horizontal from a vertical line, there was no difference in the performance of restricted and normally reared dogs.

Dogs reared under conditions of environmental restriction are inferior to normally reared dogs in learning to solve barrier problems. Fox and Stelzner (1966) reared dogs in partial social isolation beginning at 4 weeks of age for 1 week. These animals were inferior to controls in learning problem solving barrier tests, requiring many more trials to negotiate the detour. Thompson and Heron (1954) compared pure bred Scottish terriers reared in enriched or restricted environments in learning detour problems with parallel and L-shaped barriers and found that the dogs reared in restricted environments had much more difficulty than those reared in enriched environments. Thompson and Melzack (1956) reported that normally reared terriers readily learned an Umweg barrier problem for food, but restricted dogs failed to learn this problem. Similarily, Lessac and Solomon (1969) reared purebred beagles in enriched or restricted environments beginning at the age of 12 weeks for 1 year. They found that isolates took significantly longer than controls to solve the umweg barrier problem.

These authors found no difference in the response latency in a runway task when comparing beagles reared in either enriched or restricted environments.

Restricted dogs also have difficulty in problems requiring orientation. Thompson and Heron (1954) tested isolate reared dogs on orientation tests and found that the isolate reared dogs required more trials to learn than normals, for they tended to perseverate in their responses. Their purebred Scottish terriers reared until they were 7–10 months old under restricted conditions were unable to achieve criterion on a spatial delayed-response task which was readily learned by control animals.

Isolate dogs also were markedly impaired in learning a shuttle box avoidance response. Lessac and Solomon (1969) examined the learning ability of purebred beagles reared from 12 weeks of age for 1 year in a restricted environment and found them to be markedly impaired relative to animals given enriched experience in acquiring the avoidance response.

Normal dogs also are superior to restricted dogs in maze learning. Thompson and Heron (1954) examined learning in the Hebb–Williams maze in dogs reared as pets and other dogs reared under conditions of environmental restriction, and reported that the normally reared animals were superior to the restricted dogs on this task.

4. *Primates*

Several early studies using monkeys as the experimental animals indicated that isolation did not affect basic learning abilities in primates.

In an early study, rhesus monkeys were reared from birth in social isolation (Mason & Fitzgerald, 1962). These animals were able to learn an object discrimination in the WGTA, to acquire a discrimination reversal, to develop a learning set, to demonstrate form discrimination and form generalization.

Griffin and Harlow (1966) attempted to assess the effects of early social isolation upon later learning abilities. Monkeys were reared in total social isolation from birth to 3 months of age. When compared to partial social isolates in the acquisition of learning set in a WGTA, no significant differences were found as a consequence of differential rearing procedures.

Angermeier, Phelps, and Reynolds (1967) reared rhesus monkeys in isolated or enriched social environments from the age of 2 to 4 months. When these animals were later trained on a series of discrimination tasks, at 14 or 16 months of age, there was no evidence to indicate differential performance as a consequence of differential rearing procedures.

Harlow, Harlow, Schlitz, and Mohr (1971) also examined the effects of early experience upon later learning ability. Monkeys were reared in total isolation from birth until 6–9 months of age, whereas other monkeys were reared for a similar period in a socially enriched environment. When learning ability was subsequently assessed, using a series of discrimination problems in the WGTA, there was no indication that learning ability was influenced by early rearing conditions. Although the authors noted that the deprived animals did take longer to adapt to the testing apparatus, there were no differences between the rearing group in the acquisition of visual discrimination, delayed response tasks, or learning sets.

It has been suggested (Mason, 1970) that the failure to find an isolation effect in monkeys has been due to the selection of inappropriate groups as the relevant controls. As Mason noted, all of the monkeys used in the studies reviewed above were born and bred in laboratory cages and were reared under conditions that did not necessarily ensure sufficient enrichment to differentiate them from the restricted animals. Mason cites data by Anastasiou comparing the performance of jungle-born and laboratory-reared monkeys on a variety of tasks requiring a wide range of cognitive abilities. The results confirm the superiority of wild born over the laboratory-reared animals on all tasks.

Studies using chimpanzees as subjects are in good agreement with Anastasiou's findings and confirm the results of studies with other species, indicating that early rearing conditions can have marked effects upon adult learning abilities. Davenport and Rogers (1968) compared delayed response performance in chimpanzees reared in restricted environments from birth to 2 years of age with wild-born, enriched environment-reared chimpanzees, when both groups of animals were between 7 and 9 years of age. Although all animals performed more accurately on the task at the shorter delays (0 and 5 sec) the wild-born group was initially superior to the restricted animals at all testing delays. As testing continued, all animals improved, and at the end of the testing period the difference between the wild-born and restriction-reared animals was not significant at the shorter delays, although differences between the two groups at the longer delay interval (10 sec) persisted throughout the testing.

In a subsequent experiment, these differentially reared chimpanzees were compared on a discrimination learning set (Davenport, Rogers, & Menzel, 1969). Although the restriction-reared animals were able to develop learning sets, their performance was generally inferior to that of wild-born animals. The authors attributed the differences in performance primarily to the inability of the restriction-reared animals to reverse or inhibit old or irrelevant responses.

Subsequent testing of these animals on a variant of the Köhler stick problem (Menzel, Davenport, & Rogers, 1970) indicated that early experience of a general sort with instrumental tasks is necessary if animals are to profit from later opportunities for integration. Nine out of 10 wild-born chimpanzees were able to solve the stick problem on the first testing day, and all of the animals ultimately solved the problem, whereas only 1 out of 8 restriction/reared chimpanzees solved the problem on day 1, and only a very gradual improvement was noted in the other animals with subsequent testing.

VI. Conclusions

A. Issues of Development Arrest versus Deterioration

A critical question for theory and for practical applications and procedural decisions, along with the question of possibilities for remediation, is the issue: which effects of deprivation are attributable to failure of development and which are the result of a loss of behavior already present, or possible, if appropriately elicited? By several lines of evidence we know that isolation-rearing (almost always involving some sensory deprivation) and straightforward restriction of sensory input may sometimes destroy structures and behaviors that predated the deprivation procedure. In many experimental demonstrations of the effects of deprivation, the issue remains unresolved. This was pointed out by ethologists in their nature–nurture controversy with some of the English and American students of animal behavior. More recently, in their experiment showing that isolation-reared beagles suffer losses of abilities present at 12 weeks of age, Lessac and Solomon (1969) emphasize the pervasive nature of the problem. They suggest a four-group experimental design to help solve it, at the same time illustrating its use.

Investigators may contribute much by testing effects of the experimental treatments at more frequent developmental intervals. Such an approach would clarify certain ambiguities of data concerning effects of specific deprivations or enrichments, such as are involved in the use of exposures of visual patterns. Data similar to those of Dews and Wiesel on pattern deprivation within the 4–12 weeks age range of kittens could be most valuable in studies of pattern enrichment (as well as impoverishment). A demonstration of the value of early and frequent testing is the study of human infants by Weizzman, Cohen, and Pratt (1971) in which they found that at 6 weeks their infants devoted more fixation time to a familiar 3-dimensional visual display, and at 8 weeks a novel display induced longer fixation. Repeated testing of visual placing in control and experimental kittens also gave precise data on a requirement for 4–5 hr of visual pattern experience before visual placing could be elicited in approximately 4-week-old kittens (Munro, cited in Riesen, 1961).

When data from electrophysiology and from behavior correlate as well as do the development of disparity detector cells and improving depth discrimination in cats, we may be assured of a developmental effect of patterned visual experience. Conversely, we are assured of an atrophic effect when vision deteriorates and we find a drastic reduction in retinal ganglion cells with subsequent irreversible deficits, or when edge detectors are absent for lines of a specified orientation after such lines have been eliminated from the visual environment.

B. Animals Seek Stimulation

Among many and complex motivational effects of sensory deprivation, of particular significance is the seeking behavior that implies a need for the missing stimulation. Novel patterns of stimulation are sought (see Chapter VIII), and animals work avidly for specific stimulus energies. If they have had too little light they will work for light, and other forms of stimulation will not substitute (Lindsley *et al.,* 1964). When only diffused light is provided during a monkey's early weeks, and then only 1 hr daily, the diurnal activity cycle of the infant primate becomes entrained. The period of maximum activity anticipates and continues beyond the light period or may become organized around two daily half-hour light periods (Lindsley *et al.,* 1964, pp. 567–572). No experiments with the necessary control data have been executed to determine whether daily sound periods or diurnal rations of olfactory or somatosensory stimulation would suffice to entrain diurnal activity cycles in primates.

Stimulation, if it is to be sought after, may not be excessive either in energy level or complexity. Following early sensory deprivation, ordinary levels of light, sound, or other modes of stimulation are often avoided. References to painful light levels after operation for congenital cataracts recur frequently in the von Senden (1960) book. Withdrawal or disturbed behavior, hyperarousal, and, in extreme cases, even seizures have been described following the introduction of stimulation previously withheld (Riesen, 1961a; see also Chapters V and VIII). Initial hypersensitivities are best overcome by an appropriate use of optimum increments of sensory energies and perceptual patterns. These remain to be carefully worked out for any and all sense modes.

C. Remediation of Losses Once Incurred

Neural and behavioral plasticity in the older animal may be less than in the young, but we have seen examples of both gains and losses in older animals. Behavioral incapacities after sensory deprivation are often difficult to reverse, but only after extreme forms of deprivation or after critical periods of impoverishment are they irreversible. Baxter (1966), and Chow and Stewart (1972) showed in the cat that with appropriate rewards for successful use the deprived visual system may in some degree recover both function and structure. Slow recovery in the adult is in sharp contrast to initial rates of development during infancy. Even gross lesions in the infant's visual system are susceptible to recovery or to compensatory reorganization (Zilbert & Riesen, 1971; Stewart & Riesen, 1972). Individual variations in recovery rates in older organisms are as yet unexplained in spite of the repeated documentation that they are of considerable magnitude.

References

Aarons, L., Halasz, H. K. & Riesen, A. H. Interocular transfer of visual intensity discrimination after ablation of striate cortex in dark reared kittens. *Journal of Comparative & Physiological Psychology,* 1963, **56**, 196–199.

Agrawal, H. C., Fox, M. W., & Himwich, W. A. Neurochemical and behavioral effects of isolation rearing in the dog. *Life Sciences,* 1967, **6**, 71–78.

Angermeier, W. F., & Phelps, J. B. Early experience and levels of noxious stimulation in monkeys. *Psychologische Forschung,* 1971, **34**, 247–252.

Angermeier, W. F., Phelps, J. B., & Reynolds, H. H. The effects of differential early rearing upon discrimination learning in monkeys. *Psychonomic Science,* 1967, **8**, 379–380.

Annis, R. C., & Frost, B. Human visual ecology and orientation anisotropies in acuity. *Science,* 1973, **182**, 729–731.

Baxter, B. L. Effect of visual deprivation during postnatal maturation on the electroencephalogram of the cat. *Experimental Neurology,* 1966, **14**, 224–237.

Beckett, P. G. S., Frohman, C. E., Davenport, R. K., Jr., Rogers, C. M., & Gottlieb, J. S. Biologic effects of infantile restriction in chimpanzees. *Comprehensive Psychiatry,* 1963, **4**, 1–8.

Bennett, E. L., Rosenzweig, M. R., & Diamond, M. C. Time courses of effects of differential experience on brain measures and behavior of rats. In W. L. Byrne (Ed.), *Molecular approaches to learning and memory.* New York: Academic Press, 1970. Pp. 55–89.

Berger, R. J., & Meier, G. W. Eye movement during sleep and waking in infant monkeys (*Macaca mulatta*) deprived of pattern vision. *Developmental Psychobiology,* 1968, **1**, 266–275.

Blakemore, C. & Cooper, G. F. Development of the brain depends on visual experience, *Nature,* 1970, **228**, 477–478.

Chaloupka, Z., Musliveček, J., Semiginovský, B., & Hassmannová, J. The effect of afferentation in early postnatal life on the formation of temporary connections and other properties of the brain. *Activatas Nervosa Superior,* 1971, **13**, 147–148.

Chow, K. L., & Nissen, H. W. Interocular transfer of learning in visually naive and experienced chimpanzees. *Journal of Comparative and Physiological Psychology,* 1955, **48**, 229–237.

Chow, K. L., Riesen, A. H., & Newell, F. W. Degeneration of retinal ganglion cells in infant chimpanzees reared in darkness. *Journal of Comparative Neurology,* 1957, **107**, 27–42.

Chow, K. L., & Stewart, D. L. Reversal of structural and functional effects of long-term visual deprivation in cats. *Experimental Neurology,* 1972, **34**, 409–433.

Cool, S. J. Some effects of early visual environments on adult discrimination abilities in the rat. Unpublished doctoral dissertation, University of Illinois, 1966.

Cooper, R. M., & Zubek, J. P. Effects of enriched and restricted early environments on the learning ability of bright and dull rats. *Canadian Journal of Psychology,* 1958, **12**, 159–164.

Davenport, R. K., Jr., & Menzel, E. W., Jr. Stereotyped behavior of the infant chimpanzee. *Archives of General Psychiatry,* 1963, **8**, 99–104.

Davenport, R. K., Jr., & Rogers, C. M. Intellectual performance of differentially reared chimpanzees. I. Delayed response. *American Journal of Mental Deficiency,* 1968, **72**, 674–680.

Davenport, R. K., Jr., & Rogers, C. M. Differential rearing of the chimpanzee: A project survey. In G. H. Bourne (Ed.), *The chimpanzee,* Vol. 3. Basel: Karger, 1970. Pp. 337–360.

Davenport, R. K., Jr., Rogers, C. M., & Menzel, E. W., Jr., Intellectual performance of differentially reared chimpanzees: II. Discrimination learning set. *American Journal of Mental Deficiency,* 1969, **73**, 963–969.

Denenberg, V. H. Stimulation in infancy, emotional reactivity, and exploratory behavior. In D. H. Glass (Ed.), *Biology and behavior: Neurophysiology and emotion.* New York: Russell Sage Foundation, 1967. Pp. 161–190.

Dews, P. B. & Wiesel, T. N. Consequences of monocular deprivation on visual behavior in kittens, *Journal of Physiology,* 1970, **206**, 437–455,

Draper, W. A., & Bernstein, I. S. Note on the behavior of rhesus monkeys after release from a total plaster body cast. *Perceptual and Motor Skills,* 1963, **17**, 368.

Fantz, R. L. A method for studying early visual development. *Perceptual and Motor Skills,* 1956, **6**, 13–15.

Fantz, R. L. Form preference in newly hatched chicks. *Journal of Comparative & Physiological Psychology,* 1957, **50**, 422–430.

Fantz, R. L. Ontogeny of perception. In A. M. Schrier, H. F. Harlow, & F. Stollnitz, (Eds.), *Behavior of nonhuman primates: Modern research trends.* New York: Academic Press, 1965. Pp. 365–403.

Fish, S. E., & Robinson, J. S. A new coordination test of visuomotor deprived visually experienced cats. *Psychonomic Science,* 1971, **22**, 28–29.

Fitch, M. H. Development of visuomotor behaviors following monocular and binocular patterned visual deprivation in the cat. Unpublished doctoral dissertation, University of California, Riverside, 1971.

Forgays, D. G. & Forgays, J. W. The nature of the effect of free environmental experience in the rat. *Journal of Comparative and Physiological Psychology,* 1952, **45**, 322–328.

Fox, M. W., & Stelzner, D. Behavorial effects of differential early experience in the dog. *Animal Behavior,* 1966, **14**, 273–281.

Fuller, J. L. Experimental deprivation and later behavior. *Science,* 1967, **158,** 1645–1652.

Ganz, L. The role of selective receptive field in visual perception. In D. A. Hamburg,

K. H. Pribram, & A. J. Stunkard, (Eds.), *Perception and its disorders.* Williams & Wilkins, Baltimore: 1970.

Ganz L., & Fitch, M. The effect of visual deprivation on perceptual behavior. *Experimental Neurology,* 1968, **22,** 638–660.

Ganz, L., & Haffner, M. E. Permanent perceptual and neurophysiological effects of visual deprivation in the cat. *Experimental Brain Research,* 1974, **20,** 67–87.

Ganz, L., & Riesen, A. H. Stimulus generalization to hue in the dark reared macaque. *Journal of Comparative and Physiological Psychology,* 1962, **55,** 92–99.

Ganz, L., & Wilson, P. D. Innate generalization of a form discrimination without contouring eye movements. *Journal of Comparative and Physiological Psychology,* 1967, **63,** 258–269.

Gauron, E. F., & Becker, W. C. The effects of early sensory deprivation on adult rat behavior under competition stress: An attempt at a replication of a study by Alexander Wolf. *Journal of Comparative and Physiological Psychology,* 1959, **52,** 689–693.

Gluck, J. P., & Harlow, H. F. The effects of deprived and enriched rearing conditions on later learning: A review. In L. E. Jarrard (Ed.), *Cognitive processes of nonhuman primates.* New York: Academic Press, 1971. Pp. 103–119.

Goodman, L. Effect of total absence of function on the optic system of rabbit. *American Journal of Physiology,* 1932, **100,** 46–63.

Gottlieb, G. Ontogenesis of sensory function in birds and mammals. In E. Tobach, L. R. Aronson, & E. Shaw (Eds.), *Biopsychology of development.* New York: Academic Press, 1971. Pp. 67–128.

Greenough, W. T., Madden, T. C., & Fleischmann, T. B. Effects of isolation, daily handling and enriched rearing on maze learning. *Psychonomic Science,* 1972, **27,** 279–280.

Griffin, G. A., & Harlow, H. F. Effects of three months of total social deprivation on social adjustment and learning in rhesus monkeys. *Child Development,* 1966, **37,** 534–547.

Harlow, H. F., Dodsworth, R. O., & Harlow, M. K. Total social isolation in monkeys. *Proceedings of the National Academy of Sciences,* 1965, **54,** 90–97.

Harlow, H. F., Harlow, M. K., Schlitz, E. A., & Mohr, D. J. The effect of early adverse and enriched environments on the learning ability of rhesus monkeys. In L. E. Jarrard (Ed.), *Cognitive processes of nonhuman primates.* New York: Academic Press, 1971. Pp. 121–148.

Hebb, D. O. *The organization of behavior.* New York: Wiley, 1949.

Hein, A., & Diamond, R. M. Contrasting development of visually triggered and guided movements in kittens with respect to interocular and interlimb equivalence. *Journal of Comparative and Physiological Psychology,* 1971, **76,** 219–224.

Hein, A., Gower, E., & Diamond, R. Exposure requirements for developing the triggered component of the visual placing response. *Journal of Comparative and Physiological Psychology,* 1970, **73,** 188–192.

Hein, A., & Held, R. Dissociation of the visual placing response into elicited and guided components. *Science,* 1967, **158,** 390–392.

Hein, A., Held, R., & Gower, E. Development and segmentation of visually controlled movement by selective exposure during rearing. *Journal of Comparative & Physiological Psychology,* 1970, **73,** 181–187.

Held, R., & Bauer, R. Visually guided reaching in infant monkeys after restricted rearing. *Science,* 1967, **155,** 718–720.

Held, R., & Hein, A. Movement produced stimulation in the development of visually guided behavior. *Journal of Comparative & Physiological Psychology,* 1963, **56**, 872–876.

Heller, D. P. Absence of size constancy in visually deprived rats. *Journal of Comparative and Physiological Psychology,* 1968, **65**, 336–339.

Hubel, D. H. & Wiesel, T. N. Receptive fields of cells in striate cortex of very young, visually inexperienced kittens, *Journal of Neurophysiology,* 1963, **26**, 994–1002.

Hymovitch, B. The effects of experimental variations on problem solving in the rat. *Journal of Comparative and Physiological Psychology,* 1952, **45**, 313–321

Konrad, K. W., & Bagshaw, M. Effect of novel stimuli on cats reared in a restricted environment. *Journal of Comparative and Physiological Psychology,* 1970, **70**, 157–164.

Kobayashi, K., & van Hof, M. W. Shape discrimination in normal and light deprived rabbits. *Pflügers Archives,* 1970, **318**, 275. (Abstract)

Krech, D., Rosenzweig, M. R., & Bennett, E. L. Relations between brain chemistry and problem solving among rats raised in enriched and impoverished environments. *Journal of Comparative and Physiological Psychology,* 1962, **55**, 801–807.

Lessac, M. S., & Solomon, R. L. Effects of early isolation on the later adaptive behavior of beagles: A methodological demonstration. *Developmental Psychology,* 1969, **1**, 14–25.

Lindsley, D. B., Wendt, R. H., Lindsley, D. F., Fox, S. S.., Howell, J., & Adey, W. R. Diurnal activity, behavior and EEG responses in visually deprived monkeys. *Annals of the New York Academy of Science,* 1964, **117**, 564–588.

Lore, R. K. Pain avoidance behavior of rats in restricted and enriched environments. *Developmental Psychology,* 1969, **1**, 42–484.

McCall, R. B., & Lester, M. L. Differential enrichment potential of visual experience with angles versus curves. *Journal of Comparative and Physiological Psychology,* 1969, **69**, 644–648.

Monosevitz, M. Early environmental enrichment and mouse behavior. *Journal of Comparative and Physiological Psychology,* 1970, **71**, 459–466.

Mason, W. A. Informative processing and experiential deprivation: A biologic perspective. In F. A. Young & D. B. Lindsley (Eds.), *Early experience and visual information processing in perceptual and reading disorders.* Washington, D.C.: National Academy of Sciences, 1970. Pp. 302–323.

Mason, W. A., & FitzGerald, F. L. Intellectual performance of an isolation reared rhesus monkey. *Perceptual and Motor Skills,* 1962, **15**, 594.

Melzack, R. Effects of early perceptual restriction on simple visual discrimination. *Science,* 1962, **137**, 978–979.

Melzack, R. Early experience: A neurophysiological approach to heredity–environment interactions. In G. Newton & S. Levine (Eds.), *Early experience and behavior: The psychobiology of development.* Springfield, Illinois: Thomas, 1968. Pp. 65–82.

Menzel, E. W., Jr., Davenport R. K., Jr., & Rogers, C. M. The development of tool using in wild born and restriction reared chimpanzees. *Folia Primatologica,* 1970, **12**, 273–283.

Meyers, B. Discrimination of visual movement in perceptually deprived cats. *Journal of Comparative and Physiological Psychology,* 1964, **57**, 152–153.

Meyers, B., & McCleary, R. A. Interocular transfer of a pattern discrimination in pattern deprived cats. *Journal of Comparative Psychology,* 1964, **57**, 16–21.

Meyers, B. Early experience and problem solving behavior. In H. Moltz (Ed.), *The Ontogeny of vertebrate behavior.* New York: Academic Press, 1971. Pp. 57–94.

Mitchell, D. E., Freeman, R. D., Millodot, M., & Haegerstrom, G. Meridional amblyopia: Evidence for modification of the human visual system by early visual experience. *Vision Research,* 1973, **13**, 535–558

Nealey, S. M., & Riley, D. A. Loss and recovery of discrimination of visual depth in dark reared rat. *American Journal of Psychology,* 1963, **76**, 329–333

Nissen, H. W. Individuality in the behavior of chimpanzees. *American Anthropologist,* 1956, **58**, 407–413.

Nissen, H. W., Chow, K. L., & Semmes, J. Effects of restricted opportunity for tactual kinesthetic, and manipulative experience on the behavior of a chimpanzee. *American Journal of Psychology,* 1951, **64**, 485–507.

Orbach, J., & Miller, M. H. Visual performance of infrahuman primates reared in an intermittently illuminated room. *Vision Research,* 1969, **9**, 713–716.

Ordy, J. M., Massopust, L. C., & Wolin, L. R. Postnatal development of the retina, ERG and acuity in the rhesus monkey. *Experimental Neurology,* 1962, **5**, 364–382.

Rasch, E., Swift, H., Riesen, A. H., & Chow, K. L. Altered structure and composition of retinal cells in dark-reared mammals. *Experimental Cell Research,* 1961, **25**, 348–363.

Riege, W. H. Environmental influences on brain and behavior of year old rats. *Developmental Psychobiology,* 1971, **4**, 157–167.

Riesen, A. H. The development of visual perception in man and chimpanzee. *Science,* 1947, **106**, 107–108.

Riesen, A. H. Arrested Vision. *Scientific American,* 1950, **183**, 16–19.

Riesen, A. H. Plasticity of behavior: Psychological aspects. In H. F. Harlow & C. Woolsey (Eds.), *Biological and biochemical bases of behavior.* Madison: University of Wisconsin Press, 1958. Pp. 425–450.

Riesen, A. H. Excessive arousal effects of stimulation after early sensory deprivation. In P. Solomon *et al.* (Eds.), *Sensory deprivation.* Cambridge, Massachusetts: Harvard University Press, 1961. Pp. 34–40. (a)

Riesen, A. H. Studying perceptual development using the technique of sensory deprivation. *Journal of Nervous and Mental Diseases,* 1961, **132**, 21–25. (b)

Riesen, A. H. Effects of visual deprivation on perceptual function and the neural substrate. In J. de Ajuriaguerra, (Ed.), *Symposium bel air II, désafférentation expérimentale et clinique. Geneva:* George & Cie, 1965. Pp. 47–66.

Riesen, A. H. Nissen's observations on the development of sexual behavior in captive-born, nursery-reared chimpanzees. In G. H. Bourne (Ed.), *The chimpanzee,* Vol. 4. Basel, Switzerland: S. Karger, 1971. Pp. 1–18.

Riesen, A. H., & Aarons, L. Visual movement and intensity discrimination in cats after early deprivation of pattern vision. *Journal of Comparative & Physiological Psychology,* 1959, **52**, 142–149.

Riesen, A. H., Kurke, M. I., & Mellinger, J. C. Interocular transfer of habits learned monocularly in visually naive and visually experienced cats. *Journal of Comparative and Physiological Psychology,* 1953, **46**, 166–172.

Riesen, A. H., & Mellinger, J. C. Interocular transfer of habits in cats after alternating monocular visual experience. *Journal of Comparative and Physiological Psychology,* 1956, **49**, 516–520.

Riesen, A. H., Ramsey, R. L., & Wilson, P. D. The development of visual acuity in rhesus monkeys deprived of patterned light during early infancy. *Psychonomic Science,* 1964, **1**, 33–34.

Rizzolatti, G., & Tradardi, V. Pattern discrimination in monocularly reared cats. *Experimental Neurology,* 1971, **33**, 181–194.

Rosenzweig, M. R. Effects of environment on development of brain and of behavior. In E. Tobach, L. R. Aronson, & E. Shaw (Eds.), *Biopsychology of development.* New York: Academic Press, 1971. Pp. 303–342.

Rosenzweig, M. R., Bennett, E. L., & Diamond, M. C. Brain changes in response to experience. *Scientific American,* 1972, **226**, 22–29.

Sherman, S. M. Role of the visual cortex in interocular transfer in the cat. *Experimental Neurology,* 1971, **30**, 34–45.

Sherman, S. M. Development of interocular alignment in cats. *Brain Research,* 1972, **37**, 187–203. (a)

Sherman, S. M. Visual development in cats. *Investigative Ophthalmology,* 1972, **11**, 394–401. (b)

Sherman, S. M. Visual field defects in monocularly and binocularly deprived cats. *Brain Research,* 1973, **49**, 25–45.

Sherman, S. M., Hoffman, K.-P., & Stone, J. Loss of a specific cell type from the dorsal lateral geniculate nucleus in visually deprived cats. *Journal of Neurophysiology,* 1972, **35**, 532–541.

Stewart, D. L., & Riesen, A. H. Adult versus infant brain damage: Behavioral and electrophysiological effects of striatectomy in adult and neonatal rabbits. *Advances in Psychobiology* 1972, **1**, 171–211.

Sturgeon, R. D., & Reid, L. D. Rearing variations and Hebb–Williams maze performance. *Psychological Reports,* 1971, **29**, 571–580.

Tees, R. C. Effects of early auditory restriction in the rat on adult pattern discrimination. *Journal of Comparative and Physiological Psychology,* 1967, **63**, 389–393.

Tees, R. C. Effects of early visual restriction on later intensity discrimination in rats. *Journal of Comparative and Physiological Psychology,* 1968, **66**, 224–227. (a)

Tees, R. C. Effects of early restriction on later form discrimination in the rat. *Canadian Journal of Psychology,* 1968, **22**, 294–301. (b)

Tees, R. C. Luminance and luminous flux discrimination in rats after early visual deprivation. *Journal of Comparative and Physiological Psychology,* 1971, **74**, 292–297.

Thompson, W. R., & Heron, W. The effects of restricting early experience on the problem solving capacity in dogs. *Canadian Journal of Psychology,* 1954, **8**, 17–31.

Thompson, W. R., & Melzack, R. Early environment. *Scientific American,* 1956, **194**, 38–42.

Tucker, A. The effect of early light and form deprivation on the visual behavior of the chicken. Unpublished doctoral dissertation, University of Chicago, 1957.

van Hof, M. W. Orientation discrimination in normal and light deprived rabbits. *Documenta Ophthalmologica,* 1971, **30**, 299–311.

van Hof, M. W., van Hof-van Duin, J., & Kobayashi, K. Vision in rabbits and cats deprived of light after birth. *Brain Research,* 1972, **37**, 354–355.

Volokhov, A. A., & Shiljagina, N. N. (Formation of a defensive conditioned reflex to a photic stimulus after early visual deprivation.) Russian with English abstract. *Zhurnal Vysshei nervnoi deiatel nosti imeni I.P. Pavlova,* 1972, **22**, 735–742.

von Noorden, G. K., & Dowling, J. E. Experimental amblyopia in monkeys. II. Behavioral studies in strabismic amblyopia. *Archives of Ophthalmology,* 1970, **84**, 215–220.

von Noorden, G. K., Dowling, J. E., & Ferguson, D. C. Experimental amblyopia in monkeys. I. Behavioral studies of stimulus deprivation amblyopia. *Archives of Ophthalmology,* 1970, **84**, 206–214.

von Senden, M. *Space and sight* (Translation by P. Heath). London: Methuen, 1960.

Walk, R. D., & Bond, E. K. Deficit in depth perception of 90 day old dark reared rats. *Psychonomic Science,* 1968, **10**, 383–384.

Walk, R. D., & Gibson, E. J. A comparative and analytical study of depth perception. *Psychological Monographs,* 1961, **75**, 44.

Walk, R. D., Gibson, E. J., & Tighe, T. J. Behavior of light and dark reared rats on the visual cliff. *Science,* 1957, **126**, 80–81.

Weizmann, F., Cohen, L. B., & Pratt, R. J. Novelty, familiarity, and the development of infant attention. *Developmental Psychology,* 1971, **4**, 149–154.

Wiesel, T. N., & Hubel, D. H. Extent of recovery from the effects of visual deprivation in kittens deprived of vision in one eye. *Journal of Neurophysiology,* 1963, **26**, 1003–1017.

Wiesel, T. N., & Hubel, D. H. Extent of recovery from the effects of visual deprivation in kittens. *Journal of Neurophysiology,* 1965, **28**, 1060–1072.

Wilson, M., Warren, J. M., & Abbott, L. Infantile stimulation, activity and learning by cats. *Child development,* 1965, **36**, 843–853.

Wilson, P. D., & Riesen, A. H. Visual development in rhesus monkeys neonatally deprived of patterned light. *Journal of Comparative and Physiological Psychology,* 1966, **61**, 87–95.

Winsberg, G. R., & Riesen, A. H. Cytochemical changes in the nucleoproteins of macaques reared in differing visual environments. *Journal of Histochemistry and Cytochemistry,* 1966, **14**, 798–799.

Wolf, A. The dynamics of the selective inhibition of specific functions in neurosis: A preliminary report. *Psychosomatic Medicine,* 1943, **5**, 27–38.

Woods, P. J., Ruckelshaus, S. I., & Bowling, D. M. Some effects of 'free' and 'restricted' environmental rearing conditions upon adult behavior in the rat. *Psychological Reports,* 1960, **6**, 191–200.

Zalis, O. S., Zalis, A. W., Barron, K. D., & Oester, Y. T. Motor patterning following transitory sensory–motor deprivation. *Archives of Neurology,* 1965, **13**, 487–494.

Zilbert, D. E., & Riesen, A. H. A comparison of the effects of infant and adult retinal lesions upon visual acuity in the rabbit. *Experimental Neurology,* 1971, **33**, 445–458.

Zimmerman, R. R. Analysis of the discrimination learning capacities in infant rhesus monkeys. *Journal of Comparative & Physiological Psychology,* 1961, **54**, 1–10.

CHAPTER VIII

Novelty-Enhancement Effects Associated with Early Sensory–Social Isolation

Karl Konrad

Department of Psychology
Saint Mary's University

Ronald Melzack

Department of Psychology
McGill University

I. Introduction

There is convincing evidence that animals—from rat to chimpanzee—reared in sensory and social isolation show highly abnormal behavior patterns at maturity. The nature of the abnormality, however, presents a major problem. Early isolation procedures do not simply withhold experience; rather, they impose another, abnormal environment on the organism. Furthermore, emergence from this environment into the "normal" world means a drastic change from a familiar "home" into a totally novel environment.

The demonstration that the performance of rats on intelligence tests is strikingly affected by early sensory isolation (Hebb, 1949; Hymovitch, 1952) was initially interpreted to mean that an impoverished early environment diminishes problem-solving ability. Later investigators, however, began to question the simplicity of this hypothesis. In 1957, Zimbardo and Montgomery reported that isolation-reared rats explored more in a Y maze than did rats reared in an enriched environment. Their finding led them to speculate that the reported poor performance of isolation-reared rats in the Hebb–Williams intelligence-test maze might be due, at least in part, to excessive exploration of novel stimuli in the apparatus. Subsequently, Woods (1959) reported that isolation-reared rats did, in fact, engage in more exploration in the maze, and in such a way—for example, retracing the maze after solving the problem but before entering the goal box—that it seriously interfered with good maze performance. Later work by other investigators indicates that the tendency for isolation-reared mammals to "overrespond" to novel aspects of testing environments is a ubiquitous phenomenon. We refer to this effect of isolation rearing as "novelty enhancement." In what follows, we hope to show that novelty-enhancement effects are observed in the behavior of isolation-reared members of all species studied to date and in a broad range of situations, including those normally employed to study exploration, problem solving, and a range of social behaviors.

The novelty-enhancement effect of isolation-rearing implies that many aspects of most testing environments will be experienced as more novel by isolation-reared subjects than by normally reared subjects. Novelty is presumed to be enhanced for isolates because of the experience-restricted nature of their earlier life. Expectations of the world built up through the course of living in a confined, static isolation chamber are likely to be massively and continuously disconfirmed by even the modest approximation to reality provided by testing environments, with their openness, presence of objects and organisms, and continuous movement and change. Since the degree of novelty in a situation is a major determinant of behavior in that situation, part, at least, of the behavioral differences between isolates and normals may be thus explained.

A basic assumption of this hypothesis is that the differential behavior patterns of isolate and normal subjects are, in fact, on the same novelty-behavior continuum. This can be demonstrated by showing that after habituation to novelty, isolates come to behave like normal animals, and that in extreme cases of object–situation novelty, normals can display the behaviors of isolates. One would also expect that the differential behavior patterns of isolates and normals would be maintained across many different situations, all involving novel stimuli. These demonstrations may need to be made separately for each species since the function relating behavior and novelty appears to vary, except in the most general terms, from species to species. There are abundant data for the isolate chimpanzee, monkey, and dog, less for the cat and rat. Nevertheless, we feel that a good case can be made for novelty-enhancement effects on the basis of the available data.

II. Novelty Enhancement: Comparative Data

The most common method for studying the influence of early experience on later behavior is to deprive an organism of its normal environment beginning at infancy, and then to examine its behavior at maturity. This is accomplished by (1) depriving an organism of all patterned input in a modality such as vision (Riesen, 1961a, b; Wiesel & Hubel, 1965a, b), (2) restricting, or narrowing down the range of sensory experience, or (3) social isolation. Methods (2) and (3), which involve rearing animals in special isolation cages or rooms, are of major concern in this analysis. They will be considered together as "isolation" experiments, since most of the studies to be discussed involve simultaneous sensory and social isolation. Animals reared this way will be called "isolates."

A. Chimpanzee

When wild-born chimpanzees (Menzel, 1964) are presented with an unusually complex, novel object for the first time, they avoid contact with the object by attempted escape, freezing, and even, on occasion, by sleeping. As exposure to the object continues, however, behavior toward the object passes through a number of stages in the following order: threats; tentative approaches and quick retreats; brief contacts with wrist, digit, or toe; active aggression; full grasping; and play manipulations. Only after the stage of active play has been completed will subjects behave "purposively" toward the object, for example, by eating it, grooming it, or using it as a tool. If the object has no utility it will gradually come to be ignored. This is a rough description of the function relating novelty and behavior for chimpanzees. It begins with avoidance, moves to tentative threats and approaches, minimal contact, aggression, full contact, play, and finally incorporation into relevant instructional behavior (or indifference if the object lacks utility). The full novelty–behavior sequence is rarely observed among wild-born chimpanzees unless the object is unusually strange or complex. With simpler or more familiar objects, wild-born subjects begin somewhere in the middle of the sequence and advance rather quickly through manipulation and use as habituation occurs.

Among isolation-reared chimpanzees just removed from their home cage (Menzel, 1964), the novelty–behavior sequence, even for the simplest objects, is invariably entered at the first stage of complete avoidance, and progression through the sequence is accomplished at a very slow rate. Thus, when isolate and wild-born chimpanzees were tested during a 6-week period for their responsiveness to small novel objects, isolates made contacts during only 3.6% of the available time, in contrast with 54.4% for wild-born subjects (Menzel, Davenport, & Rogers, 1963a). In further tests with similar novel objects, isolates showed increasing generalization from earlier experiences and required progressively less object exposure to complete the novelty–behavior sequence. As experience with novel objects continued, the isolates became generally less fearful in all situations. It should be noted, however, that months or years were required for a significant change in fearfulness to occur.

Menzel has noted that the novelty–behavior sequence has broad relevance for understanding chimpanzee behavior. In general, there is a high probability that isolate and wild-born chimpanzees will initially respond to objects, situations, and organisms as novel things, and not as food, tools, space for locomotion, or organisms appropriate for social interaction. However, since the two groups are likely to begin in the novelty–behavior sequence at different places and move through it at different rates, wild-born chimpanzees will likely be seen to make appropriate "goal-directed" responses either exclusively, or sooner than isolate chimps. These two possibilities were seen to occur in two experiments. In the first experiment (Menzel, Davenport, & Rogers, 1963b), subjects were placed singly for 2 hr in an unfamiliar room containing barriers and manipulable objects. Wild-born subjects appeared distressed initially, but relatively quickly began to explore in the room and manipulate objects. When they slept in the room it was always after exploration and object manipulation. Isolate chimpanzees, on the other hand, spent most of the time engaged in stereotyped behaviors. They did not explore or manipulate objects, and if they slept it was apparently a sleep of avoidance. In the second experiment (Davenport, Rogers, & Menzel, unpublished data cited in Mason,

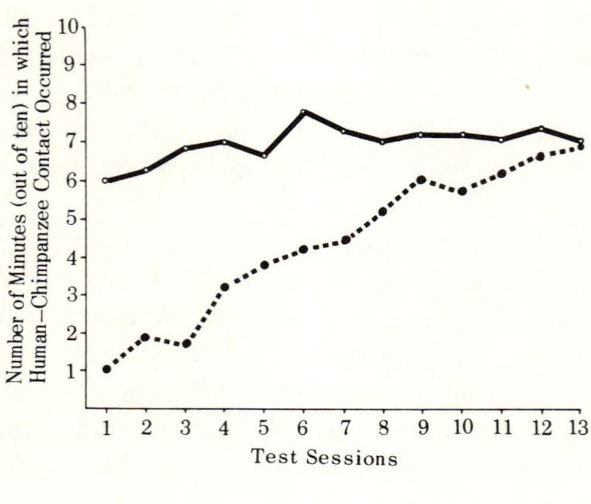

Fig. 1. Social contacts of isolate (dashed line) and wild-born (solid line) chimpanzees with a human experimenter (based on unpublished data obtained by R. K. Davenport, M. Rogers, & E. W. Menzel, cited in Mason *et al.*, 1968).

Davenport, & Menzel, 1968), isolate and wild-born chimpanzees were given the opportunity to make voluntary contact with a passive person during a 10-min period each day for 13 days. On each day after the initial 10 min, the person spent 50 min encouraging the chimpanzees to socialize by making gentle social contact. As can be seen in Fig. 1, wild-born subjects maintained a high level of social responsiveness throughout, whereas isolate subjects exhibited this level of responsiveness only after many hours of adaptation experience.

B. Monkey

The available data on novelty enhancement effects of isolation-rearing in the monkey (Mason & Green, 1962; Mason & Sponholz, 1963; Mitchell, Raymond, Ruppenthal, & Harlow, 1966; Sackett, 1965) are generally consistent with the chimpanzee data. The study by Sackett is especially interesting because it illustrates both limbs of a novelty-approach inverted "U" function, in which approach is hypothesized to increase initially as novelty decreases from extreme high values, and then to decrease again as novelty values drop to low levels and boredom sets in (Fig. 2). Sackett compared object manipulation in three groups of monkeys with differing degrees of isolation experience during early rearing: severely isolated, moderately isolated, and wild-born. The subjects were tested for 12 hr in a small wire-mesh cage on three separate occasions. On each occasion subjects were presented with a different manipulable object hanging from the center of the top of the cage. The objects ranged in "novelty" value from

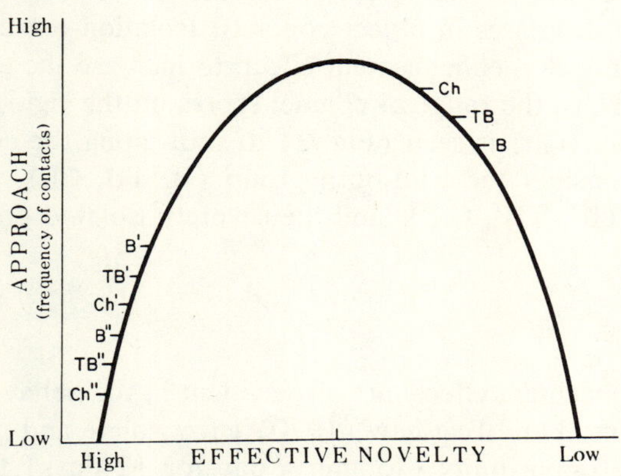

Fig. 2. Graph of the proposed relationship between approach behavior (frequency of contacts) with a manipulable object, and the effective novelty of the object. See text for explanation and definition of symbols.

simple to complex: a rigid bar, a "T" bar movable 3 in in the up–down direction, and a length of freely hanging chain. Sackett recorded both frequency and duration of object contacts. Since the frequency and duration data give essentially the same picture, we have presented only the former in Table I.

TABLE I

FREQUENCY OF CONTACTS WITH MANIPULABLE STIMULI DURING 12-HR TEST PERIODS [a]

	Degree of Rearing Isolation		
Stimulus	Severe	Moderate	Low (wild-born)
Rigid bar	36	301	601
T bar	21	101	1202
Chain	2	57	2010

[a] From Sackett (1965).

Consider the results of Table I in the context of Fig. 2, which illustrates the relationship between degree of object novelty and approach behavior. In the figure, novelty is labeled "effective novelty" since we conceive of it as being a function of stimulus parameters (for example, complexity) and subject–experience parameters (for example, the richness of the early environment). These two factors are exhibited in Sackett's results. With increasing object complexity, approaches (object contacts) increase for wild-born subjects. For isolation-reared subjects, who appear to be operating on the left-side of the curve, increases in stimulus complexity are associated with decreases in object contacts. Isolation-rearing is presumed, because of the novelty–enhancement effect, to increase the effective novelty of all objects. Thus, the range of contact scores on the rigid bar (B), T bar (TB), and chain (Ch) is seen (Fig. 2) to shift along the curve from right to left as we consider the wild-born group (B, TB, Ch), the moderately isolated group (B′, TB′, Ch′), and the severely isolated group (B″, TB″, Ch″).

C. CAT

Novelty enhancement effects are also evident in the behavior of isolation-reared cats. Konrad and Bagshaw (1970) gave isolate and normally reared control cats the opportunity (15 min a day for 12 days) to enter an unfamiliar room, to explore it, and to play with twisted pipe cleaners placed on the floor. The results of this experiment, in terms of latency to enter, and exploration and play times, are presented in Fig. 3. The novelty–behavior

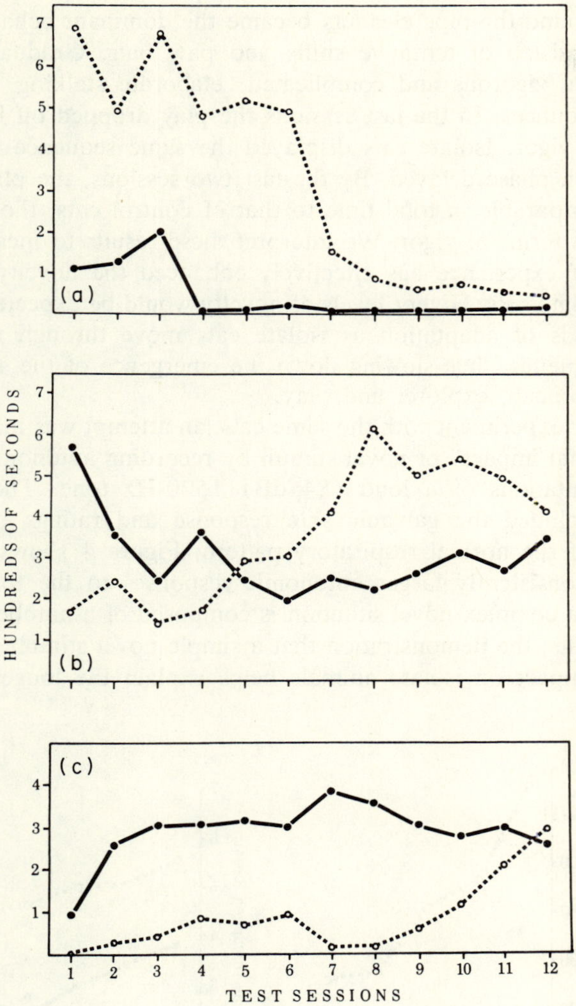

Fig. 3. Mean latency (A), exploration (B), and play (C) scores for isolate and control cats during successive testing sessions: dashed lines, isolate; solid lines, control. (From Konrad & Bagshaw, 1970.)

sequence was roughly the same for both groups of cats, but differed in timing for the two groups. Control cats delayed entering the room during the early sessions; threafter latencies dropped to about 15 sec. After entering the room in the early sessions, the predominant behavior of control cats was systematic exploration—initially around the perimeter of the room and then in the central portions. In subsequent sessions, play behavior centering around the pipe cleaners became the dominant behavior. At first the play consisted of tentative sniffs and paw bats. Gradually the play became more vigorous and complicated: elaborate stalking, wild rushes, leaps, and pounces. In the last sessions the play dropped off both in total time and in vigor. Isolate cats displayed the same sequence of behavior, but with each phase delayed. By the last two sessions, the play of isolate cats was comparable in total time to that of control cats, though still not equivalent in terms of vigor. We interpret these results to mean that early restriction of experience has effectively enhanced the novelty of the test room for isolate cats. Higher levels of novelty would be expected to require longer periods of adaptation as isolate cats move through the novelty–behavior sequence, thus slowing down the emergence of the sequence behaviors: approach, explore, and play.

In another experiment with the same cats, an attempt was made to assess the "emotional impact" of novel stimuli by recording autonomic responses to 50 presentations of a loud (84 dB) 1500-Hz tone. The autonomic measures included the galvanic skin response and ratings of degree of disruption of the normal respiratory pattern. Figure 4 shows that isolate cats made consistently larger autonomic responses to the tone presentations. Since a complex novel situation is composed of a number of discrete novel elements, the demonstration that a simple novel stimulus has greater emotional impact on isolate animals helps explain the longer periods of

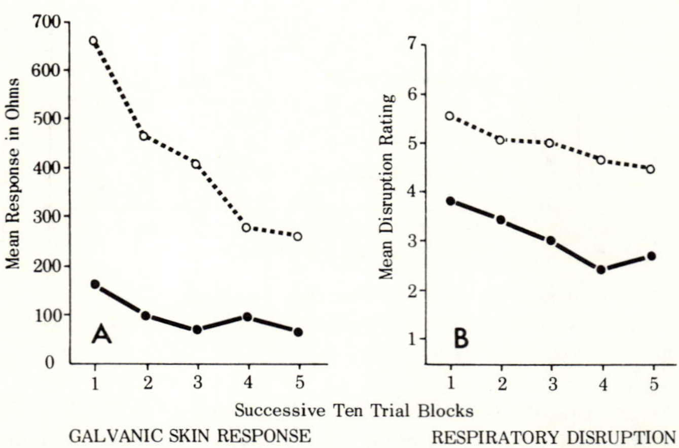

Fig. 4. Mean GSR (A) and respiratory disruption (B) responses elicited by tone presentations in isolate and control cats: dashed lines, isolate; solid lines control. (From Konrad & Bagshaw, 1970.)

habituation required by isolates before approaching and dealing with complex novel situations.

D. Dog

Similar novelty enhancement effects have been observed in dogs. Isolate Scottish terriers were found (Thompson & Heron, 1954a) to be more active than pet-reared controls in exploring a room which contained several partitions. Our interpretation is that isolate animals found the essentially empty room more novel, and therefore more worthy of extended exploration, than did the control terriers. Consistent with this point of view are several incidental findings in the same experiment: severely isolated dogs explored more than slightly isolated, and younger (less experienced) dogs in both groups explored more than older (more experienced) dogs.

These observations, and similar data (Fig. 5A) obtained by Melzack (1968) with beagles, are in apparent contradiction with results obtained

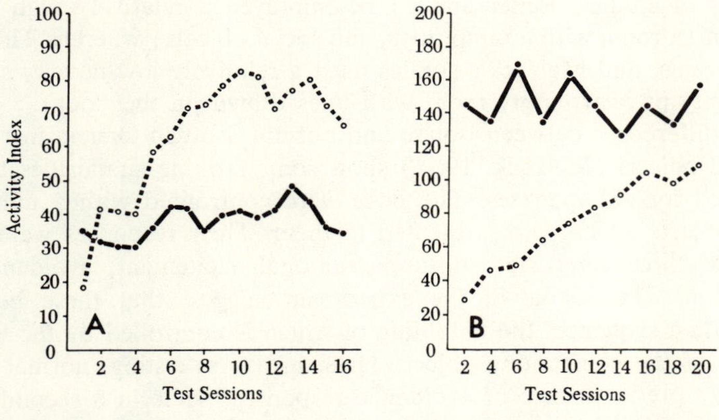

Fig. 5. Development of activity in isolate and control beagles after release from rearing cages (solid lines, control): (A) activity in an empty room (dashed line, isolate) (from Melzack, 1968); (B) activity in a novel arena (dashed line, isolate combined) (adapted from Fuller and Clark, 1966).

by Fuller and Clark (1966), who tested isolate and control beagles in a novel, room-like "arena" over a number of days (Fig. 5B). Each subject's latency to enter the arena, activity in the arena, and contacts with arena objects—toys, another dog, a human experimenter—were recorded. By the second session, all normally reared beagles had entered and were active in the arena. Isolate beagles, on the other hand, were slow to enter the arena, and 40% had still not entered by the end of the experiment. Because of their delayed emergence, isolate dogs did not approach normal levels of arena activity until the last testing sessions (see Fig. 5B), nor did they make as many object contacts in the arena as normal dogs. In addition, when object contacts were made by isolates, they tended to be less vigorous than those of normal subjects. In their conclusions, Fuller and Clark (1966) suggest that the abnormal behavior of their isolation-reared beagles is due to ". . . a blocking of approach and contactual responses by pre-emptive aversive reactions to unfamiliar stimuli."

The apparent contradiction between Thompson and Heron's (1954a) and Melzack's (1968) observations that isolate dogs (scotties and beagles) explore more than control dogs, and Fuller and Clark's (1966) report that isolate beagles explore less than control beagles may be resolved if we consider the inverted "U" curve of Fig. 2. Fuller and Clark's test situation may have produced data for both groups on the left side of the curve (control > isolates), whereas Melzack's test situation may have produced data for both groups on the right side (control < isolate). This interpretation is consistent with the nature of the test situations employed in the two sets of studies. Fuller and Clark employed a relatively high novelty situation (a room with a ramp, toys, and social objects) whereas Thompson and Heron's, and Melzack's studies used a relatively low-novelty situation (an empty or near empty room with lines drawn on the floor).

The differences between isolate and normal Scottish terriers in response to novel objects (Melzack, 1954) show some striking similarities to those described for chimpanzees. The dogs were confronted with a number of novel objects which were presented to them. Their responses were classified into three categories: diffuse emotional excitement, avoidance, and aggression. The results of the experiment suggest that these behaviors constitute a sequence, the unfolding of which is controlled by the effective novelty of the confronting object. Thus, in a first testing, normal terriers showed a predominance of avoidance responses, while in a second testing with the same objects 10 months later, the responses were distributed about equally in the avoidance and aggression categories. In the case of isolate terriers, responses were concentrated in the diffuse emotional excitement category on first testing, and in the avoidance category, on second testing.

Similarly, the social behavior of isolation-reared terriers may be affected by novelty factors (Melzack & Thompson, 1956). When isolate terriers were introduced to a strange dog, they responded with diffuse emotional excitement: excited, rapid movement near the social object, with short, jerky, to-and-fro movements. In the same situation, normal dogs exhibited well-organized social curiosity: sniffing, following, threats, etc. When confronted with the experimenter playing the role of a "friendly man," the isolate dogs again showed primarily diffuse emotional excitement, whereas normal terriers responded with appropriate, organized friendly responses. When the experimenter played the role of a "timid man" who withdrew whenever the dog approached—a human behavior pattern probably novel even for normally reared dogs—both restricted and control dogs exhibited diffuse emotional excitement.

E. Rat

It has already been noted that isolation-reared rats spend more time than control rats in exploring a Y maze (Zimbardo & Montgomery, 1957). It is possible, then, that the poor performance by isolates in the Hebb–Williams maze (Hebb, 1949; Hymovitch, 1952) may be due to inappropriate exploration in the maze (Woods, 1959). In Woods' experiment, the subjects were given eight trials on each of six problems in a Hebb–Williams maze. Figure 6A shows average errors over the eight trials for all six

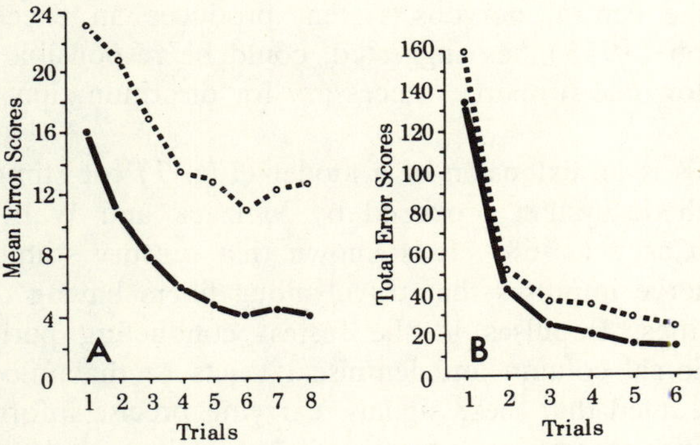

Fig. 6. Maze performance of isolate and control animals (dashed lines, isolate, and solid lines, control): (A) Rats, points on curve obtained by averaging error scores on each trial over problems 1–6 (adapted from Woods, 1959); (B) Scottish terriers; points obtained by averaging error scores on each trial over problems 1–18 (adapted from Thompson & Heron, 1954b).

problems combined. As in the case of Scottish terriers (Thompson & Heron, 1954b; see Fig. 6B), both groups learn (that is, eliminate errors) at the same rate, but isolate subjects show inferior performance throughout —perhaps due to a tendency to engage in inappropriate exploration in a test environment whose novelty is enhanced for isolation-reared subjects.

In summary, the failure of isolate animals of many species to approach and interact with novel objects and situations before experiencing prolonged exposure to them underscores the critical role of novelty habituation as a general precondition to all other purposeful behavior. This role is likely to be obscured in normally reared animals whose extensive experience during the course of development provides them with sufficient novelty habituation to deal purposefully with a broad range of objects, foods, habitats, and social partners, with only a minimum of additional habituation experience. Only on rare occasions is their behavior likely to be conspicuously controlled by the novelty characteristics of objects and situations.

III. Novelty Enhancement: An Information Processing Approach

The novelty enhancement concept is the basis of a physiological model to account for the effects of early isolation. Melzack (1965) has proposed that: (1) the sensory inputs evoked by novel stimuli in isolation-reared animals are not filtered or selected by memories of the significances of the stimuli (normally acquired in early experience), so that (2) the total input bombarding the central nervous system produces an excessive arousal which, as Hebb (1955) has suggested, could be responsible for the correspondingly low cue properties necessary for discrimination and adaptive response.

This analysis is an extension of a model (Fig. 7) for stimulus selection in the somesthetic system proposed by Melzack and Wall (1965) and Melzack and Casey (1968). It is known that sensory stimulation of the skin evokes nerve impulses that travel along fibers having different conduction velocities. Impulses in the fastest conducting peripheral fibers traverse the dorsal column and lemniscal tracts to thalamic and cortical areas. It is assumed that these signals, carrying precise information about the stimulus, do not evoke "sensation," but activate "phase sequences" corresponding to earlier experience, which are then able to control information selection (via centrifugal fibers) at lower synaptic levels of the more slowly conducting fiber systems. In this way, past experience would be able to influence the selection of the particular patterns that subserve perception and response while other patterns are inhibited or otherwise filtered out. Thus, the "phase sequence," developed on the basis of prior experience, is conceived to be actively engaged in information selection in the early stages of sensory transmission rather than passively evoked to subserve perception per se.

The model, then, suggests that memories of earlier experience normally exert control over information selection at successive synaptic levels of sensory pathways. As a result of severe restriction of early experience,

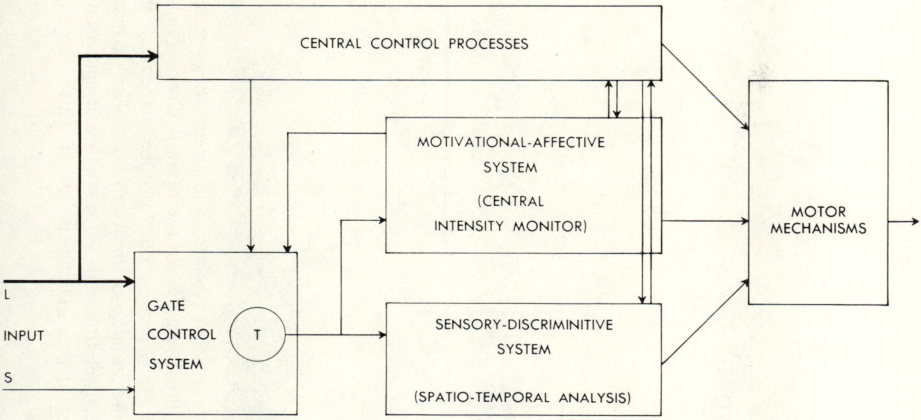

Fig. 7. Conceptual model of the sensory, motivational, and central control determinants of pain. The output of the T cells of the gate control system projects to the sensory–discriminative system (via neospinothalmic fibers) and the motivational–affective system (via the paramedial ascending system). The central control trigger (comprising the dorsal-column and dorsolateral projection systems) is represented by a line running from the large fiber system to central control processes; these, in turn, project back to the gate control system, and to the sensory–discriminative and motivational–affective systems. All three systems interact with one another, and project to the motor system. (From Melzack & Casey, 1968.)

most stimuli in a totally new environment have no meaning (phase sequences representing prior associations) to provide a basis for selective filtering of the sensory input. Consequently, all inputs, irrelevant as well as relevant, would reach the brain where they could bombard the neural systems that produce sensory and emotional arousal. In the extreme, the excessive arousal might produce complete disruption of organized, adaptive behavior. In lesser degrees, the excessive arousal would place animals at the earlier stages of the novelty-behavior sequence, for example, escape–freezing instead of approach; exploration–manipulation rather than play; and play instead of means–end behavior.

This analysis is supported by physiological observations (Melzack & Burns, 1965) of isolate and control beagles with implanted subcortical and cortical recording electrodes. When isolate dogs were first permitted to look at a novel environment through their open cage doors, their reticular and cortical EEGs showed a striking shift from predominantly low to high frequences (indicating high levels of EEG arousal), and a shift back to low frequencies only after the door was closed. The EEGs of control dogs showed brief shifts to higher frequencies, but never to the extent observed

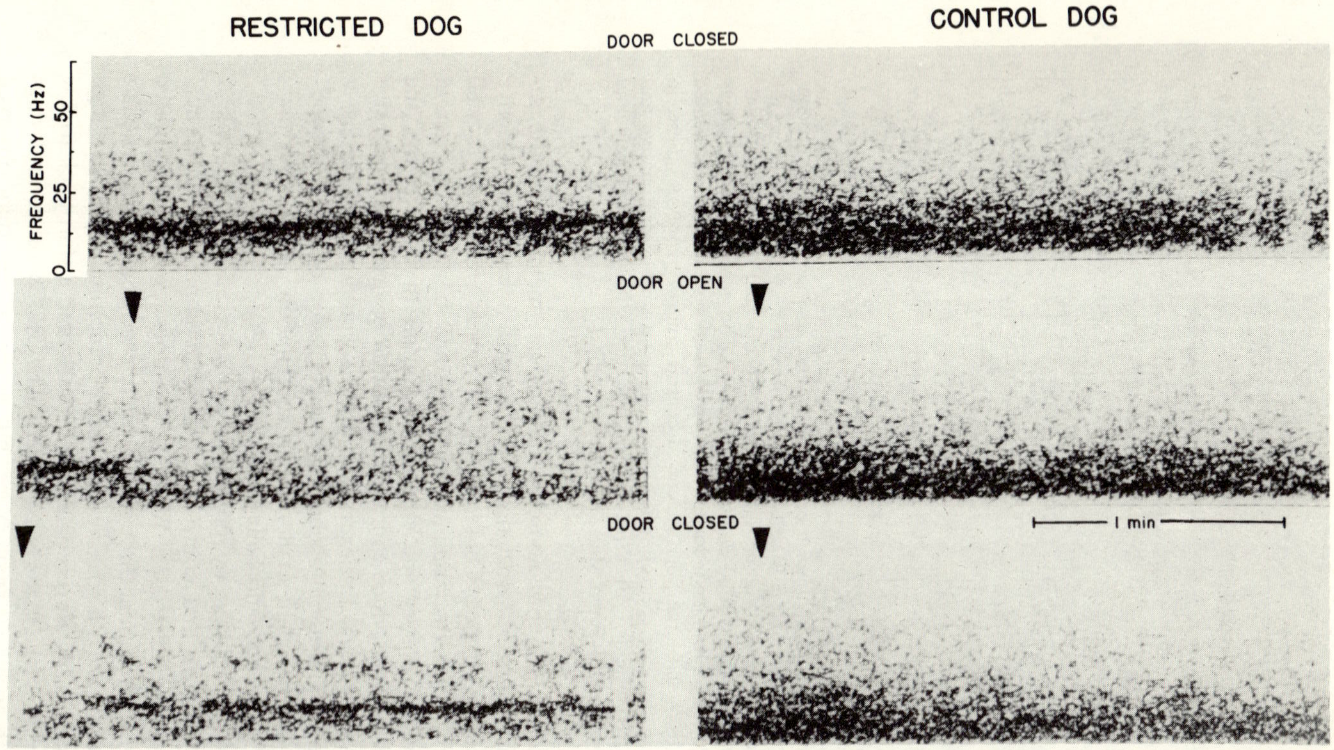

Fig. 8. Spectrographic frequency analysis of EEG changes in the reticular formation of restricted (isolate) and control dogs produced by presentation of a novel environment. The EEG recorded from the restricted dog in its home cage while the door is closed (top) shows predominantly low-frequency activity, with a strong, dominant frequency of about 15 Hz. When the door is opened (center), the dominant frequency disappears and there is a relative increase in the higher frequencies for the duration of the open door. The dominant low-frequency activity returns only after the door is closed (bottom). The EEG from the control littermate shows a broad spectrum of low frequencies that remains relatively unchanged by the presentation of the novel cage. Arrows indicate points at which the cage door was opened and closed. (From Melzack & Burns, 1965.)

in the isolate dogs, returning to predominantly low frequency activity before removing the novel stimulus (Fig. 8). The EEG changes observed in the isolate dogs gradually decreased in magnitude during successive presentations until they approached the brief, low-magnitude shifts observed in the control dogs. The isolate dogs' EEG, however, as long as 6 months after release from restriction, continued to show a greater density in the high frequency end of the EEG spectrum, particularly from frontal cortical areas, than that observed in their control littermates. Even more striking was the variability of their EEG records, which showed shifts in activity from moment to moment, compared with the more stable, homogeneous records of the control dogs. An apparently similar phenomenon was observed by Konrad and Bagshaw (1970) who found that the incidence of "spontaneous" galvanic skin responses was seven times greater in isolate cats than in control cats when subjects were placed in a novel testing environment. On the basis of these two findings, we propose that when an isolation-reared animal is suddenly confronted with highly novel surroundings, the nervous system attempts to maintain tolerable levels of arousal by "gating out" or blocking novel stimuli. Periodically, the blocking process may be relaxed (or fail), permitting arousing novel stimuli to have access to the central nervous system and concomitantly producing spontaneous EEG shifts or galvanic skin responses. The processes of blockade and relaxation would provide organisms with a mechanism for coming to terms with a novel environment at a less than precipitous rate.

It has also been observed (Melzack & Burns, 1965) that responses evoked in the reticular formation by clicks show marked changes in amplitude and wave form (averaged evoked responses, Fig. 9) when a novel environment was presented to the isolate dogs. Analysis of the cumulative amplitudes of successive evoked responses (cumulative response records, Fig. 9) showed that these changes may continue for the duration of the presentation period and return to their former amplitude range only after the novel stimulus is removed. Evoked cortical responses were generally diminished in amplitude when the cage door was opened or closed, but did not exhibit the changes in wave form observed in the reticular responses. The control dogs, in contrast, showed little change in response amplitude that was coincident with the presentation of the novel cage. Although response amplitude changes were observed, they occurred "spontaneously" and were not locked to changes in environment, which characteristically occurred in the isolate dogs. If the magnitude of change in the cumulative evoked response records is ranked for all dogs, the largest effects produced by presentation of the novel cage occur in the isolate dogs, with no overlap between the two groups. Comparable changes were observed when light flashes were presented. It would be wrong to assume

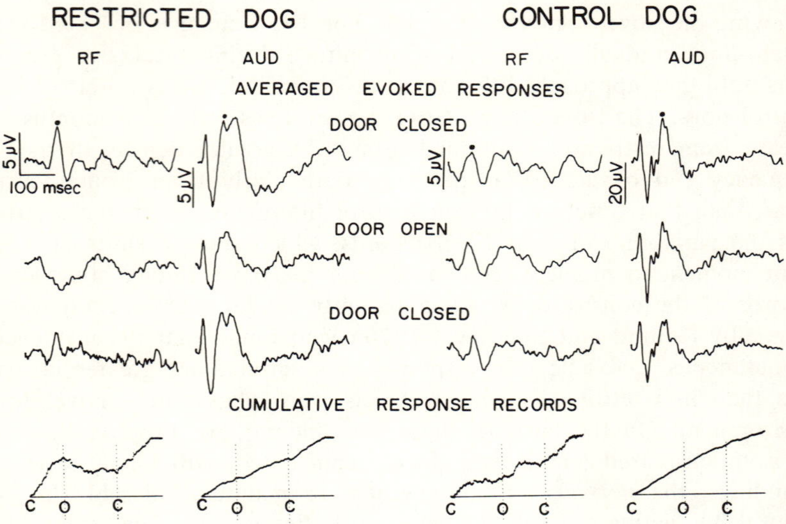

Fig. 9. Effects of presentation of a novel environment on responses evoked by clicks in the reticular formation and cortex: isolate, left, and control, right. Top: averages of 100 evoked responses. Bottom: cumulative records, in which the voltages at the point indicated by the dot above the averaged evoked responses at the top are added algebraically, so that the cumulative voltage growth is displayed as it builds up during successive evoked responses. The bottom left record, for example, indicates successive, large, relatively uniform evoked-response amplitudes when the door is closed; opening the door (O) produces a change in polarity of response (so that successive voltages are subtracted from the cumulative total), or a marked decrease of evoked response amplitude (so that the cumulative record is relatively flat). When the door is closed (C), high-amplitude evoked responses again appear. The record from the reticular formation of the control dog shows variability in evoked response amplitude, but it is not locked to presentation and removal of the unfamiliar cage. (From Melzack & Burns, 1965.)

that these evoked responses are the signal for auditory or visual perception. But it is reasonable to suppose that they represent part of the total sensory information subserving perception. It may be concluded, then, that processing of sensory information in isolation-reared dogs, during the high arousal states produced by an unfamiliar environment, differs from that in normal dogs showing more moderate levels of arousal.

IV. Novelty Enhancement: Interaction with Other Effects of Isolation Rearing

Several abnormal characteristics of the behavior of isolates, such as behavior stereotypy and social–sexual incompetence, cannot be classified as novelty-enhancement effects. Some are, at least in part, due to a failure in the normal weaning process or the lack of opportunity for normal peer–peer interactions. Even in these cases, however, there appear to be important interactions with the novelty enhancement arousal effects characteristic of isloation-reared animals.

A. Behavior Stereotypy

Stereotyped behavior patterns are prominent in the behavior of isolation-reared chimpanzees and monkeys, and can be classified into three categories: (1) repetitive movements, such as rocking, swaying, and head banging, (2) sucking of body parts, usually the digits of the hands or feet, and (3) self-clasping. Mason *et al.* (1968) have suggested that stereotypes arise from a disruption in the normal development of mother–infant relations as a result of rearing in isolation. Sucking and clasping responses in primate infants are directed toward aspects of the mother's body. The mother also provides abundant kinesthetic stimulation for her clinging infant as she travels about. As the infant matures, the mother normally extinguishes these various forms of reflex attachment to her person (Hinde & Spencer–Booth, 1967). Isolation-reared infants, in contrast, can direct sucking and clasping responses only toward themselves. Moreover, they must also produce their own movement stimulation by rocking, swaying, and so forth. Once these stereotypies are established, they may persist indefinitely in the absence of the normal extinguishing agent (the mother) —especially if the responses serve as "comforters" in high arousal situations, as suggested by the fact that stereotypies are frequently displayed by isolate primates when they are confronted with unfamiliar objects or surroundings (Mason *et al.*, 1968).

The suggestion that the stereotyped behavior patterns observed in isolate primates reflect a high level of arousal led Fitz-Gerald (1964), working in collaboration with Mason and Berkson, to manipulate the arousal level by means of pharmacological agents. She found that barbiturates, which are known to lower the level of central nervous system arousal, lowered the frequency of stereotyped response patterns and, under certain conditions, produced increased interaction with environmental objects. On the other hand, amphetamine, which increases arousal, produced increases in stereotyped responses and concomitant decreases in selective responses to environmental stimuli.

Characteristic of the stereotyped response is its repetitiveness, as though there were a failure of some mechanism to inhibit the response pattern once it is triggered. It is conceivable that the elevated arousal levels that disrupt the selection of relevant sensory patterns from the total input may also result in selection failure on the motor output side. Thus, natural response tendencies or particular acquired responses might continue even when they are irrelevant and impede the organism in its adaptive responses to the environment. This conception could explain the persistent position habits acquired by isolate beagles during visual discrimination training (Melzack, 1965). Isolate beagles also exhibited "superstitious" behavior sequences in the course of learning a simple problem, for example, one dog turned a complete circle before each press on a panel, and again before consuming each food reward. In the same panel-pressing problem, isolates took much longer to extinguish than did normals (see Fig. 10).

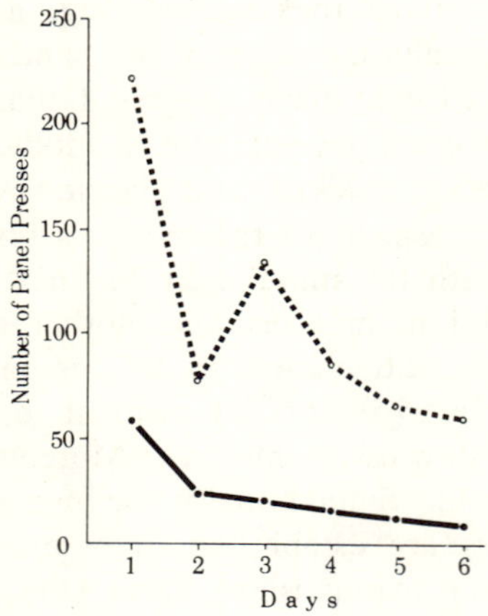

Fig. 10 Number of panel presses made by isolate and control dogs during six extinction periods. (From Melzack, 1965.)

B. Social–Sexual Incompetence

Many primate species are highly gregarious and live most of their lives in a social group. The harmony of these groups appears to depend on a system of social relationships which are maintained by subtle forms of species-specific communication: vocalizations, facial gestures, body postures, and sequences of these forms (Altmann, 1967). Although the particular forms of communication may be species-specific, their appropriate use is by no means automatic, and proficiency in their interpretation and use seems to depend heavily on early, prolonged socialization experience (Mason, 1960, 1961). Isolation-reared primates are understandably lacking in early socialization experience, and it is not surprising that they are, in fact, socially inept as adults (see Mason *et al.,* 1968). In addition, Miller, Caul, and Mirsky (1967) have demonstrated that isolate monkeys perform poorly, compared to wild-born monkeys, in a cooperative shock-avoidance learning situation in which success is dependent on appropriate "sending" and "receiving" of facial gesture information.

An interesting illustration of the way in which early experience and maturational factors may interact to produce competent social learning is provided by Sackett (1966). He observed that isolation-reared infant rhesus monkeys show marked fear of photographs of adult monkey threat gestures beginning at about 2.5 months of age. The degree of fearfulness produced by the pictures increases rapidly to a peak at 3.5 months, then diminishes slowly. Here, then, is an instance in which maturational processes set the stage for a particular kind of learning to occur. Under normal circumstances, the species-specific threat gesture and the accompanying innate fear response would occur in the context of other social responses such as chasing, fights, and so on. Failure for particular learning to occur at this specific stage of maturation may result in a subsequent loss of ability to discriminate and utilize these cues. As a result, when an isolation-reared monkey is confronted as an adult with a social conflict situation, gestures, and other social cues may have no particular significance, and the isolate may fail to behave appropriately. The resulting state of confusion could be expected to enhance the level of the isolate's arousal, which, in turn, might disrupt or lower the probability of its discriminating other relevant cues in the environment. This sequence describes a "vicious circle" in which failure to appreciate relevant information (on the basis of prior experience) leads to excessive arousal, which, in turn, interferes with mechanisms, both innate and acquired, that would normally act in the selection of cues for adaptive response.

Harlow (1965) and Mason (1960) have observed that isolation rearing also has disastrous effects on the adult heterosexual behavior of rhesus monkeys. The difficulties of isolate monkeys seem to be of two sorts: motivational and technical. Isolates sometimes respond to potential sexual partners with such inappropriate motivations as fear, aggression, or playfulness. In normal animals these constitute early stages in the sequence of behavior patterns elicited by novel objects. These data suggest, then, that the absence of the appropriate motivational behavior in isolate rhesus monkeys in sexual situations may be associated with the enhanced novelty consequences of isolation rearing. However, even when isolates appear to be sexually motivated, they still fail to manage the mechanics of copulation —putting the right things in the right places at the right times. This technical failure may well stem from the fact that isolate monkeys are deprived of opportunities for normal peer interactions during their development: Harlow (1965) has shown that the mechanics of rhesus monkey sexual behavior are normally established during development in the context of peer–peer play interactions. It is interesting to note that although isolate chimpanzees may sufler from the same lack of heterosexual experience as isolate monkeys, the outcome in terms of successful copulation may be different. In pairings between isolate male chimpanzees and sophisticated female partners, sexual encounters were often successful because the experienced females were able to compensate for the technical deficiencies of the isolate males (Mason *et al.,* 1968).

C. Failure to Select Relevant Sensory Information

Isolation-reared animals also show abnormal behavior toward nonsocial sensory inputs. Isolate Scottish terriers frequently failed to respond normally to low- or medium-level noxious stimulation, such as a flaming match or pin prick. They usually oriented toward the site of stimulation or withdrew reflexively, but rarely squealed or showed other signs of sustained emotional disturbance which were observed in control dogs (Melzack & Scott, 1957). The behavior of restricted beagles to noxious stimuli was in some respects not as abnormal as that observed in the scottie, but nevertheless revealed a pattern that has many similarities (Melzack, 1968). Isolate beagles also had difficulty learning a simple visual discrimination and in utilizing it during reversal training (Melzack, 1962). Moreover, they appeared to take little notice of auditory stimuli, such as lion roars or cock crows, which elicited a marked disruption in ongoing behavior in normal control dogs (Melzack, 1965).

These data are best explained in terms of the novelty–enhancement concept. The high levels of arousal produced by emergence into a totally new environment, in which all inputs are novel and unusual, would be expected to interfere with the ability to select the cues necessary for adaptive response. Even the poor performance by isolate scotties on maze problems (Thompson & Heron, 1954b) may be attributed to a failure to discriminate the relevant cues in the maze rather than to a cognitive deficit per se (Melzack, 1965). The novelty enhancement concept is further supported by Lessac and Solomon's (1969) observation that beagle puppies are able to avoid electric shock but, after isolation-rearing for several months, are unable to perform avoidance responses. The isolation-rearing, in other words, disrupted a behavior pattern which the dogs had previously been capable of performing. A result such as this is best explained in terms of novelty–enhancement arousal effects.

V. The Nature of Sensory Social Isolation

The novelty enhancement concept must be considered within the framework of heredity–environment interactions. Isolation-reared animals not only demonstrate the contributions of early experience, but also the genetic contributions to behavior. It is difficult to imagine a more homogeneous environment than an isolation cage or room. Yet there are marked differences from animal to animal, even in isolate dogs from the same litter. One beagle, for example, may be so active that he has whirling fits, while a littermate appears "normal" until a stimulus calls out excessive excitement that differentiates him from the control dogs (Melzack, 1965). With environment held so constant, this variability of behavior can only be attributed to genetic contributions.

The behavioral differences between isolate scotties and beagles (Melzack, 1968) are consistent with observations that each breed tends to show characteristic responses to fear-producing objects (Mahut, 1958) and that rearing methods have different effects in different breeds (Freedman, 1958). Interspecies differences among mammals are just as striking. The novelty enhancement arousal of isolate dogs (Melzack & Thompson, 1956) is generally manifested in diffuse, gross bodily activity, while isolate monkeys and chimpanzees (Mason *et al.,* 1968) show more specific behavior patterns that can be related to particular stereotyped activities acquired during isolation.

The data obtained with species ranging from rat to chimpanzee suggest that the novelty-evoked behavior patterns in isolate and control animals lie on the same continuum. There is evidence that isolates, after habituation to novelty, show behavior patterns that approximate those of normal controls. Thus, a study (Davenport & Rogers, 1968) with delayed response tasks shows that wild-born chimpanzees initially performed better than isolates after either short or long delays but, by the end of the experiment, wild-born animals were better only on the task involving the longest delay. This suggestion is further supported by the observation that normally reared animals sometimes show behavior that is qualitatively similar to that observed in isolates. Scotties raised in homes, for example, show diffuse emotional excitement like that exhibited by restricted dogs when they are confronted with a social stimulus (a "timid" man) for which they have no ready response (Melzack & Thompson, 1956). It is significant, moreover, that when control beagles that had been raised on a farm were placed in laboratory cages, they exhibited an extremely high level of behavioral excitement that subsided only after weeks or months (Melzack, 1968).

A radical change in environment, whether it be from an isolation cage or from a farm, confronts the organism with stimuli that have little or no meaning, and prior experience is relatively useless in determining the relevance or irrelevance of social and physical stimuli. Under such conditions, experience fails to make its normal contribution to selection and filtering processes at the early stages of information transmission, so that all inputs reach the brain and produce excessive arousal. Hebb (1949, 1955) has described some of the behavioral abnormalities that accompany extreme arousal: disorganized behavior patterns ranging from "freezing" responses to irrelevant and aimless activity; failure to discriminate and respond adaptively to relevant cues in the environment; and disruption of higher central nervous system processes such as utilization of relevant memory stores, attention, perception, and so forth. These kinds of behavior are characteristic of isolation-reared animals released into a totally new environment.

Acknowledgments

The work in this chapter was supported by contract DAHC-15-68-C-0396 from the Advanced Research Projects Agency. We are grateful to the following investigators for permission to adapt their data for several figures in this paper: R. K. Davenport, Jr., C. M. Rogers, and E. W. Menzel (Fig. 1); J. L. Fuller and L. D. Clark (Fig. 5B); P. J. Woods (Fig. 6A); W. R. Thompson and W. Heron (Fig. 6B).

References

Altmann, S. A. (Ed.) *Social communication among primates.* Chicago: University of Chicago Press, 1967.

Davenport, R. K., Jr., & Rogers, C. M. Intellectual performance of differentially reared chimpanzees: I. Delayed Response. *American Journal of Mental Deficiency,* 1968, **72**, 674–680.

Fitz-Gerald, F. L. The effects of drugs upon stereotyped behavior in young chimpanzees. Unpublished doctoral dissertation, McGill University, 1964.

Freedman, D. G. Constitutional and environmental interactions in rearing four breeds of dogs. *Science,* 1958, **127**, 585–586.

Fuller, J. L., & Clark, L. D. Effects of rearing with specific stimuli upon postisolation behavior in dogs. *Journal of Comparative and Physiological Psychology,* 1966, **61**, 258–263.

Harlow, H. F. Sexual behavior in the rhesus monkey. In F. A. Beach (Ed.), *Sex and behavior.* New York: Wiley, 1965. Pp. 234–265.

Hebb, D. O. *The organization of behavior.* New York: Wiley, 1949.

Hebb, D. O. Drives and the C. N. S. (conceptual nervous system). *Psychological Review,* 1955, **62**, 243–254.

Hinde, R. A., & Spencer-Booth, Y. The behavior of socially living rhesus monkeys in their first two and a half years. *Animal Behavior,* 1967, **15**, 169–196.

Hymovitch, B. The effects of experimental variations on problem solving in the rat. *Journal of Comparative and Physiological Psychology,* 1952, **45**, 313–328.

Konrad, K. W., & Bagshaw, M. The effect of novel stimuli on cats reared in a restricted environment. *Journal of Comparative and Physiological Psychology,* 1970, **70**, 157–164.

Lessac, M. S., & Solomon, R. L. Effects of early isolation on the later adaptive behavior of beagles: A methodological demonstration. *Developmental Psychology,* 1969, **1**, 14–25.

Mahut, H. Breed differences in the dog's emotional behavior. *Canadian Journal of Psychology,* 1958, **12**, 35–44.

Mason, W. A. The effects of social restriction on the behavior of rhesus monkeys: I. Free social behavior. *Journal of Comparative and Physiological Psychology,* 1960, **53,** 582–589.

Mason, W. A. Effects of age and stimulus characteristics on manipulatory responsiveness of monkeys raised in a restricted environment. *The Journal of Genetic Psychobiology,* 1961, **99,** 301–308.

Mason, W. A., Davenport, R. K., Jr., & Menzel, E. W., Jr. Early experience and the social development of rhesus monkeys and chimpanzees. In G. Newton & S. Levine (Eds.), *Early experience and behavior.* Springfield, Illinois: Charles C Thomas, 1968. Pp. 440–480.

Mason, W. A., & Green, P. C. The effects of social restriction on the behavior of rhesus monkeys: IV. Response to a novel environment and to an alien species. *Journal of Comparative and Physiological Psychology,* 1962, **55,** 363–368.

Mason, W. A., & Sponholz, R. R. Behavior of rhesus monkeys raised in isolation. *Journal of Psychiatric Research,* 1963, **1,** 299–306.

Melzack, R. The genesis of emotional behavior: An experimental study of the dog. *Journal of Comparative and Physiological Psychology,* 1954, **47,** 166–168.

Melzack, R. Effects of early perceptual restriction on simple visual discrimination. *Science,* 1962, **137,** 978–979.

Melzack, R. Effects of early experience on behavior: Experimental and conceptual considerations. In P. H. Hoch & J. Zubin (Eds.), *Psychopathology of perception.* New York: Grune & Stratton, 1965. Pp. 271–299.

Melzack, R. Early experience: A neuropsychological approach to heredity-environment interactions. In G. Newton & S. Levine (Eds.), *Early experience and behavior.* Springfield, Illinois: Charles C Thomas, 1968. Pp. 65–82.

Melzack, R., & Burns, S. K. Neurophysiological effects of early sensory restriction. *Experimental Neurology,* 1965, **13,** 163–175.

Melzack, R., & Casey, K. L. Sensory, motivational and central control determinants of pain: A new conceptual model. In D. R. Kenshalo (Ed.), *The skin senses.* Springfield, Illinois: Charles C Thomas, 1968. Pp. 423–439.

Melzack, R., & Scott, T. H. The effects of early experience on the response to pain. *Journal of Comparative and Physiological Psychology,* 1957, **50,** 155–161.

Melzack, R., & Thompson, W. R. Effects of early experience on social behavior. *Canadian Journal of Psychology,* 1956, **10,** 82–90.

Melzack, R., & Wall, P. D. Pain mechanisms: A new theory. *Science,* 1965, **150,** 971–979.

Menzel, E. W., Jr. Patterns of responsiveness in chimpanzees reared through infancy under conditions of environmental restriction. *Psychologische Forschung,* 1964, **27,** 337–365.

Menzel, E. W., Jr., Davenport, R. K., Jr., & Rogers, C. M. The effects of environmental restriction upon the chimpanzee's responsiveness to objects. *Journal of Comparative and Physiological Psychology,* 1963, **56,** 78–85. (a)

Menzel, E. W., Jr., Davenport, R. K., Jr., & Rogers, C. M. Effects of environmental restriction upon the chimpanzee's responsiveness in novel situations. *Journal of Comparative and Physiological Psychology,* 1963, **56,** 329–334. (b)

Miller, R. E., Caul, W. F., & Mirsky, I. A. Communication of affects between feral and socially isolated monkeys. *Journal of Personality and Social Psychology,* 1967, **7,** 231–239.

Mitchell, G. D., Raymond, E. J., Ruppenthal, G. C., & Harlow, H. F. Long-term effects of total social isolation upon behavior of rhesus monkeys. *Psychological Reports,* 1966, **18,** 567–580.

Riesen, A. H. Excessive arousal effects of stimulation after early sensory deprivation. In P. Solomon, P. E. Kubzansky, P. H. Liederman, J. H. Mendelson, R. Turnbull, & D. Wexler (Eds.), *Sensory deprivation.* Cambridge, Massachusetts: Harvard University Press, 1961. Pp. 34–40. (a)

Riesen, A. H. Stimulation as a requirement for growth and function in behavioral development. In D. W. Fiske & S. R. Maddi (Eds.), *Functions of varied experience.* Homewood: Dorsey Press, 1961. Pp. 57–80. (b)

Sackett, G. P. Manipulatory behavior in monkeys reared under different levels of early stimulus variation. *Perceptual and Motor Skills,* 1965, **20**, 985–988.

Sackett, G. P. Monkeys reared in isolation with pictures as visual input: evidence for an innate releasing mechanism. *Science,* 1966, **154**, 1468–1473.

Thompson, W. R., & Heron, W. The effects of early restriction on activity in dogs. *Journal of Comparative and Physiological Psychology,* 1954, **47**, 77–82. (a)

Thompson, W. R., & Heron, W. The effects of restricting early experience on the problem-solving capacity of dogs. *Canadian Journal of Psychology,* 1954, **8**, 17–31. (b)

Wiesel, T. N., & Hubel, D. H. Comparison of the effects of unilateral and bilateral eye closure on cortical unit responses in kittens. *Journal of Neurophysiology,* 1965, **28**, 1029–1040. (a)

Wiesel, T. N., & Hubel, D. H. Extent of recovery from the effects of visual deprivation in kittens. *Journal of Neurophysiology,* 1965, **28**, 1060–1072. (b)

Woods, P. J. The effects of free and restricted environmental experience on problem-solving behavior in the rat. *Journal of Comparative and Physiological Psychology,* 1959, **52**, 399–402.

Zimbardo, P. G., & Montgomery, K. C. Effects of "free-environment" rearing upon exploratory behavior. *Psychological Reports,* 1957, **3**, 589–594.

CHAPTER IX

Interpretations and Implications

Austin H. Riesen

Department of Psychology
University of California, Riverside

I. Function and Structural Development of the Nervous System

Behavioral precision, complex perceptual organization, and the development of fine structures of the nervous system depend upon functional demands from the environment. The effects of function on fine structures are selective. How, why, and wherefore these effects come about remain largely to be determined, but recent progress is remarkable after a century of little more than surmises (and even denials that function affects structure: Burr, 1930; Goodman, 1932).

Stimulation contributes to shaping the rapidly growing nervous system anatomically and physiologically under the overall guidance of a genetic code. The gene-determined heritage is most clearly revealed in anatomical and physiologic systems and in behaviors that are observable prior to functional demands. Embryogenesis, neurophysiological events, and behaviors in naïve organisms are species characteristic. Their organizations are revealed in young animals at birth, or hatching, or by short-term sensory deprivation experiments. Chapter VI by Ganz reviews behavioral organizations so discovered. Fischer (1972) presents findings on innate determinants of following behavior in newly hatched chicks. Innate behavioral organizations set the base lines upon which more refined behaviors in auditory or visual space, and new approach, avoidance, and choice responding become elaborated. Essential contributing factors include nutritional processes, intrinsic maturational changes, spontaneous neural activity, and exploratory behavioral tendencies, all of which interact with physiologic processes that are activated by sensory events. Future research must reveal in detail how these interactions take place and what degrees of possible interchangeability the various growth-supporting factors may possess, as well as the limits of sequential flexibilities. Behavioral development is said to be orderly, yet variability is tolerated. What developmental costs may attend deviations from optimal orders and combinations of events? When behavioral remediation is desirable are there clearly understood alternatives during later stages in a life cycle? Evidence described in earlier chapters of this book suggests cautious optimism. Much work remains before the alternatives can be reliably achieved. Even the biochemical and hormonal misfortunes of early childhood are not leading inevitably to irrevocable impairments.

II. Neural Metabolic Processes in Sensory Deprivation

A. Nutrition and Stimulation Yield Semiindependent Outcomes

Are nutrition and stimulation additive or interchangeable in the support of neural growth? Until we have more specific knowledge of the effects of protein deprivation on neural fine structures, this question will be difficult to answer. Behavioral effects are to some extent additive and subtractive (Levitsky & Barnes, 1972), but this does not necessarily imply common mechanism.

In the offspring of rat mothers that were fed a deficient diet (50% of ad-lib feeding quantities) during gestation and lactation, later maze performance was significantly impaired, even when the young had been provided after weaning with a standard ad-lib diet. Tanabe (1972) studied the effects of postweaning environmental enrichment on the maze performance of undernourished Wistar rats and reports an alleviation. However, the offspring of normally fed mothers showed a similar gain in performance following enrichment of the postweaning environment. Tanabe (1972) concludes, therefore, that "although enrichment will serve to remediate a maze performance deficit, it is not specifically a therapy for deficits caused by maternal food deprivation [p. 224]."

The additive effects of sensory stimulation and adequate nutrition upon learning ability and brain development are not unexpected. Interpretations of the behavioral data remain uncertain at the present time, however.

Learning deficits are not invariably found following early undernutrition and when present are associated with changes in activity levels and in food motivation. These complicate any assessment of the structure–function relationships. Early undernourishment clearly has such widespread consequences in retarded neural development (Cragg, 1972; Dobbing, Hopewell, & Lynch, 1971; Neville & Chase, 1971) that multiple and complex effects upon behavioral parameters are the only outcome reasonably to be expected.

A final point of emphasis must be that neonatal malnutrition produces permanent deficits and is therefore paralleled by the severest forms of sensory deprivation. Various measures of neural structure show a permanent failure of recovery after neonatal food restriction (Culley & Lineberger, 1968; Dobbing, *et al.* 1971; Howard & Granoff, 1968) or following prolonged early stimulus deprivation (Brattgård, 1952; Riesen, 1970). The amount of functional recovery that may at times be achieved in spite of these measurable deficits in structure must be a continuing challenge to the neurosciences as to the worker in remedial education.

B. Growth Hormones and Neuropsychological Development

The role of growth hormone in the development of the nervous system is so basic that we may ask whether effects of the dietary and functional demand variables discussed in Section A (p. 278) are mediated by hormone action. Since many of the stimulus-deprivation studies have employed reduced illumination, which in turn may affect hormonal balance, the question deserves careful evaluation and more experimental study than it has received thus far.

On the basis of current evidence, the three factors—growth hormone, nutrition, and neural stimulation—can best be considered as interacting but largely separable factors capable of exercising their influences on development independently. To what extent one may substitute for another depends upon the specific effects on growth or on behavioral development that are measured. Equally important is the exact period during development that one or more of these experimental variables are introduced. A full review of the relevant studies will not be attempted here.

The capacity of substitution of growth hormone for a deficiency in nutrition in rats during pregnancy in the prevention of decreased cerebral weight, cerebral DNA, and cerebral protein has been demonstrated by Zamenhof, van Marthens, and Grauel (1971). A parallel substitutive action of prenatally administered bovine growth hormone for the effects of environmental isolation on learning capacity (Lashley III maze and shuttle box avoidance learning) was reported by Ray and Hochhauser,

(1969). Growth hormone did not improve the abilities of animals reared under environmental enrichment. The authors suggested that a ceiling effect in the behavioral measures under the enrichment condition may have limited performance so that only the improvement due to growth hormone following environmental impoverishment was revealed. Mechanisms of physiological action remain to be determined for both types of effect.

C. Hypersensitivity, Seizures after Sensory Deprivation

In Chapter IV, Sharpless has examined the general problem and possible mechanisms in stimulus deprivation supersensitivity. At the behavioral level as well as in neurophysiological preparations this is a highly significant area of concern and clearly of fundamental importance. Seizures consequent to sensory restriction have more often than otherwise been treated as nuisance side effects (Fitch, 1971; Riesen, 1961). As Sharpless points out (p. 141) in Section IV,D, the fundamental role of disuse potentiation in epilepsy is indicated by studies of the effect of exercise on isolated slabs of cortex. Normal levels of regular functioning are by implication the required condition for avoiding epileptiform seizures in neural systems. Echlin and McDonald (1954) are credited with first calling attention to the parallel between supersensitivity of partially isolated cortical slabs and focal cortical epilepsy. A series of studies has by now left little doubt about the role of stimulation in maintaining normal levels of neuronal activity (Rutledge, 1969). Sensory deprivation increases the likelihood that physiological and anatomical conditions for seizurelike discharges will develop in mammalian central nervous systems.

III. Competition for Synaptic Space

A. Evidence from Function in Support of the Hypothesis

Behavioral effects of visual deprivation suggest that transmission of visual information fails somewhere along the pathway to central integrating systems. Reduced dendritic branching and lowered counts of dendritic spines support the hypothesis that such failure occurs primarily in Layers III and IV of the occipital cortex. Electrophysiological evidence, as cited earlier (Chapter V), that Y cells of the lateral geniculate nucleus cease to function and that binocular cells of the visual cortex fail to develop or are lost leaves us with the clear implication that transmission is impaired at many levels. All such evidence can be explained by the hypothesis of synaptic failure, either through failure of development, or atrophy, or both.

Under the condition of monocular deprivation, behavioral (Dews &

Wiesel, 1970; Fitch, 1971) and electrophysiological evidence, and the evidence from morphological studies of local regions of the lateral geniculate nucleus, have shown that one eye and its pathways survive at the expense of the other. This has brought the suggestion from Hubel and Wiesel that synaptic spaces normally involved in cortical projections from one eye are taken over by afferents from the other eye.

B. Changes in Size and Number of Synapses

A number of stimulus reduction techniques have been used in preparing animals for studies of the ultrastructure of cortical synapses. These have included suturing of the lid of one eye (Fifková, 1970a, b) and comparing synapses of the right and left visual cortices, and rearing animals under the EC or the IC conditions and again examining numbers and dimensions of synapses of the visual cortex (Møllgaard, Diamond, Bennett, Rosenzweig, & Lindner, 1971; West & Greenough, 1972). These and several other studies, including dark-versus light-rearing, are in agreement insofar as they all show a change in which increases of synaptic dimensions are associated with reduced numbers of synapses per unit volume of neural tissue. In cortical Layers I–IV, synapses become larger with increased stimulation of either visual origin or multisensory origin.

This result—increase in synaptic dimensions with a reduction in numbers of synapses—does correspond to the hypothesis of competition for synaptic space, with greater stimulation correlating with growth of individual synapses and disappearances of synapses that fail to grow. Not yet known is whether the larger synapses are indeed the organelles that are responsible for neuronal firing, in units, for example, that respond to the nondeprived eye after monocular deprivation.

Complicating the structure–function relations are data indicating that in deep layers of the visual cortex (Cragg, 1967) and in the lateral geniculate nucleus (Cragg, 1969) the initial exposure of dark-reared rats to light stimulation increases the numbers of synapses. Whether larger synapses or greater numbers are associated with an increase in efficiency of functional pathways appears to depend upon the nature and locus of the interconnections under scrutiny.

IV. What Structures Interact with Which Functions?

Future research must tell us much more in detail what specific roles are being carried by simple cells, complex, Y cells, X cells, cortical and subcortical tracts (as in vision or in learning of a specific kind), and by systems that provide for interactions between levels or between sensory, limbic, and motor integrating centers. By selective sensory deprivation, progress in the analysis of such structure–function relations may be expected to continue. Results of recent years are such that we may be justified in expecting a rising rate of discoveries.

At the level of single cells, we now speak of "feature detectors" and of units that respond to locations in the third dimension. At the level of specific sensory modalities we can begin to point to the education of one sense by another. Early experience contributes to refinements of function (and presumably of structure) at both levels. To examples of previous chapters should be added a study by Rileigh and Odom (1972), demonstrating that rhythm and duration in a visual sequence are inaccurately perceived (poorly reproduced) by 10-year-old deaf children. Beats and short time durations are "salient" in the auditory but not in the visual sense mode. By age 15 years, the deaf no longer lag behind in this ability (Fig. 1). Other visual tasks show similar evidence for the facilitation by early auditory experience. Are there dendritic structures or memory molecules that develop as correlated neural changes? Electrophysiological correlates may be found before the anatomic.

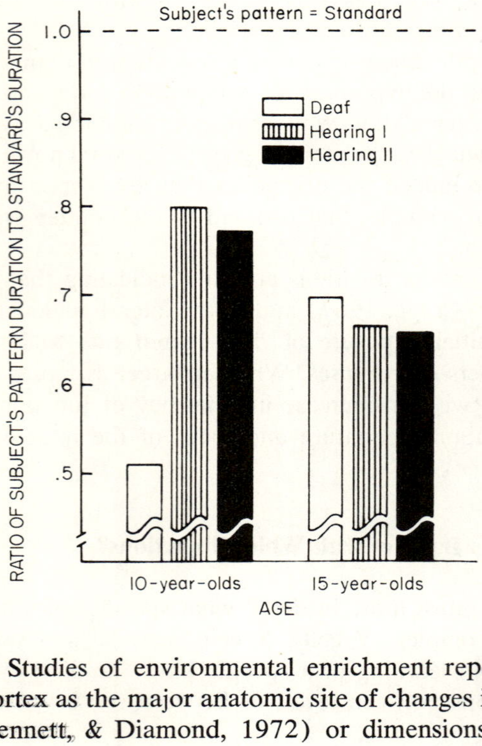

Fig. 1. Accuracy of reproduction of the duration of a visually presented pattern by deaf and hearing children at two age levels. Both duration and rhythms were less accurately reproduced by 10-year-old deaf children. Hearing II represents a test done under white noise. (From Rileigh & Odom, 1972.)

Studies of environmental enrichment repeatedly implicate the posterior cortex as the major anatomic site of changes in brain chemistry (Rosenzweig, Bennett, & Diamond, 1972) or dimensions of synapses (West & Greenough, 1972). This supports Lashley's long-standing claims for a nonvisual function of the visual cortex. Since the changes occur even in blinded rats, and in seeing rats after visual stimulation, the occipital cortex is implicated as a multimodal integrating area as well as a visual information processing system. Selective sensory deprivations should make possible the identification of cortical layers, cell types, and synaptic populations within the posterior cortex that carry information from nonvisual stimulation. Well-tested procedures of single unit recording and degeneration after deafferentation should be used in conjunction with studies of dendritic spines and synapses.

Of all sensory systems thus far studied, the somatosensory are the most neglected, probably because they are difficult to isolate. Somatosensory deprivation has been regarded as a major component (artifact?) in studies of social isolation (Prescott, 1971). Are the social–aggressive behaviors, the impairment in problem solving, and the motor stereotypes of social isolation experiments the result of somatosensory deprivation during critical periods in infancy? Prescott makes a case for such a view. Restrictions of movement and of bodily contact are difficult to separate from social isolation procedures, but this must be attempted if we are to understand the severe and long-lasting consequences of developmental deprivations.

A very different proposal for explaining social isolation behaviors is offered by Sackett (1970). Instead of assuming that a denervation sensitivity results in hyperirritability as does Prescott, Sackett believes that social isolates fail to develop inhibitory control. The monkey mother is seen as the most important source of opportunities by the infant to learn an inhibitory mode, being especially important at 4–6 months in rhesus monkeys. Automated teaching devices could provide graded amounts of experience in inhibitory responding with or without "adequate" somatosensory stimulation in a multidimensional experiment to test the theories of Prescott and Sackett.

V. Sensory–Motor and Motor–Sensory Integrations

As fundamental as the problem of intersensory or cross-modal integrations of Section IV (p. 281) are the innate and the experience-modified integrations between motor and sensory events. The studies of Held, Hein, and others have contributed major facts and principles in this area of human and animal behavior development. Disconnections or rearrangements of motor and sensory events have systematic consequences. Behavior in space and under sensory guidance clearly has an initial basis in innately organized neural pathways. Refinements of these have been dealt with in the chapters by Ganz, and by Riesen and Zilbert. There remains a vast area for neuroscience research to provide a better understanding of how skills of locomotion and manipulation are developed and maintained. Memories of such skills are paradoxical in their degree of permanence, their modifiability, and their fragility. What are the storage mechanisms?

VI. Discriminative Responding to Complex Sensory Patterns

Readiness to discriminate patterns that are internally complicated requires prior experience with sensory patterns. The basic fact as a principle was seen in experiments with animals deprived of pattern vision or reared with much reduced auditory stimulation (Chapter VI,pp. 195–197; Chapter VII, pp. 221–252).

What relation to the patterns later to be discriminated should characterize the patterns of earlier experience? Would some patterns interfere? Would the frequent repetition of similar patterns be the most efficient use of earlier perceptual learning time or would too much repetition hinder later recognition, as the habituation principle would require? We are still far from an ability to specify optimum schedules of experience for rapid learning of complex sensory patterns. However, a beginning has been made that shows some early exposure patterns serve better than others. Reinforcement histories associated with patterned experiences are also in need of systematic experimentation.

One approach to the evalutaion of factors associated with repeated exposures of visual patterns has made use of a difficulty of discrimination dimension. Using previous evidence from discrimination learning studies with rats, Oswalt (1972) gave different groups of rat pups experience with visual forms that were known to be of three different degrees of difficulty for normally reared albino rats. The forms were exposed on walls of living cages from before eye opening to age 50 days. Control groups were exposed to flat white panels. All animals lived 4 to a cage. Animals that were exposed to and later learned to respond discriminatively to easy (horizontal versus vertical striations) or medium difficulty (U and inverted U) forms received no benefit from their earlier experience. The group exposed to difficult forms (circle versus triangle) was the only group whose later learning performance was significantly facilitated (314 as compared with 246 correct trials in a total of 450). This result fits well into the series of studies of more severe visual deprivation as surveyed in Chapters VI and VII. The evidence can also be used to broaden the generality of a series of studies (by Cool, and by McCall and Lester) showing the importance of early experience with angles.

On the basis of experimental findings cited above and incorporating the principle of novelty enhancement (Chapter VIII), we may conclude that pattern discriminations are facilitated by experience with complex patterns, by introducing variations in patterns between exposure and test, and by moving during ontogenesis from simpler (easier) to increasingly more complex (more difficult) patterns.

References

Brattgård, S. O. The importance of adequate stimulation for the chemical composition of retinal ganglion cells during early postnatal development. *Acta Radiologica, Supplementum 96,* 1952, 180.

Burr, H. S. Hyperplasia in the brain of amblystoma. *Journal of Experimental Zoology,* 1930, **55**, 171–191.

Cragg, B. G. Changes in visual cortex on first exposure of rats to light. Effect on synaptic dimensions. *Nature,* 1967 **215**, 251–253.

Cragg, B. G. The effects of vision and dark-rearing on the size and density of synapses in the lateral geniculate nucleus measured by electron microscopy. *Brain Research,* 1969, **13**, 53–67.

Cragg, B. G. The development of cortical synapses during starvation in the rat. *Brain,* 1972, **95**, 143–150.

Culley, W. J., & Lineberger, R. O. Effect of undernutrition on the size and composition of the rat brain. *Journal of Nutrition,* 1968, **96**, 375–381.

Dews, P. B., & Wiesel, T. N. Consequences of monocular deprivation on visual behavior in kittens. *Journal of Physiology,* 1970, **206**, 437–455.

Dobbing, J., Hopewell, J. W., & Lynch, A. Vulnerability of developing brain: VII. Permanent deficit of neurons in cerebral and cerebellar cortex following early mild undernutrition. *Experimental Neurology,* 1971, **32**, 439–447.

Echlin, F., & McDonald, J. The supersensitivity of chronically isolated and partially isolated cerebral cortex as a mechanism in focal cortical epilepsy. *Transactions of the American Neurological Association,* 1954, **79**, 75–79.

Fifková, E. The effect of monocular deprivation on the synaptic contracts of the visual cortex. *Journal of Neurobiology,* 1970a, **1**, 285–294.

Fifková, E. Changes of axosomatic synapses in the visual cortex of monocularly deprived rats. *Journal of Neurobiology,* 1970b, **2**, 61–71.

Fischer, G. J. Sound stimuli and following in a domestic fowl: Frequency, rate, and duration. *Journal of Comparative and Physiological Psychology,* 1972, **81**, 183–190.

Fitch, M. H. Development of visuomotor behaviors following monocular and binocular patterned visual deprivation in the cat. Unpublished doctoral dissertation, University of California. Riverside, 1971.

Goodman, L. Effect of total absence of function on the optic system of rabbit. *American Journal of Physiology,* 1932, **100**, 46–63.

Howard, E., & Granoff, D. M. Effect of neonatal food restriction in mice on brain growth, DNA and cholesterol, and on adult delayed response learning. *Journal of Nutrition,* 1968, **95**, 111–121.

Levitsky, D. A., & Barnes, R. H. Nutritional and environmental interactions in the behavioral development of the rat: Long-term effects. *Science,* 1972, **176**, 68–71.

Møllgaard, K., Diamond, M. C., Bennett, E. L., Rosenzweig, M. R., & Lindner, B. Quantitative synaptic changes with differential experience in rat brain. *International Journal of Neuroscience,* 1971, **2**, 113–128.

Neville, H. E., & Chase, H. P. Undernutrition and cerebellar development. *Experimental Neurology,* 1971, **33**, 485–497.

Oswalt, R. M. Relationship between level of visual pattern difficulty during rearing and subsequent discrimination in rats. *Journal of Comparative and Physiological Psychology,* 1972, **81**, 122–125.

Prescott, J. W. Early somatosensory deprivation as an ontogenetic process in the abnormal development of the brain and behavior. In E. I. Goldsmith & J. Moor-Jankowski (Eds.), *Medical primatology* 1970. Basel, Switzerland: Karger, 1971. Pp. 357–375.

Ray, O. S., & Hochhauser, S. Growth hormone and environmental complexity effects on behavior in the rat. *Developmental Psychology,* 1969, **1**, 311–317.

Riesen, A. H. Excessive arousal effects of stimulation after early sensory deprivation. In P. Solomon, P. E. Kubzansky, P. H. Leiderman, J. H. Mendelson, R. Trumbull, & D. Wexler (Eds.), *Sensory deprivation: A symposium,* Cambridge, Massachusetts: Harvard University Press, 1961, Pp. 34–40.

Riesen, A. H. Effects of visual environment on the retina. In F. A. Young & D. B. Lindsley (Eds.), *Early experience and visual information processing in perceptual and reading disorders.* Washington, D. C.: National Academy of Sciences, 1970. Pp. 249–260.

Rileigh, K. K., & Odom, P. B. Perception of rhythm by subjects with normal and deficient hearing. *Developmental Psychology,* 1972, **7**, 54–61.

Rosenzweig, M. R., Bennett, E. L., & Diamond, M. C. Brain changes in response to experience. *Scientific American,* 1972, **226**, 22–29.

Rutledge, L. T. Effect of stimulation on isolated cortex. In H. Jasper, A. Ward, & A. Pope (Eds.), *Basic mechanisms of the epilepsies.* Boston: Little, Brown, 1969. Pp. 349–355.

Sackett, G. P. Innate mechanisms, rearing conditions, and a theory of early experience effects in primates. In M. R. Jones (Ed.), *Miami symposium on the prediction of behavior, 1968: Effects of early experience.* Coral Gables, Florida: University of Miami Press, 1970. Pp. 11–53.

Tanabe, G. Remediating maze deficiencies by the use of environmental enrichment. *Developmental Psychology,* 1972, **7**, 224.

West, R. W., & Greenough, W. T. Effect of environmental complexity on cortical synapses of rats: Preliminary results. *Behavioral Biology,* 1972, **7**, 279–284.

Zamenhof, S., van Marthens, E., & Grauel, L. Prenatal cerebral development: Effect of restricted diet, reversal by growth hormone. *Science,* 1971, **174**, 954–955.

Author Index

A

Aarons, L., 177, 196, 209, 215, 227, 230, 246, 250
Abbott, L., 241
Adey, W. R., 159, 166, 167, 245, 249
Aghajanian, G. K., 47, 82
Agin, D., 104, 119
Agranoff, B. W., 93, 119
Agrawal, H. C., 109, 237, 246
Albuquerque, E. X., 126, 147
Aldsogius, H., 69, 85
Allison, A. C., 37, 82, 117, 119
Altman, J., 14, 49, 66, 67, 77, 78, 82
Altmann, S. A., 270, 274
Anderson, W. J., 14, 49, 66, 77, 78, 82
Angermeier, W. F., 238, 242, 246
Angerrne, J. B., 115, 119
Annis, R. C., 225, 246
Ansberry, M., 164
Appel, S. H., 101, 119
April, R., 140, 151
Aprison, M. H., 109, 121
Arduini, A., 68, 79, 82
Aref'eva, A. M., 103, 123
Ariëns, E. J., 132, 147
Auerbach, E., 100, 124, 158, 168
Aumann, K., 132, 152
Axelrod, J., 131, 149
Axelsson, J., 126, 133, 147

B

Bachelard, H. S., 95, 122
Baggio, G., 14, 55, 61, 64, 85, 106, 120
Bagshaw, M., 235, 249, 258, 259, 260, 267, 275
Bahr, G. F., 103, 119
Bailey, H. L., 14, 49, 64, 87
Ball, W., 174, 206
Bárány, R., 184, 206
Barelare, B., 2, 7
Barlow, H. B., 68, 87, 160, 164
Barnes, R. H., 278, 285

Barr, M. L., 14, 28, 35, 61, 65, 73, 82, 83, 100, 115, 120
Barron, D. H., 17, 33, 82
Barron, K. D., 234, 252
Bateson, P. P. G., 93, 101, 119, 121
Batkin, S., 164
Bauer, J. A., 202, 203, 204, 208
Bauer, R., 228, 248
Baxter, Bruce L., 104, 119, 154, 159, 165, 172, 173, 174, 177, 187, 206, 215, 230, 246
Beatty, N., 143, 151
Becker, W. C., 232, 248
Beckett, P. G. S., 238, 246
Benhamida, C., 13, 34, 71, 82
Bennett, E. L., 10, 11, 14, 25, 48, 49, 62, 66, 67, 78, 79, 82, 84, 85, 86, 88, 117, 118, 122, 235, 239, 240, 246, 249, 251, 281, 282, 286
Beránek, R., 133, 140, 147
Berger, H., 9, 14, 15, 39, 58, 82
Berger, R. J., 219, 246
Berl, S., 144, 147
Berman, A. J., 204, 209
Berman, N., 162, 165
Berman, S., 158, 166
Bernstein, I. S., 234
Bertaccini, G., 97, 111, 120
Bertram, E. G., 14, 61, 65, 82
Bianchi, C. P., 135, 147
Bishop, P. O., 160, 165, 167
Black, R., 144, 149
Blakemore, C., 161, 165, 171, 206, 225, 246
Bloom, F. E., 14, 47, 82
Bodian, D., 14, 90
Bonaventure, N., 154, 165
Bond, E. K., 203, 204, 210, 217, 252
Bondy, S. C., 24, 50, 82, 93, 114, 116, 119
Bower, T. G. R., 174, 175, 206
Bowling, D. M., 236, 239, 252
Bowman, W. C., 133, 147
Bowsher, D., 19, 35, 82
Bradley, K., 145, 147
Brattgård, S. O., 14, 41, 42, 55, 82, 99, 102, 103, 116, 119, 279, 285
Brazovskaya, F. A., 118, 119
Bronshtein, A. A., 116, 124
Broomhead, S., 106, 123
Broughton, J. M., 175, 206
Brown, D. A., 138, 147
Brown, G. L., 139, 147
Bullock, T., 145, 147
Burke, W., 13, 43, 58, 68, 83
Burns, B. D., 13, 83, 142, 147
Burns, S. K., 163, 166, 265, 266, 267, 268, 275
Burr, H. S., 227, 285

C

Cadell, T. E., 186, 208
Callison, D. A., 157, 165
Cannon, W. B., 125, 132, 134, 138, 139, 147
Caputto, R., 117
Carrier, O., 131, 135, 147
Carrier, S. C., III, 101, 120
Carta, F., 15, 41, 54, 87, 102, 105, 106, 122
Casey, K. L., 264, 265, 275
Castle, P., 175, 186, 187, 210
Caul, W. F., 271, 276
Caviness, J. A., 174
Cervoni, P., 139, 150
Chaloupka, Z., 217, 246
Chang, H. C., 108, 119
Chang, H. T., 68, 83
Chase, H. B., 13, 38, 39, 83
Chase, H. P., 279, 286
Chein, S., 139, 147
Cheng, M., 151
Chopra, S. P., 94, 123
Chornock, F. W., 150
Chow, K. L., 14, 15, 40, 42, 44, 55, 58, 59, 77, 83, 88, 94, 99, 100, 102, 103, 113, 114, 119, 123, 165, 171, 172, 188, 191, 194, 206, 207, 209, 213, 219, 220, 221, 222, 223, 230, 231, 233, 246, 247, 250
Chu, N.-S., 142, 143, 144, 147
Clark, L. D., 261, 262, 274
Cogan, D. G., 187, 207
Cohen, L. B., 244, 252
Cohen, L. H., 95, 120
Cohen, S. A., 130, 147
Cole, L., 3, 4, 7

Coleman, P. D., 44, 47, 56, 63, 73, 83, 159, 167
Collier, B., 109, 120
Colonnier, M., 13, 22, 24, 27, 34, 76, 83, 88
Cook, W. H., 28, 37, 73, 83, 100, 115 120
Cool, S. J., 224, 247
Cooper, G. F., 161, 165, 206, 225, 246
Cooper, R. M., 240, 247
Cornwell, Anne C., 104, 120, 154, 165
Cosenza, C., 14, 66, 84
Cowan, W. M., 10, 11, 19, 31, 75, 83, 88
Cragg, B. G., 14, 25, 30, 47, 53, 79, 83, 279, 281, 285
Creutzfeldt, O. D., 144, 147
Cross, H. A., 183
Crozier, W. J., 69, 83
Culley, W. J., 279, 285
Curtis, D. R., 112, 120
Cynader, M., 162, 165

D

Daniels, J., 151
Das, G. D., 14, 49, 66, 67, 77, 78, 82
Davenport, R. K., Jr., 238, 243, 244, 246, 247, 249, 256, 257, 269, 271, 272, 273, 274, 275, 276
Davis, C. M., 2, 6
Davis, F. N., 116, 119
Davis, J. M., 101, 121
Davis, R., 109, 112, 116, 120
Davis, W., 101, 119
Dearnaley, D. P., 139, 147
DeBold, R. C., 94, 101, 120
Deffenu, G., 97, 111, 120
DeLong, G. R., 17, 27, 83, 114, 120
Denenberg, V. H., 235, 247
Dennis, M. J., 127, 147, 149, 150
de Oliveira, Castro G., 79, 83
Desmedt, J., 141, 148
de Vos, M., 97, 120
Dervar, A. J., 101, 120
Dews, P. B., 189, 190, 207, 213, 220, 221, 222, 229, 247, 280, 285
Diamond, J., 14, 83, 126, 128, 148
Diamond, M. C., 14, 48, 49, 50, 62, 66, 67, 78, 79, 82, 84, 85, 88, 89, 235, 239, 240, 246, 281, 282, 286
Diamond, R. M., 177, 179, 198, 199, 206, 207, 215, 220, 226, 248
D'Monte, B., 94, 123
Dobbing, J., 279, 285
Dodsworth, R. O., 237, 248
Dolley, D. H., 14, 84
Domino, E. F., 142, 148
Donaldson, H. H., 15, 31, 84
Donovan, A., 113, 120
Doty, R., 141, 148
Dowling, J. E., 167, 229, 231, 251
Downer, J. L. deC., 94, 97, 98, 100, 105, 122
Drachman, D. B., 148
Drake, C. G., 68, 84
Draper, W. A., 234, 247
Draskoczky, P. R., 138, 150
Duffy, F., 164, 166
Duncan, J. A., 142, 143, 148, 151
Dzidzishvili, N. N., 13, 14, 28, 54, 84, 158, 165

E

Eayrs, J. T., 5, 6
Eccles, J. C., 140, 148
Echlin, F., 141, 142, 143, 148, 151, 280, 285
Edwards, B. J., 181, 208
Eldred, E., 140, 152
Ellingson, R. J., 157, 167
Emmelin, N., 131, 132, 148
Erulkar, S. D., 36, 88, 116, 123
Ervin, F. R., 4, 6, 10, 88
Estéban, M. E., 27, 47, 75, 90
Eterovic, V.A., 117, 120
Eysel, U. Th., 156, 165

F

Fairhurst, A. S., 149
Falk, J. L., 4, 6
Fantz, R. L., 4, 7, 172, 173, 175, 176, 183, 191, 207, 214, 215, 217, 247
Faro, M. D., 117, 120
Fautrez, J., 97, 100, 120, 124
Feltz, A., 148

Fentress, J., 141, 148
Ferchmin, P. A., 117, 120
Ferguson, D. C., 167, 229
Ferguson, J., 144, 148
Fifková, E., 14, 15, 23, 47, 48, 51, 52, 53, 71, 72, 73, 84, 100, 120, 158, 165, 281, 285
Firshein, W., 101, 120
Fish, S. E., 227, 247
Fishbach, G. D., 130, 140, 147, 148, 150
Fischer, G. J., 277, 285
Fitch, M. H., 69, 84, 154, 165, 171, 172, 177, 189, 190, 191, 193, 194, 207, 215, 219, 220, 221, 222, 223, 230, 247, 248, 280, 281, 285
Fitz-Gerald, F. L., 242, 249, 269, 274
FitzHugh, R., 68, 87
Fleischmann, T. B., 239, 248
Fleming, W. W., 130, 131, 132, 135, 148, 149
Flynn, J. T., 155, 156, 165, 166
Foerster, O., 18, 84
Foley, J. P., Jr., 177, 207
Forgays, D. G., 239, 247
Forgays, J. W., 239, 247
Fourment, A., 157, 158, 165, 167
Fox, M. W., 44, 58, 84, 165, 237, 241, 246, 247
Fox, S. S., 159, 166, 167, 245, 249
Franguelli, R., 15, 41, 54, 87, 102, 105, 106, 122
Frank, G. B., 126, 148
Franken, L., 141, 148
Freedman, D. G., 273, 274
Freedman, S. J., 201, 208
Freeman, R. D., 161, 164, 165, 167, 183, 208, 225, 250
Frohman, E. E., 238, 246
Frost, B., 225, 246
Fuller, J. L., 236, 237, 247, 261, 262, 274
Furchogott, R., 139, 150

G

Gaedt, Chr., 156, 165
Gagel, O., 18, 84
Ganz, L., 69, 84, 154, 158, 165, 171, 172, 177, 189, 190, 191, 192, 194, 197, 207, 214, 215, 219, 220, 221, 223, 226, 230, 247, 248
Garcia, A. M., 100, 120
Garcia, J., 4, 7
Gardner, L. I., 5, 7
Garey, L. J., 24, 29, 71, 84
Gauron, E. F., 228, 232, 248
Gay, A. J., 98, 100, 107, 120
Geffen, L. B., 139
Gellis, S. S., 187, 207
Ghetti, B., 13, 24, 29, 31, 71, 84, 85
Gibson, E. J., 172, 174, 177, 180, 181, 182, 183, 187, 191, 210, 215, 217, 252
Gibson, W. C., 22, 37, 85
Glass, J. D., 158, 165
Glees, P., 19, 30, 85
Glisson, S., 44, 58, 84
Globus, A., 10, 13, 14, 23, 28, 33, 47, 54, 59, 62, 63, 66, 75, 78, 79, 85
Glow, P. H., 108, 120
Gluck, J. P., 238, 248
Gordon, J., Jr., 16, 26, 89
Gorman, J. J., 187, 207
Goswamy, S., 154, 165
Gottlieb, G., 248
Gottlieb, J. S., 232, 238, 246
Gower, E. C., 177, 178, 198, 199, 206, 207, 220, 226, 248
Goel, B. K., 94, 123
Gogel, W. C., 4, 7
Goldby, F., 18, 31, 85
Goldfarb, J., 140, 141, 148
Gomirato, G., 14, 55, 61, 64, 85, 106, 120
Goodman, L., 14, 15, 39, 44, 55, 85, 216, 248, 277, 285
Grafstein, B., 104, 120, 141, 148
Granit, R., 63, 79, 85
Granoff, D. M., 279, 285
Grant, G., 69, 85
Grauel, L., 279, 286
Gray, E. G., 14, 23, 24, 83, 85
Graymore, C., 95, 121
Green, J. R., 143, 148
Green, P. C., 257, 275
Green, R. D., III, 131, 132, 135, 136, 138, 148, 152
Greenough, W. T., 61, 62, 66, 90, 239, 248, 281, 282, 286

Griffin, G. A., 242, 246
Griffitsh, G. M., 13, 38, 39, 88
Groth, H., 164
Guillery, R. W., 157, 166
Guth, L., 129, 134, 149
Gutmann, E., 134, 135, 149
Gyllensten, L., 13, 38, 39, 41, 47, 50, 51, 79, 85, 86, 94, 112, 114, 115, 116, 118, 121

H

Haddara, M. A. H., 19, 27, 86
Hadorn, J., 134, 152
Haegerstrom, G., 225, 250
Haffner, M. E., 158, 165, 194, 207, 230, 248
Halasz, H. K., 215, 246
Halpern, L. M., 141, 142, 143, 144, 148, 149, 151
Hamasaki, D. I., 155, 156, 166
Hamberger, C. A., 14, 60, 64, 86
Hamlyn, L. H., 13, 17, 34, 85, 86
Hámori, J., 23, 29, 86, 87
Hanzliková, V., 134, 135, 149
Harlow, H. F., 237, 238, 242, 243, 248, 257, 271, 272, 274, 276
Harlow, M. K., 237, 243, 248
Harris, A. J., 127, 147, 149, 150
Harris, C. S., 200, 207
Harris, T. M., 131, 135, 149
Harter, M. R., 159, 166
Hartman, C. G., 177, 210
Hasan, M., 19, 30, 85
Hassler, R., 14, 53, 73, 84
Hassmannová, J., 246
Hayhow, W. R., 13, 43, 58, 68, 83
Hebb, C. O., 109, 121, 143, 149
Hebb, D. O., 188, 207, 238, 248, 253, 263, 264, 274
Hechst, B., 31, 44, 86
Hein, A., 162, 165, 177, 178, 179, 182, 198, 199, 200, 201, 202, 205, 206, 207, 208, 215, 220, 226, 228, 229, 248
Held, R., 175, 178, 179, 182, 186, 187, 197, 198, 200, 201, 202, 203, 204, 205, 206, 207, 208, 210, 215, 228, 229, 248
Heller, D. P., 185, 209, 217, 249
Hellström, B., 103, 113, 121, 154, 166
Henry, G. H., 160, 165
Herman, T. S., 4, 6
Heron, W., 125, 149, 188, 209, 241, 242, 251, 261, 262, 263, 272, 276
Hertting, G., 131, 149
Herz, R., 135, 149
Hess, A., 13, 15, 28, 86, 108, 109, 121
Hess, E. H., 4, 5, 7
Himwich, W. A., 109, 121, 237, 246
Hinde, R. A., 269, 274
Hines, M., 175, 177, 208
Hirsch, H. V. B., 161, 166, 171, 208
Hirsch, J. C., 13, 82
Hník, P., 134, 140, 147, 149
Hochberg, J. E., 169, 170, 208
Hochhauser, S., 279, 286
Hoffman, K.–P., 40, 89, 156, 167, 230, 251
Hogan, J. A., 4, 7
Holloway, R. L., 14, 61, 67, 86
Holt, L. E., Jr., 2, 7
Hopewell, J. W., 279, 285
Horn, G., 93, 101, 119, 121
Horoupian, D. S., 31, 84,
Housepian, E. M., 143, 150
Howard, E., 279, 285
Howe, H., 14, 90
Howell, J. N., 135, 149, 159, 166, 245, 249
Hubel, D. H., 14, 15, 16, 42, 56, 57, 74, 77, 86, 90, 91, 105, 121, 156, 160, 161, 166, 167, 168, 171, 172, 177, 183, 189, 190, 191, 194, 199, 200, 208, 210, 219, 220, 221, 249, 252, 255, 276
Hudgins, P. M., 131, 135, 149
Hydén, H., 14, 60, 61, 64, 86, 93, 121
Hymovitch, B., 239, 249, 253, 263, 274

I

Iida, T., 96, 97, 98, 106, 110, 121
Illera, A. J., 23, 24, 86
Ingolia, R. L., 104, 120
Inman, O., 44, 58, 84
Inoue, F., 126, 148

Ireland, K. F., 5, 6
Isaacson, A., 135, 149

J

Jaffe, J., 125, 149
Jasper, H., 144, 148
Jenden, D., 149
Johns, T. R., 129, 149
Johnson, R. E., 14, 66, 84
Jones, E. G., 32, 36, 71, 86
Jones, R., 129, 149
Jones, W. H., 30, 86, 117, 121
Jung, R., 118, 121
Jurevics, H. A., 131, 135, 147

K

Kandel, E. R., 145, 151
Kang, B. S., 158, 166
Karli, P., 154, 165
Karlsson, J. O., 104, 122
Karlsson, U., 110, 122
Karmel, B. Z., 182, 191, 210
Karstens, A., 132, 152
Katz, B., 128, 149
Kemp, J. M., 32, 36, 74, 75, 76, 86
Kirpekar, S. M., 139, 150
Kobayashi, K., 215, 216, 249
Kocher, R. A., 14, 49, 65, 86
Koelle, G. B., 107, 122, 128, 152
Koelle, G. W., 107, 109, 122
Koenig, H., 102, 122
Konrad, K. W., 235, 249, 258, 259, 260, 267, 275
Korr, I. M., 128, 150
Kozak, W., 140, 150
Krech, D., 10, 11, 14, 25, 48, 49, 67, 82, 84, 86, 117, 118, 122, 240, 249
Krip, G., 152
Krnjević, K., 142, 143, 144, 149, 150
Kruger, L., 23, 87
Kuffler, S. W., 68, 87, 127, 137, 138, 146, 147, 149, 150
Kupfer, C., 15, 27, 29, 37, 42, 57, 87, 94, 96, 97, 98, 100, 105, 122
Kurke, M. I., 172, 180, 188, 208, 209, 215, 231, 250

L

Laminar, D. C., 148
Lange, P. W., 93, 121
Langer, S. Z., 138, 139, 150, 151
Larsell, O., 16, 26, 87
Lashley, K. S., 175, 177, 181, 208
Law, F., 49, 67, 84
Leaf, R. C., 101, 120
Lee, L. Y., 108, 119
Legein, C. P. J. J. M. M., 154, 167
Le Gros, Clark, W. E., 14, 17, 22, 31, 43, 59, 87
Lessac, M. S., 213, 237, 241, 242, 244, 249, 272, 275
Lester, M. L., 224, 249
LeVay, S., 22, 30, 87
Levick, W. R., 68, 87
Levi-Montalcini, R., 13, 18, 32, 87
Levitsky, D. A., 278, 285
Li, T. H., 108, 119
Liberman, R., 95, 107, 122
Lindberg, J., 13, 38, 39, 85
Lindner, B., 49, 67, 84, 88, 281, 286
Lindner, I., 22, 28, 55, 87
Lindsley, D. B., 159, 166, 245, 249
Lindsley, D. F., 159, 166, 167, 245, 249
Lineberger, R. O., 279
Liu, C. N., 14, 49, 64, 87
Lockhard, J., 144, 149
Loeser, J., 69, 87
Loewy, A. D., 13, 18, 34, 87
Lombroso, C., 164, 166
Lømo, T., 129, 150
Lore, R. K., 234, 249
Lowry, O. H., 94, 122
Lux, H. D., 144, 147
Lynch, A., 279, 285

M

Mac Neill, M., 67, 87
Madden, T. C., 239, 248
Mahut, H., 273, 275
Maletta, G. J., 53, 87, 105, 109, 111, 122
Mallart, A., 148
Malmfors, T., 50, 51, 79, 85, 86, 94, 112, 114, 115, 118, 121
Mann, G., 10, 11, 14, 65, 87

Maraini, G., 15, 41, 54, 87, 102, 105, 106, 122
Margolis, F. L., 26, 50, 82, 93, 119
Marty, R., 157, 166
Mason, W. A., 237, 238, 242, 243, 249, 256, 257, 269, 270, 271, 272, 273, 275
Massopust, L. C., 185, 208, 219, 250
Matthews, M. R., 13, 18, 19, 30, 33, 71, 75, 88
McCall, R. B., 224, 249
McCleary, R. A., 189, 197, 200, 208, 223, 230, 249
McDonald, J., 141, 142, 148, 280, 285
McGinnis, J. M., 185, 208
McIlwain, H., 95, 122
McIntyre, A. K., 139, 148
McIsaac, R. J., 126, 147
McMahan, U. J., 21, 27, 76, 88, 127, 150
McMurtry, J. C., 144, 147
Meier, G. W., 219, 246
Meisami, E., 163, 166
Mellinger, J. C., 172, 188, 189, 190, 191, 209, 215, 230, 250
Melzack, R., 163, 166, 188, 208, 234, 236, 241, 249, 251, 261, 262, 264, 265, 266, 267, 268, 270, 272, 273, 275
Mendelson, J. H., 10, 88
Menzel, E. W., Jr., 238, 243, 244, 247, 249, 255, 256, 257, 269, 271, 272, 273, 275, 276
Meyers, B., 189, 197, 200, 208, 223, 227, 230, 238, 249
Mikeladze, A. L., 14, 62, 65, 88
Miledi, R., 126, 128, 134, 148, 149, 150
Milledot, M., 164, 165, 225, 250
Miller, M. H., 226, 250
Miller, R. E., 271, 276
Mirsky, I. A., 271, 276
Mitchell, D. E., 225, 250
Mitchell, D. M., 164, 165
Mitchell, G. D., 257, 270
Mitchell, J. F., 109, 120
Modern, F., 132, 150
Mohr, D. J., 243, 248
Møllgaard, K., 79, 88, 281, 286
Monosevitz, M., 236, 249
Montgomery, K. C., 253, 263
Moore, M. K., 175, 206
Morelos, B. S., 114, 119
Mouren-Mathieu, A. M., 23, 24, 34, 76, 88
Mowbray, J. B., 186, 208
Muller, R., 140, 148
Murray, J. G., 139, 150
Murray, M., 104, 120
Muslivěck, J., 246

N

Nachman, M., 3, 4, 7
Nealey, S. M., 181, 182, 208, 217, 250
Nelson, P. G., 140, 151
Neville, H. E., 279, 286
Newell, F. W., 14, 59, 83, 114, 119, 172, 207, 213, 247
Nichols, W. N., 107, 109, 122
Nikara, T., 160, 167
Nissen, H. W., 188, 191, 206, 231, 233, 238, 247, 250
Noell, W. K., 95, 120, 158, 166
Norrlin, M.–L., 50, 51, 79, 85, 86, 94, 112, 115, 118, 121

O

Odom, P. B., 282
Oester, Y. T., 129, 151, 234, 252
Orbach, J., 226, 250
Ordy, J. M., 185, 208, 219, 250
Oswalt, R. M., 284, 286
Otani, T., 145, 151

P

Palmer, L. A., 162, 167
Palmer, P., 29, 42, 87, 96, 97, 98, 122
Patton, R. G., 5, 7
Penman, J., 13, 18, 37, 88, 117, 122
Pepeu, G., 97, 111, 120
Perry, W. L. M., 133, 150
Pettigrew, J. D., 160, 161, 164, 166, 167, 183, 208
Phelps, J. B., 238, 242, 246
Phillis, J. W., 112, 122, 142, 150
Pigon, A. A., 14, 61, 64, 86

Pinching, A. J., 13, 20, 25, 32, 33, 76, 88
Pincus, G., 69, 83
Pinneo, L. R., 68, 79, 82
Pinsky, C., 152
Pollack, J. G., 155, 166
Potter, L. T., 134, 150
Powell, T. P. S., 13, 19, 20, 21, 22, 23, 24, 25, 29, 30, 33, 34, 36, 71, 74, 75, 76, 84, 86, 88, 116, 123
Pratt, R. J., 244, 252
Prescott, J. W., 283, 286
Purpura, D. P., 143, 150

R

Race, J., Jr., 15, 27, 39, 51, 90, 114, 123
Rackensperger, W., 156, 166
Rademaker, G. G. J., 177, 208
Ramsey, R. L., 187, 194, 209, 250
Ranck, J., 151
Raper, C., 133, 147
Rasch, E., 14, 40, 42, 58, 88, 94, 99, 100, 102, 103, 113, 123, 172, 209, 213, 250
Ray, O. S., 279, 286
Raymond, E. J., 257, 276
Reading, H. W., 101, 120
Reas, H. W., 132, 150
Recordon, E., 13, 38, 39, 88
Reid, L. D., 239, 251
Reiffenstein, R., 143, 144, 150
Reinert, H., 133, 150
Reuter, J. H., 154, 167
Reynolds, H. H., 242
Rhodes, H., 49, 67, 84
Richardson, K., 103, 106, 123
Richter, C. P., 2, 7
Riege, W. H., 235, 240, 250
Riesen, A. H., 10, 14, 40, 42, 44, 47, 54, 56, 58, 59, 63, 73, 77, 83, 88, 89, 91, 94, 99, 100, 102, 103, 104, 113, 114, 119, 123, 124, 154, 155, 159, 165, 167, 172, 173, 174, 176, 177, 183, 187, 188, 189, 190, 191, 194, 195, 196, 197, 207, 209, 210, 213, 214, 215, 218, 219, 221, 222, 223, 224, 227, 230, 231, 238, 245, 246, 247, 248, 250, 251, 252, 255, 276, 279, 280, 286
Rileigh, K. K., 282, 286
Riley, D. A., 182, 208, 217, 250
Rizzolatti, G., 219, 220, 221, 222, 223, 250
Robb, R., 164, 166
Robbins, N., 140, 141, 148, 150, 151
Robert, E., 129, 151
Robinson, J. S., 227, 247
Rock, I., 185, 209
Rodieck, R. W., 63, 89
Rogers, C. M., 238, 243, 244, 246, 247, 249, 256, 273, 274
Röhlich, P., 79, 89
Roland, A. L., 15, 27, 39, 51, 90, 114, 123
Rose, G. H., 157, 167
Rose, S., 93, 94, 101, 103, 106, 108, 119, 120, 121, 123
Rosenberg, P., 143, 151
Rosenblueth, A., 125, 132, 134, 138, 139, 147
Rosenblum, L. A., 183, 209
Rosenquist, A. C., 162, 167
Rosenthal, J., 129, 150
Rosenzweig, M. R., 10, 11, 14, 27, 48, 49, 62, 66, 67, 78, 79, 82, 84, 85, 86, 88, 89, 117, 118, 122, 235, 239, 240, 246, 249, 251, 281, 282, 286
Rothballer, A., 131, 151
Rowley, W. F., 18, 34, 91
Rozin, P., 3, 7
Ruckelshaus, S. I., 236, 239, 252
Ruiz de Pereda, G., 13, 34, 71, 82
Ruiz-Marcos, A., 19, 26, 89
Ruppenthal, G. C., 257, 276
Russell, J. T., 181, 208
Rutledge, L. T., 141, 142, 143, 144, 147, 148, 151, 280, 286

S

Sackett, G. P., 257, 271, 276, 283, 286
Saffran, E., 14, 49, 66, 79, 89
Sanderson, K. J., 15, 40, 55, 89, 156, 167
Sandow, A., 135, 149
Sankova, E. I., 103, 123
Santori, M., 15, 41, 54, 87, 102, 105, 106, 122

Sasaki, K., 145, 151
Sastry, P., 141, 148
Satinsky, D., 112, 123
Satterberg, J. A., 69, 84, 154, 165, 171, 194, 207
Schaefer, T. J., 74, 90
Schaeppi, U., 131, 151
Schapiro, S., 14, 62, 64, 75, 89
Scheibel, A. B., 10, 11, 13, 14, 23, 28, 33, 47, 54, 62, 63, 75, 77, 85, 89
Scheibel, M. E., 10, 11, 77, 89
Scheibler, T. H., 96, 97, 98, 106, 110, 121
Scherrer, J., 157, 158, 165, 167
Schiff, W., 174, 209
Schimke, R. T., 14, 41, 55, 89, 96, 97, 107, 123
Schlitz, E. A., 243, 248
Schmidt, J. L., 132, 148
Schüpbach, P., 14, 39, 50, 89
Scott, S., 101, 119
Scott, T. H., 272, 275
Seeman, P., 135, 152
Seiler, N., 123
Sellinger, O. Z., 144, 147
Semiginovsky, B., 246
Semmes, J., 233, 250
Shabadash, A. L., 49, 89
Sharpless, S. K., 104, 120, 125, 130, 131, 141, 142, 144, 148, 149, 151, 154, 165
Sherman, S. M., 15, 40, 55, 89, 156, 162, 167, 230, 231, 251
Shiljagina, N. N., 217, 251
Shlaer, R., 161, 167
Sidman, R. L., 17, 27, 83, 114, 115, 119, 120
Siegel, J., 159, 167
Silberberg, D. H., 98, 100, 107, 120
Silver, A., 109, 121, 143, 144, 149, 150
Singh, V. B., 93, 106, 118, 123
Sinha, A. K., 106, 123
Siou, G., 22, 28, 89, 109, 123
Sjöstrand, J., 104, 122
Slagle, R. W., 14, 49, 66, 79, 89
Smith, C. B., 139, 151
Smith, C. J., 160, 165
Smith, K. U., 177, 178, 184, 209, 210
Smith, M. C., 13, 18, 37, 88, 117, 122
Smith, P. S., 63, 89
Sokoll, M. D., 129, 151
Solomon, R. L., 213, 237, 241, 242, 244, 249, 272, 275
Somjen, G. G., 145, 147
Sonesson, B., 151
Sotelo, C., 23, 32, 89
Spalding, D. A., 169, 170, 172, 180, 209
Spehlmann, R., 141, 151, 159, 167
Spencer-Booth, Y., 269, 274
Spencer, J. W., 157, 165
Spencer, W. A., 140, 145, 151
Spiegel, E. A., 141, 151
Spinelli, D. N., 161, 166, 171
Sponholz, R. R., 257, 275
Stavraky, G. W., 68, 84, 125, 237, 139, 151
Stelzner, D., 237, 241, 247
Stephenson, R. P., 132, 151
Sterling, P., 162, 167
Sternschein, E., 64, 89
Stewart, D. L., 14, 15, 42, 55, 77, 83, 165, 171, 194, 207, 219, 220, 221, 222, 223, 230, 246, 247, 251
Stone, J., 40, 89, 156, 167, 230, 251
Struck, G., 144, 147
Sturgeon, R. D., 239, 251
Suitt, C. D., 159, 166
Svanidze, E. K., 103, 104, 105, 113, 123
Swan, A. B., 109, 121
Swift, H., 14, 40, 58, 88, 94, 99, 100, 102, 103, 113, 123, 172, 209, 213, 250
Szekely, E. G., 141, 151
Szenthágothai, J., 22, 29, 36, 76, 89, 143, 151

T

Talwar, G. P., 93, 94, 106, 118, 123
Tanabe, G., 278, 286
Taub, E., 201, 204, 209
Tauber, E. S., 185, 209
Taylor, J., 131, 135, 136, 152
Tebecis, A. K., 112, 122
Tees, R. C., 217, 232, 251
Terry, R. J., 15, 16, 26, 27, 39, 51, 89, 90, 123
Tewari, H. B., 118, 124

Thesleff, S., 126, 128, 129, 133, 147, 149, 151, 152
Thienes, C., 132, 150
Thomas, D. B., 30, 74, 86, 117, 121
Thompson, J. W., 139, 150
Thompson, W. R., 90, 188, 209, 234, 236, 241, 242, 251, 261, 262, 263, 272, 273, 275, 276
Thorndike, E., 180, 210
Thorpe, W., 135, 152
Tighe, T. J., 181, 210, 217, 252
Timiras, P. S., 53, 87, 105, 109, 111, 122, 163, 166
Tinklepaugh, O. L., 177, 210
Tischner, K., 19, 28, 85
Titova, L. K., 116, 124
Török, L. J., 79, 89
Torvik, A., 17, 35, 63, 74, 90, 117, 124
Tower, S. S., 14, 90
Towson, M., 95, 121
Tradardi, B., 219, 220, 221, 222, 223, 250
Trendelenburg, U., 130, 131, 132, 138, 139, 150, 151, 152
Triggle, C., 143, 144, 150
Tronick, E., 174, 206
Trychin, S., 182, 191, 210
Tsai, T. H., 139, 151
Tsang, Y. C., 16, 25, 73, 90
Tucker, A., 217, 251
Tyagi, H. R., 118, 124

U

Umrath, K., 15, 17, 22, 26, 27, 40, 54, 55, 56, 58, 87, 90
Usami, E., 104, 124
Utley, J. D., 116, 124

V

Valverde, F., 14, 19, 23, 24, 25, 44, 47, 50, 71, 72, 73, 75, 89, 90
Vander Eeken, H., 97, 100, 124
Van der Loos, H., 15, 30, 90
Van der Mark, F., 154, 167
Van Hof, M. W., 104, 124, 154, 167, 216, 249, 251
Van Hof-Van Duin, J., 215, 216
Van Marthens, E., 279, 286
Van Niel, S., 143, 148
Varma, D. R., 138, 152
Vazquez, A. J., 142, 152
Vesper, J., 156, 166
Vickerson, F. H. L., 138, 152
Vinnikov, Ya. A., 116, 124
Volkmar, F. R., 14, 61, 66, 90
Volle, R. L., 138, 152
Volokohov, A. A., 217, 251
Von Bach, L., 82
Von Noorden, G. K., 167, 229, 231, 251
Von Senden, M., 173, 209, 245, 251
Vrbová, G., 129, 149
Vukovich, K. R., 14, 62, 64, 75, 89
Vyskočil, F., 133, 147

W

Walberg, F., 24, 36, 90
Walk, R. D., 171, 172, 174, 177, 180, 181, 182, 183, 187, 191, 203, 204, 210, 215, 217, 252
Walker, J. H., 28, 37, 73, 83, 100, 115, 120
Walker, V. S., 158, 166
Wall, P. D., 264, 275
Walsh, E. G., 109, 121
Ward, A., 144, 149
Waser, P. G., 134, 152
Watanabe, S., 144
Watson, J. B., 175, 177, 208
Watson, J. R., 164
Warkentin, J., 177, 178, 184, 210
Warren, J. M., 241, 252
Waugh, K. T., 180, 210
Wawrzyniak, M., 110, 124
Weber, A., 135, 149
Weiskrantz, L., 58, 90, 172, 210
Weizmann, F., 244, 252
Wendt, R. H., 159, 166, 167, 245, 249
West, R. W., 281, 282, 286
Westerman, R., 140, 150
Westman, J., 24, 35, 90
Westrum, L. E., 20, 22, 23, 32, 76, 90
Whitby, L. G., 131, 149
White, B. L., 174, 175, 186, 187, 210
White, C. T., 159, 166
White, L. E., Jr., 20, 30, 90

Wickelgren, B. G., 162, 167
Wiesel, T. N., 14, 15, 16, 42, 56, 57, 74, 77, 86, 90, 91, 105, 121, 156, 160, 161, 166, 167, 168, 171, 172, 177, 183, 189, 190, 191, 194, 199, 200, 207, 208, 210, 213, 219, 220, 221, 222, 229, 247, 249, 252, 255, 270, 281
Wilkinson, P. N., 150
Williams, W. O., 68, 87
Wilson, M., 241, 252
Wilson, P. D., 77, 91, 172, 173, 174, 176, 177, 183, 187, 194, 209, 120, 218, 219, 226, 248, 250, 252
Windle, W. F., 117, 120
Wiśniewski, H. M., 13, 24, 29, 31, 71, 84, 85
Witzke, F., 148
Wiu, S. Y., 14, 49, 66, 79, 89
Wolf, A., 232, 252
Wolff, P. H., 210
Wolin, L. R., 185, 219, 250
Woods, P. J., 236, 239, 252, 254, 263, 276
Woolsey, T. A., 15, 32, 90

Y

Yakovlev, V. A., 116, 124
Yasargil, G. M., 14, 83
Yellin, H., 140, 152
Yinon, U., 100, 124, 158, 168
York, D. H., 112, 122
Youmans, W., 132, 152
Young, I. J., 18, 35, 91

Z

Zalis, A. W., 234, 252
Zalis, O. S., 234, 252
Zamenhof, S., 279, 286
Zetterström, B., 103, 113, 121, 154, 166, 168
Zilbert, D. E., 246, 252
Zimbardo, P. G., 253, 263, 276
Zimmerman, R. R., 219, 252
Zubek, J. P., 67, 87, 240, 247

Subject Index

A

Acetylcholine, 126, 127, 129, 132–136, 138–139, 142, 143, 145, 146
Acetylcholinesterase
and neural transmitters, 107–112
and presynaptic activity, 50
Alpha-glycerophosphate dehydrogenase, 98
Amblyopia ex anopsia, 229–231
Amphibians
neurochemistry of, 118
presynaptic activity, 16, 23, 26, 32, 65
Astigmatisms, 163–164
Auditory cortex, 32, 36, 50, 67, 79
Auditory deprivation, 164, 232, 282, 284
Auditory system, 116
Axonal transport, 104

B

Binocular pattern deprivation, *see also* Pattern deprivation
depth perception, 180–184
looming response, 174
open field behavior, 172–174
optokinetic response, 184–187
reaching behavior, 174–177
recovery, 172–173, 183–184, 187–188
visual placing, 177–180, 200, 221
Birds
neurochemistry, 116
presynaptic activity, 39, 50, 65
Blood supply, *see* Vascularity
Brain specific proteins, 118
Bridgeman, Laura, 15–16, 31

C

Cannon's Law, 125, 137–139
Cats
binocular pattern deprivation, 172, 173, 177–179, 182, 184
early sensory environments, 219–223, 225, 226–227, 229–231, 235–236, 241
electrophysiological changes, 159–161
monocular deprivation, 190–193

Cats (*continued*)
neurochemistry, 96–99, 102–103, 111–113, 117
novelty enhancement, 258–260, 267
presynaptic activity, 17–19, 22–23, 24, 28–29, 34–37, 40–44, 55–58, 61, 63–69, 74
visuo-motor deprivation, 196–201
Caudate nucleus, 34, 74, 76
Cells, *see also individual cell types*
electrophysiological changes, 156
loss of, 16–18, 27–28, 40–41, 53, 55, 59
proliferation of, 66, 77
soma, 18–19, 22, 26, 28, 32–35, 38, 40–44, 49, 51, 55–61, 64, 77
Cerebellum, 21, 26, 29, 34, 49, 50, 65, 76–77
Cerebral cortex
disuse sensitization, 141–146
presynaptic activity, 31, 50, 76
Cerebral palsy, 117
Chicks
binocular pattern deprivation, 180–181
early sensory environment, 217
innate stimulus preferences, 5
presynaptic activity, 18, 26, 32, 50
Chimpanzee
binocular pattern deprivation, 172
early sensory environment, 218, 231, 233, 238, 243
neurochemistry, 99, 102, 105, 113
novelty-enhancement, 255–257, 273
presynaptic activity, 40–41, 59
visuo-motor deprivation, 195
Cochlear nucleus, 18, 22, 32, 36
Contracture response, 134–135
Cortex, *see individual cortical areas*
Cortical responses, 157–162
Corticospinal tract, 33
Critical period, 2, 6, 16, 74

D

Dark adaptation, 41, 63, 117–118
Dark discharge, 68
Deafferentation, *see also Transneuronal degeneration*
presynaptic activity, 10, 15–40, 73, 75–76, 81
Deiters' nucleus, 64
Dendritic branching, 19, 22, 26, 31–35, 44, 56, 59, 61, 63, 66–67, 73, 76
Dendritic length, 20, 44, 47, 56, 61, 63, 73
Dendritic spines, 19–25, 26–29, 32–35, 44–47, 50, 53, 61–62, 65–66, 71–77
Dendritic volume, 22, 33
Denervation supersensitivity, 125–127, 129, 131, 134–135, 145–146
Disuse potentiation, 137, 139, 140, 146
Disuse supersensitivity
in autonomic effector organs, 45, 46, 130–132
changes in coupling, 134–136
in neurons, 136–146
receptor proliferation, 132–136
reversibility, 132
in skeletal muscle, 128–129, 145–146
DNA of lateral geniculate, 100
Dogs
early sensory environment, 234–237, 241–242
electrophysiological changes, 157, 163
neurochemistry, 108
novelty enhancement, 265–267, 273
presynaptic activity, 17, 29, 44, 58, 65
DOPA, 111–112
Ducks, early sensory environment of, 232

E

Electroencephalogram arousal, 163
Electroretinogram
in darkrearing, 154–155
in monocular lid suturing, 154–155
Enrichment, sensory
effect on brain weight, 49
effect on dendrites, 61–62
genetic factors, 238–241, 243
presynaptic activity, 48–49, 60–62, 64–67
studies of, 6
Epilepsy, *see* Seizures
Esotropia, 164, 231
Excitation-contraction coupling, 135–136, 146
Exotropia, 231–232

Exploratory behavior, 212, 235–236, 241, 245

F

Fear, *see* Innate aversion
Frontal cortex, 66, 106
Function-structure relations, 277–283

G

Ganglion cells, 17–18, 40–41, 55–56, 59, 65, 68
Gerbils, 66
Glial cells, 17, 19, 23, 24, 25, 27, 29, 34, 41, 49, 61, 64, 71, 73, 76, 77, 118
Glycolysis
  in LGN, 96
  in retina, 94–96
Golgi, 19, 21, 23, 27, 31, 33, 36, 39, 44, 58, 62, 64, 75–76
Growth, effects of environment and inheritance on, 1–5
Growth hormone, 279–280
Guinea pig
  neurochemical studies, 108
  presynaptic activity, 28, 49, 64

H

Humans
  acuity, 225
  alcohol, 18, 37
  binocular pattern deprivation, 174–176, 185–187
  congenital absence of eye, 38–39
  with corneal opacities, 31, 44
  deafness, 282
  electrophysiological changes, 159, 163–165
  LGN after enucleation, 22, 25, 31
  presynaptic activity, 15–16, 18–19, 22, 24–25, 31, 37, 38–39, 44
  spinothalamic tractotomy, 19, 37
Hypersensitivity, 68–69, 245, 280, *see also* Disuse supersensitivity

I

Individual variation, 62–63
Inferior olive, 24, 36–37, 74
Information processing
  congruence of, 11–12, 42, 62, 69
  in isolates, 264–268
  overload, 11, 14–15, 69, 77
Innate aversion, 181–184, 237, 255, 262
Innate competence, 169–170, 173, 177, 181–183, 185, 187–188, 192, 206, 284
Interocular transfer, 220, 230–231, 287
Isolation
  behavior stereotypy, 269–270, 283
  comparative data, 255–264, 273
  fear, as a result of, 237, 255, 262
  genetic factors, 236, 273
  hyperactivity, 237
  information processing, 264–268, 274
  learning capacity, 279
  losses of abilities, 244
  physiological correlates, 265–268
  problem solving, 241–244
  recovery, 254
  social behavior, 238, 255–257, 260, 262–263
  social–sexual incompetence, 238, 270–272

J

Jamming *see* Information processing, overload

L

Lactate dehydrogenase, 96
Learning, 10, 220, 222–228, 230–231, 279, 284–285
Leucine, 41, 54, 102, 105–106
LGB, 27–31, 38, 51–53, 55, 57–58, 65
LGN
  electrophysiological changes, 155, 156
  neurochemistry, 96–98, 100, 105, 107–112, 114–115
  presynaptic activity, 27, 30, 31, 51, 54, 56–57, 59
Light deprivation
  acuity, 216

Light deprivation (*continued*)
depth perception, 215–217
guided reaching, 215, *see also* Pattern deprivation, guided placing
intensity discrimination, 215, 217
pattern discrimination, 216–217
postnatal, 215
recovery, 246
visual placing, 177–180, 215–216
Lysine, 106

M

Malate dehydrogenase, 97
Maturational competence, 178, 187
Mice
neurochemistry, 108, 112, 115
presynaptic activity, 19, 26–27, 32, 38–39, 41, 44–47, 50–51, 66, 79
Microtubules, 31, 33
Monkeys
binocular pattern deprivation, 172–173, 175, 182–183, 185–186
early sensory environment, 218–219, 226, 228–230, 231–234, 237–238, 242–243
neurochemistry, 97–98, 100, 107, 117
novelty enhancement, 257–258, 273
presynaptic activity, 18–19, 24, 29–31, 42–44, 47, 62, 63, 77
visuo-motor deprivation, 202–204
Monocular deprivation
acuity, 229, 231
alternating, 231
amblyopia, 229–231
depth perception, 190–191
electrophysiological changes, 154–158, 160, 162–163, 281
interocular transfer, 230–231, 281
neurochemistry, 102, 110
open field response, 189–190
optokinetic response, 191–194
presynaptic activity, 26–31, 38, 41, 42, 47, 50–57, 69, 71, 77
recovery, 42, 77, 189–191, 193–194, 230
Motor deprivation, *see* Visual–motor deprivation
Myelination, 98, 112, 114

N

Nativism *vs.* Empiricism, 169–170, 173, 188, 200–203
Neocortex, 67
Nervous system, development of, 277–279, 283
Neurons
of autonomic ganglia, 138–139
disuse and denervation effects, 126–127, 133, 136–146
isolated cortex, 141–146
and norepinephrine, 139
spinal neurons, 139–141
of sympathetic ganglia, 133, 146
Nissl substance, 15, 18, 28, 30, 34–35, 39, 42, 49, 56, 58, 60–61, 64, 65, 100–101, 113, 116
Novelty enhancement
arousal effects, 163, 272, 274
comparative studies, 255–264
early sensory environment, 212
genetic differences, 273
information processing, 264–268, 274
Nuclear volume, 16, 22, 50–51, 58–59
Nucleoprotein, 49, 55, 60–61, 64
Nutrition, 278–280

O

Occipital cortex, 49, 62, 66, 118
Olfactory system, 17, 20–21, 23, 32–33, 37, 71, 116
Optic lobes, 16, 26, 116
Optic nerve, 22, 26–27, 38–39, 58
Optic track, 27

P

Pain, 62, 64–65, 234
Pattern deprivation
acuity, 218, 220–222, 225
depth perception, 180–184, 218, 220–221
eye movements, 226
form discrimination, 217, 222–226
guided placing, 177–180, 215–216, 220–221, 226
intensity discrimination, 219, 222
limited pattern discrimination, 224–225

Pattern deprivation (*continued*)
line orientation, 225
optokinetic responding, 222
presynaptic activity, 39, 50–55, 57–59, 62–63
stroboscopic environment, 226, 241, 284
Pattern evoked responses, 159
Phosphatases, 106, 118
Phylogenetic comparisons
electrophysiology, 154–155
presynaptic activity, 18, 26–37, 38, 40–42, 50–59, 62–66, 71–72, 154–155, 206
visual orientation, 206
Pontine nucleus, 37, 74
Postsynaptic structure, 16, 20, 23, 24–25, 29, 32–34, 62, 64, 76
Presynaptic action potentials
decreased sensory input, 50–65
increased sensory input, 64–65
Presynaptic structure, 10–13, 29, 32, 52–53, 65, 71
Problem-solving behavior, 213, 235, 238, 243–244
Protein synthesis, 102–106, 118, *see also* RNA
Pyramidal cells, 26, 32, 36–37, 50, 52, 54, 56, 66, 76
Pyridine nucleotide, 98

R

Rabbits
early sensory environment, 216, 234
electrophysiological changes, 154, 157–158
neurochemistry, 95–97, 99, 102, 104, 107–110, 115
presynaptic activity, 15, 17–18, 21–23, 28–29, 33–34, 39–42, 44, 47, 50, 52, 54–55, 64, 75
Rats
binocular pattern deprivation, 181
early sensory environment, 217, 224, 232, 235, 238–240
electrophysiological changes, 157–158, 163
neurochemistry, 95–96, 99, 101–103, 105–110, 117
novelty enhancement, 263
nutrition, 278, 284
presynaptic activity, 16, 20, 23, 27, 32, 33, 40–41, 47, 49, 51–54, 60–62, 64, 66, 67, 69, 72–73, 76–78
Reafference hypothesis, 198
Receptor proliferation, 132–136
Reticular formation, 112, 117
Retina
glycolysis in, 2–4, 26,
inner plexiform layer, 94–95, 97, 99–103, 106–107, 109, 112–114
loss of ganglion cells, 113
malate dehydrogenase activity, 97
neurochemistry, 102–103
presynaptic activity, 38, 40–41, 51, 55, 57–59, 63, 65, 68–69, 71, 79
RNA
of cortex, 99–101
of LGN, 100
of retina, 42, 50, 54, 56, 59, 99–100
of sensory nucleus, 50, 58–59, 61, 64

S

S–100 protein, 118
Seizures, 141–146, 163, 280
Single cell responses, 160–162
Somatosensory cortex, 15, 24, 66, 67, 69
Somatosensory deprivation, 233–234, 283
Somatosensory system, 117
Spinal cord, 18, 35, 37, 64, 65
Squid, 104
Stellate cells, 19, 24, 44, 47, 54, 56, 63, 66–67, 73–74
Stereotyped behavior, 236–238
Stimulus preferences, 3–4
Stimulus-response suppression hypothesis, 202–206
Stimulus seeking, 245
Strabismus, 164, 231
Stress, 48, 62, 64–65
Sulfhydrl groups, 103–105
Superior colliculus
electrophysiological changes, 162
presynaptic activity, 15–16, 27–28, 31, 38, 39, 51, 53, 54, 55, 57, 59

Superior colliculus (*continued*)
protein changes, 104, 108–111, 114
Synapses, 12, 22, 37, 39, 44, 47–48, 51–53, 61–62, 73, 75–76, 78, 108, 110, 280–281

T

Transneuronal degeneration, 10–11, 13, 16–23, 29, 33, 71, 73, 75–76

V

Vascularity, 114, 116, 118
Visual acuity, *see* Pattern deprivation
Visual cortex
electrophysiology, 157–162, 281–283
neurochemical changes, 101, 105–106, 109, 111–112, 115–117
presynaptic activity, 15–16, 19, 22–23, 24, 27, 39–42, 44, 47–49, 51–59, 64, 66, 69, 73, 79
Visual evoked potentials, 157–159
Visual–motor deprivation
decorrelated feedback, 204–206, 229
discrimination ability, 195–197
guided reaching, 228–229
looming response, 195
movement discrimination, 227
optokinetic response, 195
orientation in space, 195, 197
placing response, 199–200
recovery, 200
visual depth, 228
visual placing, 228
Visual placing, *see* Pattern deprivation, guided placing, Visual–motor deprivation

X

X cells, 156

Y

Y cells, 156

A
B 5
C 6
D 7
E 8
F 9
G 0
H 1
I 2
J 3